Menarche

Menarche

The Transition from Girl to Woman

Edited by
Sharon Golub
College of New Rochelle

LexingtonBooks
D.C. Heath and Company
Lexington, Massachusetts
Toronto

Library of Congress Cataloging in Publication Data

Main entry under title:
  Menarche, the transition from girl to woman.

  Outgrowth of the Fourth Interdisciplinary Menstrual Cycle Research
Conference on Menarche held June 12-13, 1981 at the College of New
Rochelle and sponsored by the Society for Menstrual Cycle Research and the
College of New Rochelle.
  Includes index.
  1. Menarche—Congresses. I. Golub, Sharon. II. Interdisciplinary
Menstrual Cycle Research Conference on Menarche (4th : 1981 : College of
New Rochelle). III. Society for Menstrual Cycle Research. IV. College of New
Rochelle. [DNLM: 1. Menarche. WP 540 M547]
RJ145.M46   1982   612′.662   82-48105
ISBN 0-669-05982-x

To my mother and the memory of my father, with love

Contents

Contents

Figures

Tables

Preface and
Acknowledgments

Menarche is a landmark event in every woman's life. Yet in our culture both the experience and the language associated with it are veiled in secrecy. Last spring, a sociology professor with whom I teach told me that she asked a question about menarche on a final exam and found that half the women in the class did not know the meaning of the term. I have had other, similar experiences. This hush-hush attitude is not universal. In some cultures menarche is celebrated with great joy and ritual feasting. Colin Turnbull, in his book *The Forest People*, reports that among the Pygmies of the Congo the menarcheal girl is considered "blessed with the blood." Everyone is told the good news and it is a time of gladness for the whole people, one of the happiest in their lives. In contrast, in our culture menarche is more likely to be treated as a hygienic crisis.

This book is an outgrowth of an interdisciplinary research conference on menarche that was sponsored by the Society for Menstrual Cycle Research and the College of New Rochelle and was supported by a grant from TAMPAX Incorporated. The society believed that it was time to focus attention on women's first experience with menstruation. The conference brought together people from a variety of disciplines who have done research regarding the onset of menstruation and provided these scientists and scholars with an opportunity to present and discuss their work and to learn what people in other fields were doing. This communication across disciplines was an important aim of the conference and is an aim of this book as well.

Contributors to this book represent the physical and social sciences, medicine, nursing, education, and the humanities. In writing their chapters, authors were asked to keep in mind the fact that they were addressing not only people in their own areas of specialization. Therefore, although the chapters differ in their complexity, all of the work discussed is accessible to students and nonspecialists as well as to researchers in the field. The book should prove useful to undergraduate and graduate students studying the physiology and psychology of adolescence, female development, human sexuality, health education, women's studies, medicine, social work, and nursing.

The book consists of eight topical sections with each section further divided into chapters describing relevant research. Each section is concerned with one aspect of menarche. These are: physiological, psychological, educational, sexual, literary, clinical and psychiatric. In the epilogue there is a discussion of the implications of the research presented both for further research and for women's health.

Until quite recently menarche has received little attention in the scientific literature and perhaps even less in the humanities. It is hoped that the ideas and findings presented here will serve as an impetus for further research. There is a need to recognize menarche as a very significant event in women's lives and to assess its impact on the physical and psychosexual development of young women.

Acknowledgments

The Fourth Interdisciplinary Menstrual Cycle Research Conference on Menarche, from which this book developed, was made possible by a grant from TAMPAX Incorporated, which is gratefully acknowledged. The conference was held at the College of New Rochelle and I am indebted to the many people at the college whose help was so freely given. I would especially like to express my gratitude to Sr. Dorothy Ann Kelly, O.S.U., president of the College of New Rochelle, for her continuous encouragement and support. Special thanks also go to Fred Smith and Rosemary Lewis, the librarians who saw to it that I got every reference regarding menarche that crossed their desks or computers, and to Mimi Fitzgerald for some clever library-detective work. The National Planning Committee, comprised of Jeanne Brooks-Gunn, Alice Dan, Inge Dyrenfurth, Mary Anna Friederich, Effie Graham, and Mary Parlee, was wonderful. Their ideas helped to shape the conference. Thanks are also due to the conference contributors and participants who brought their work, their ideas, and their enthusiasm to the meetings, giving us some provocative papers and lively discussion.

Part I
Physiological
Factors Influencing
Menarche

Introduction to Part I

The onset of menstruation and the subsequent maintenance of menstrual functioning are affected by many factors, among them: heredity, endocrine function, nutrition, physical activity, light, illness, stress, and even the season of the year—girls most often have their first menstrual periods in the late fall or early winter (Science News 1980). Another factor that is thought to affect menarcheal timing and is mentioned from time-to-time throughout this book is the secular trend: the increases in height and weight and earlier ages at menarche that have been reported in many populations throughout the world. For instance, the average age of menarche in the United States is now 12.8 years. One hundred years ago it was about 15.5 to 16. The secular trend appears to be related to improvements in nutrition and health care. And some authors claim that the secular trend in the United States has stopped, there having been no changes in menarcheal age for the last thirty years (Zacharias and Rand 1978).

In the following chapters attention is focused on three major physiological influences on menarche: nutrition, hormones, and genetics. First, Rose Frisch discusses the relationship between puberty, fatness, and fertility. In particular she notes the body and hormonal changes occurring at puberty and their relation to nutrition. Elsewhere, Frisch has suggested that "reproduction requires energy"—both pregnancy and lactation require extra calories—and this energy may come from the fat stored by the sixteen-to-eighteen-year-old girl (Frisch 1980). In this chapter, Frisch proposes that a critical minimum weight for height is necessary to trigger and maintain regular ovulation and menstruation. Further, she suggests that when the proportion of body fat falls below a certain height-weight ratio, ovulation ceases. She supports her hypothesis with a discussion of her research with animals, dancers, and athletes. Frisch also points out the relationship between body fat and the reproductive hormones, indicating that adipose tissue may be an additional source of estrogen.

Inge Dyrenfurth's chapter discusses the endocrine aspects of menarche in depth. She describes the rhythmic endocrinological changes that go on throughout women's lives, noting that various hormones dominate or recede in importance at different times in the life cycle. Using graphs and illustrations to clarify complex material, Dyrenfurth explains the importance of the adrenal and ovarian hormones at the time of puberty and during the reproductive years. Emphasizing continuity as well as change, she points out that the endocrine activity occurring at puberty follows the hormonal events of childhood and precedes that of later life. She also calls attention to the interaction occurring between the different hormones and between hormones and other things. For example, Dyrenfurth describes the interrelatedness of the reproductive hormones, other endocrine glands, and environmental influences such as nutrition and light, in bone and calcium metabolism.

Some studies have indicated a relationship between genetic factors and age at menarche. For example, significant correlations have been found between girls' menarcheal ages and those of their mothers (Chern, Gatewood, and Anderson 1980; Zacharias and Rand 1978). In the next chapter, Madeleine Goodman and her colleagues describe research in which they attempt to tease out the differential influence of genetic and environmental factors (such as the secular trend) on age at menarche, height, and weight. Goodman et al. looked at a large population of Caucasian, Japanese, and Chinese women living in Hawaii. In studying these women, who were born between 1900 and 1940, they were able to compare racial groups with the same climatic and socioeconomic backgrounds, attempting to see if there were racially determined genetic differences. The authors found secular trends toward earlier age at menarche in all three groups, with a more rapid rate of decline among the Oriental women. In general, there was little ethnic group heterogeneity in such biological variables as the age of menarche or the effect of age at menarche on adult weight and height. However, there were some racial differences in variables that are influenced by individual preferences such as time spend breast-feeding or number of live births. This chapter also demonstrates the advantages of such sophisticated statistical techniques as path analysis in getting at causal factors.

References

Chern, M.M., Gatewood, L.C., and Anderson, V.E. 1980. The inheritance of menstrual traits. In A. Dan, E.A. Graham, C.P. Beecher, eds., *The menstrual cycle: A synthesis of interdisciplinary research* vol. 1. New York: Springer.

Frisch, R. 1980. Fatness, puberty, and fertility. *Natural History* 89:16-27. *Science News*. 6 September 1980. 118:150.

Zacharias, L., and Rand, W.M. 1978. American girls: Their growth and development. *National Elementary Principal* 28:29-34.

1

Fatness, Menarche, and Fertility

Rose E. Frisch

Undernutrition delays sexual development in girls and boys, (Frisch 1972; Frisch and McArthur 1974; Tanner 1962) as in other mammals (Kennedy and Mitra 1963; Hammond 1955). Some factor other than chronological age therefore controls the pubertal process. Undernutrition, chronic or acute, also causes the cessation of established reproductive ability in the human female (Frisch and McArthur 1974) and male (Keys 1950), as well as in other mammals (Hammond 1955).

Frisch and McArthur (1974) found that the onset and maintenance of regular menstrual function in women are each dependent on the maintenance of a minimum weight for height, apparently representing a critical fat storage. These findings imply that a particular body composition of fat/lean or fat/body weight may be an important determinant for female reproductive ability.

Data from both nonanorectic and anorectic female patients show that a loss of body weight in the range of 10 to 15 percent of normal weight for height, which represents a loss of about one-third of body fat, results in amenorrhea. Data from obese women show that excess fatness also causes amenorrhea. Too little fat or too much fat therefore turns off sexual function in the human female (Frisch 1977a).

The recent findings that aromatization of androgens to estrogen takes place in adipose tissue, in female breast fat and abdominal fat (Nimrod and Ryan 1975), in the omentum (Perel and Killinger 1979), and in the fatty marrow of the long bones (Frisch, Canick, and Tulchinsky 1980b), suggest that adipose tissue may be a significant extragonadal source of estrogen. Body weight, hence fatness, also influences the direction of estrogen metabolism to the most potent or least potent forms (Fishman, Boyar, and Hellman 1975). The high percentage of fat, about 24 percent at menarche and about 26 to 28 percent in the average (165 centimeters, 57 kilograms) U.S. woman at the completion of her growth, thus may influence reproductive ability directly (Frisch 1976).

Studies in premenopausal and postmenopausal women indicate that excess body weight is associated with a diminished capacity of serum sex-hormone binding globulin (SHBG). The diminished SHBG in turn is correlated with an elevated percentage of serum estradiol in the free state (that is, not bound to serum estradiol or albumin). These changes in body-fat composition also may influence reproductive performance by regulating the

5

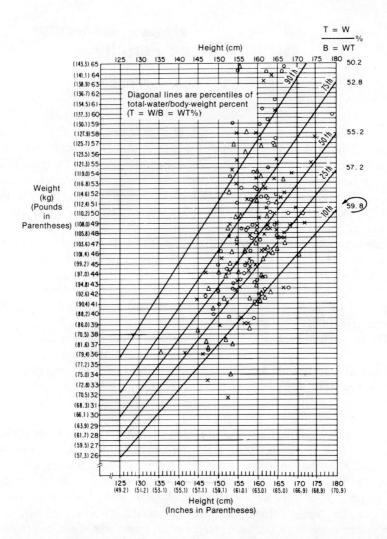

Legend: The minimal weight necessary for a particular height for onset of menstrual cycles is indicated on the weight scale by the 10th-percentile diagonal line of total-water/body-weight percent, 59.8 percent, as it crosses the vertical height lines. *Height growth of girls must be completed, or approaching completion.* For example, a fifteen-year-old girl whose completed height is 160 centimeters (63 inches) should weigh at least 41.4 kilograms (91 pounds) before menstrual cycles can be expected to start. Reprinted from Frisch and McArthur 1974, with permission from *Science.*

Source: Frisch, R.E., and McArthur, J.W. Menstrual cycles: Fatness as a determinant of minimum weight for height. *Science,* 13 September 1974, 185:949-951, figures 1 and 2. Copyright 1974 by the American Association for the Advancement of Science.

Figure 1-1. Minimal Weight for Height Necessary for Onset of Menstrual Cycles

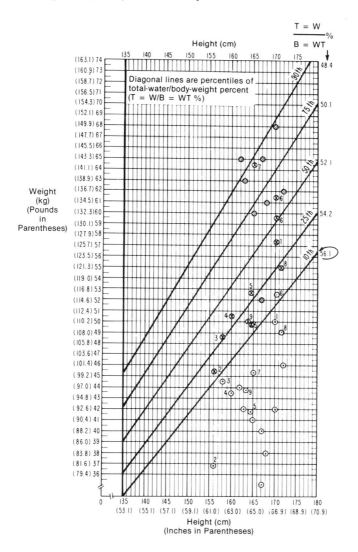

Legend: The minimal weight necessary for a particular height for restoration menstrual cycles is indicated on the weight scale by the 10th-percentile diagonal line of total-water/body-weight percent, 56.1 percent, as it crosses the vertical height line. For example, a twenty-year-old woman whose height is 160 centimeters should weigh at least 46.3 kilograms (102 pounds) before menstrual cycles would be expected to resume. Reprinted from Frisch and McArthur 1974, with permission from *Science*.

Source: Frisch, R.E., and McArthur, J.W. Menstrual cycles: Fatness as a determinant of minimum weight for height. *Science*, 13 September 1974, 185:949-951, figures 1 and 2. Copyright 1974 by the American Association for the Advancement of Science.

Figure 1-2. Minimal Weight for Height Necessary for Restoration of Menstrual Cycles

availability of estradiol to the brain and other target tissues (Nisker, Hammond, and Siiteri 1980).

Body-Weight Changes and Gonadotropin Secretion

Endrocrine studies of undernourished, nonanorectic subjects being refed showed that the mean initial serum follicle-stimulating hormone (FSH) concentration was within the limits of normal for young women of reproductive age, but the serum luteinizing (LH) concentration and the vaginal maturation scores were low. As weight was regained, serum LH concentration increased and the vaginal-maturation score rose. After weight gain to levels close to the normal range, spontaneous menses occurred but were anovulatory in 70 percent of the cases. Regular ovulatory cycles began with continued weight gain (McArthur et al. 1976).

The findings that: (a) urinary and plasma gonadotropins are low in underweight patients with or without anorexia nervosa; (b) the response to luteinizing hormone-releasing hormone (LH-RH) is diminished when body weight is low and is restored when body weight returns to the normal range (Boyar et al. 1974; Palmer et al. 1975; Warren et al. 1975); (c) a normal response to clomiphene citrate occurs only after body weight returns to the normal range (Marshall and Frasier 1971), suggest that a central-nervous-system signal affects hypothalamic function and, thus, the secretion of gonadotropins by the anterior pituitary.

Vigersky et al. (1977) concluded from temperature regulation and hormone data of nonanorectic women with secondary amenorrhea that hypothalamic dysfunction may be caused by weight loss itself. Thermoregulation at 10°C and 49°C was abnormal and correlated with the percentage below ideal body weight. Peak plasma LH hormone-level response to LH-RH was delayed in these subjects and the delay was correlated with percentage below ideal body weight.

Body Temperature, Food Intake, Ovulation, and Flushing

Wakeling and Russell (1970) have observed that basal temperature is reduced and temperature regulation is impaired in anorectic girls. These authors report that the central body temperature of anorectic patients rises in response to a standard meal, whereas in normal subjects central body temperature remains constant. The importance to the human female of a normal lack of such a response to a meal is suggested by the phenomenon of *flushing* in animals (Coop 1966): Flushing is the increase in the rate of twinning in sheep resulting from short term (for example, a week), high caloric feeding before mating to the ram. The well-nourished, human female fortunately does not normally superovulate in response to a high caloric intake, like a large steak dinner, although, interestingly, there is evidence for some residual flushing effect even in human beings. The rate of human dizygotic twinning, but not monozygotic twinning, fell during wartime restrictions in nutrition and the rate returned to normal after the return of a normal food supply (Bulmer 1970).

Delayed Menarche and Amenorrhea of Dancers and Athletes

High energy outputs, in addition to low nutritional intake would be expected to affect menstrual periodicity, if a critical amount of fat is necessary in relation to the amount of muscle mass. Ballet dancers (Frisch, Wyshak, and Vincent 1980; Warren 1980) and atheletes (Dale, Gerlach, and Wilhite 1979; Frisch et al. 1981) in fact have a delayed age of menarche and a high incidence of irregular cycles and amenorrhea. Some dancers and athletes who began their training at ages nine or ten years still had not had menarche at ages eighteen to twenty years.

Does intense exercise cause delayed menarche and amenorrhea of athletes, or do late maturers choose to be athletes? To answer this question, Frisch et al. (1981) studied the age of menarche and changes in menstrual periodicity of twenty-one college swimmers and seventeen runners, mean age 19.1 ± 0.2 years in relation to the age of initiating training, physical indices, and stress indices. The mean age of menarche of all the athletes, 13.9 ± 0.3 years was significantly later ($p < 0.001$) than that of the general population, 12.8 ± 0.5. However, the mean menarcheal age of the eighteen athletes whose training began *before* menarche was 15.1 ± 0.5 years, whereas the mean menarcheal age of the twenty postmenarcheal-trained athletes was 12.8 ± 0.2 years ($p < 0.001$). The latter mean age was similar to that of the college controls (12.7 ± 0.4 years) and the general population. Each year of premenarcheal training delayed menarche by five months. Of the premenarcheal-trained athletes, only 17 percent had regular cycles; 61 percent were irregular; and 22 percent were amenorrheic. In contrast, 60 percent of the postmenarcheal-trained athletes were regular, forty percent were irregular, and none were amenorrheic. During intense training, the incidence of oligoamenorrhea and amenorrhea increased in both groups. Six swimmers with amenorrhea and oligoamenorrhea averaged low-normal gonadotropins, prolactin, and estrogen. Progesterone was follicular phase level. Testosterone, free testosterone, and androstenedione were in the normal range. Serum T_4, T_3, RT_3, and TSH for these swimmers were also in the normal range. Top-rank athletes had increased muscularity and decreased adiposity, determined by physical measurements, including ultrasound measurement of subcutaneous fat thickness (Frisch et al. 1981).

One swimmer was an exceptionally interesting subject in relation to stress. This top-rank 17.5 year-old swimmer who began training at age 7.5 years, had had menarche at 15.4 years. She was oligoamenorrheic at the start of the study with a cycle interval of five months. She was very lean: her height was 169.2 centimeters, weight 48.9 kilograms (108 pounds), which is 82.5 percent of ideal weight, and 2.1 kilograms below the critical weight for her height found necessary for regular cycles (Frisch and McArthur 1974). After two months of training and no menses, this swimmer, whose tension score was high on a Profile Moods State Test, suddenly reported a four-day period. On inquiry she reported she had gained five pounds (2.3 kilograms) "on purpose, by eating a lot of carbohydrate," to see if she would have a cycle. She lost the five pounds by the next month, also on purpose, and had no more cycles (Frisch et al. 1981).

In addition to the rise in the lean-mass/fat ratio that accompanies serious athletic training, metabolic or hormone changes, such as changes in plasma insulin that have been reported for men athletes (Wahren 1979) may also affect the regulation of menstrual cyclicity in these very active women through central nervous signals to the hypothalamus.

Initial Findings: Weight at Puberty

The idea that relative fatness is important for female reproductive ability followed from our first findings that the events of the adolescent growth spurt, particularly menarche in girls, were each closely related to an average critical body weight. The mean weight at menarche for U.S. girls was 47.8 ± 0.5 kilograms, at the mean height of 158.5 ± 0.5 centimeters at the mean age of 12.9 ± 0.1 years (Frisch and Revelle 1971). (This mean age includes girls from Denver, who have a slightly later age of menarche than the rest of the population due to the slowing effect of altitude on growth rate.)

Since individual girls have menarche at all different weights and heights, the notion of an average critical weight of 47 kilograms for early and late maturing girls at menarche was analyzed in terms of the components of body weight at menarche (Frisch 1976). Body composition was investigated because total body water (TW) and lean body weight (LBW, TW/0.72) are more closely correlated with metabolic rate than is body weight, since they represent the metabolic mass as a first approximation. Metabolic rate was considered important since Kennedy hypothesized a food intake-lipostat-metabolic signal to explain his findings on weight and puberty in the rat (Kennedy and Mitra 1963; Kennedy 1969).

The greatest change in estimated body composition of both early and late maturing girls during the adolescent growth spurt was a large increase in body fat, from about 5 to 11 kilograms, a 120 percent increase, compared to a 44 percent increase in lean body weight. There was thus a change in ratio of LBW to fat from 5:1 at initiation of the spurt to 3:1 at menarche (Frisch 1976).

Total Body Water as Percent of Body Weight, (TW/BWt%): An Indicator of Fatness

Total body water as percent of body weight (TW/BWt%) is a more important index than the absolute amount of total water because it is an index of fatness (Friis-Hansen 1956) (see table 1-1). Percentiles of total-water/body-weight percent, which are percentiles of fatness, were made at menarche and for the same girls, at age eighteen years, the age at which body composition was stabilized (Frisch 1976). From clinical data, we found that 56.1 percent of total water/body weight, the tenth percentile at age eighteen years, which is equivalent to about 22 percent fat of body weight, indicated a minimal weight for height necessary for the restoration and maintenance of menstrual cycles. For example, a twenty-year-old woman whose height is 160 centimeters (63 inches) should weigh at least 46.3 kilograms (102 pounds) before menstrual cycles would be expected to resume (see figure 1-2).

Table 1-1

Ratio of Total Body Water to Body Weight as an Index of Fatness: Comparison of an Eighteen-Year-Old Girl and a Fifteen-Year-Old Boy of the Same Height and Weight

	Girl *(Age 18)*	*Boy* *(Age 15)*
Height (centimeters)	165.0	165.0
Weight (kilograms)	57.0	57.0
Total body water (TBW) (liters)	29.5	36.0
Lean body weight (kilograms) (TBW/0.72)	41.0	50.0
Fat (kilograms)	16.0	7.0
$\dfrac{\text{Fat}}{\text{Body Weight}}$ percent	28.0%	12.0%
$\dfrac{\text{Total Body Water}}{\text{Body Weight}}$ percent	51.8%	63.0%

Source: Estimated by equations of Mellits and Check (1970). See also Frisch (1976) *Human Biology* 48 and Frisch (1981) *New England Journal of Medicine* 305.

Note: Fat/body weight percent = $100 - (\text{TW/BWt\%})/0.72$.

The weights at which menstrual cycles ceased or resumed in postmenarcheal patients ages sixteen and older were about 10 percent heavier than the minimal weights for the same height observed at menarche (Frisch and McArthur 1974) (see figure 1-1).

For example, a fifteen-year-old girl whose completed height is 160 centimeters should weigh at least 41.4 kilograms before menstrual cycles can be expected to start (see figure 1-1).

The body-composition data showed that both early and late maturing girls gained an average of 4.5 kilograms of fat from menarche to age eighteen years. At age eighteen years mean fat was 16.0 ± 0.3 kilograms, 27 percent of body weight of 57.1 ± 0.6 kilograms. Reflecting this increase in fatness, the total-water/body-weight percent decreases from 55.1 ± 0.2 percent at menarche (12.9 ± 0.1 years) to 52.1 % ± 0.2 percent (SD 3.0) at age eighteen years (Frisch 1976).

Body Composition and LH Secretory Patterns

Boyar et al, (1974) found that the type of LH secretory pattern, prepubertal or pubertal, is closely correlated with the extent of loss or gain of body weight. Comparison of total-water/body-weight percent (TW/BWt%), with the normal values found at adolescence, menarche, and age eighteen years shows that a prepubertal body composition is correlated with a prepubertal LH secretory pattern, and a pubertal body composition is correlated with a pubertal LH secretion (Frisch 1977a).

The main function of the 16 kilograms of fat stored on an average by both early and late maturers by age eighteen years may be to provide easily mobilized energy for a pregnancy and for lactation; the 144,000 calories would be sufficient for a pregnancy and three-months' lactation (Frisch and McArthur 1974; Frisch 1976). Since infant survival is correlated with birth weight (Frisch 1972), and birth weight is correlated with the prepregnancy weight of the mother, the regulation of female body size and body composition at menarche has obvious selective advantages for the species. In prehistoric times, when food supplies were scarce, or fluctuated seasonally, stored fat would have been important for successful reproduction.

Other factors, such as emotional stress, affect the maintenance or onset of menstrual cycles. Therefore, menstrual cycles may cease without weight loss and may not resume in some subjects even though the minimum weight for height has been achieved. Also, the Frisch-McArthur standards apply as yet only to Caucasian U.S. females and European females, since different races have different critical weights at menarche and it is not yet known whether the different critical weights represent the same critical body composition of fatness (Frisch and McArthur 1974).

Effects of Weight Loss on Male Fertility

Studies on the effects of weight loss on male reproductive ability show that undernutrition also affects male fertility, but the pattern of effects is different for men than for women. In men, caloric reduction and weight loss affects libido first, then the amount of prostate fluid, then sperm mobility and sperm longevity. A larger weight loss, 25 percent of body weight is necessary, before sperm production is affected (Keys et al. 1950). These changes returned to normal in reverse order with nutritional rehabilitation.

Experimental Evidence: Early First Estrus of Rats on a High-Fat Diet

When rats were fed a high-fat (HF) diet, the fat being substituted isocalorically for carbohydrate, the HF-diet rats had estrus significantly ($p < 0.001$) earlier than did the low-fat (LF) diet rats. Confirming and extending Kennedy's findings (Kennedy and Mitra 1963) the caloric intake per 100 gram body weight of the HF- and LF-diet rats did not differ at vaginal opening or at first estrus, whereas the two groups differed significantly at both events in age, absolute food intake, relative food intake, and absolute caloric intake (Frisch, Hegsted and Yoshinaga 1975b).

Carcass analysis at first estrus showed that the HF- and LF-diet rats had similar body compositions, although their ages and body weights differed significantly (Frisch, Hegsted and Yoshinaga 1977b).

Nutrition, Disease, and Fertility

The findings on minimal weights for heights necessary for the onset and maintenance of menstrual cycles (Frisch and McArthur 1974) suggested that environmental factors, such as nutrition and disease, could affect the time of attainment and level of function of each reproductive event in the female, thus affecting the length of the reproductive span and reproductive efficiency. For example, undernourished girls would be expected to have later menarche, a longer period of adolescent sterility, a higher incidence of irregular and anovulatory cycles than normal, amenorrhea when weight loss is in the range of 10 to 15 percent of body weight, higher pregnancy wastage; longer lactational amenorrhea, and therefore, longer birth intervals, and a shorter time to menopause (Frisch 1978) (see figures 1-3 and 1-4).

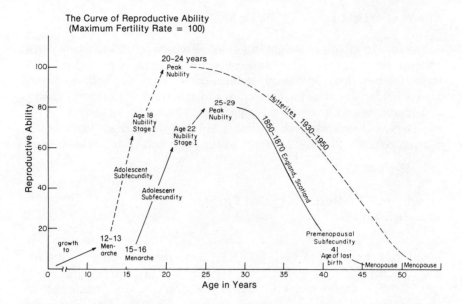

The Curve of Reproductive Ability
(Maximum Fertility Rate = 100)

Legend: The midnineteenth-century curve of female reproductive ability (variation of the rate of childbearing with age) compared to that of the well-nourished, noncontracepting modern Hutterites. The Hutterite fertility curve results in an average of ten to twelve children; the 1850-1870 fertility curve in about six to eight children. Reprinted with permission from Frisch 1978, in *Science*.

Source: Frisch, R.E. Population, food intake, and fertility. *Science*, 6 January 1978, 199: 22-30, figure 1. Copyright 1978 by the American Association for the Advancement of Science. Reprinted with permission.

Figure 1-3. Reproductive Ability Curve

British historical data from the nineteenth century on nutrition, growth, age specific fertility, and the ages of reproductive events show that slow growth to maturity of women and men due to undernutrition, hard work, and disease is actually correlated with a reproductive span that is shorter and less efficient than that of a well-nourished population. The submaximally nourished females and males are identifiable by a later average age of completion of growth, twenty to twenty-one years, and twenty-three to twenty-five years, respectively, compared to that of contemporary, well-nourished females and males who complete their growth by ages sixteen to eighteen years, and twenty to twenty-one years, respectively (Frisch 1978).

Historical Data on Age of Menarche and Amenorrhea

The average age of menarche in midnineteenth-century Britain was 15.5 to 16.5 years (Wyshak and Frisch 1982); menarcheal age also differed by social

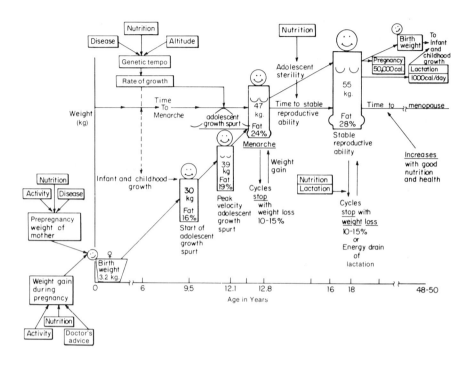

Legend: The biological determinants of female reproductive ability. Each reproductive milestone can be affected by environmental factors, as shown. The maintenance of regular ovulatory cycles is related to a critical fatness level, and is thus directly affected by undernutrition and energy-draining activities, such as lactation and physical work. Reprinted from Frisch 1975, with permission from *Social Biology*.

Source: Frisch, R.E. Demographic implications of the biological determinants of female fecundity. *Social Biology*, 1975, 22:18. Reprinted with permission.

Figure 1-4. Biological Determinants of Female Reproductive Ability

class, upper-class women having menarche 0.5 to one year earlier on average than working-class women. Undernutrition and hard living were the explanations given for the class differences and for the great variability in age of menarche, which ranged from ten to twenty-six years in the working class. A girl who did not have menarche by age seventeen or eighteen years was considered in a weak state of health. U.S. girls who had menarche at 11.5 or 12.5 years in 1871 were considered to be cases of precocious puberty (Harris 1871). The average age of menarche in 1877 was about 14.8 years (Wyshak and Frisch 1982). The average age of menarche in the United States is now about 12.8 years (Zacharias, Rand, and Wurtman 1976), as it has been for the last three decades (Wyshak and Frisch 1982).

About half of all married women between the ages of twenty and forty-five years were reported to have "diseases of the uterus," which included amenorrhea. The main causes given for amenorrhea were those which "impair the constitutional tone and impoverish the blood": poor diet, disease, particularly tuberculosis and chlorosis (anemia), unsuitable employment, and cold and damp. Doctors noted that working-class women were underweight and amenorrheic because of poverty; upper-class women because of their desire to be fashionably thin. Stress ("violent fits of passion") was also noted as a cause of amenorrhea (Frisch 1978).

The greater risks of pregnancy for an undernourished woman were also understood historically. A century ago, when undernourishment was widespread, Dr. J.M. Duncan told the Royal College of Physicians that although sterility of women was often curable, "a good argument may be made out for not curing it, in many cases at least," because an undernourished mother puts herself and her fetus at risk (Frisch 1978; Frisch, Wyshak, and Vincent 1980d). Of course, as today, it was assumed that pathologic causes of sterility were excluded.

Summary

While the reproductive system is slowly maturing, the growing body also changes, not only in size, and proportions, but in the relative proportions of the tissues, neural, bone, muscle, and fat (Frisch 1980a). The role of estrogen in modulating food intake (Wade 1975), and fat storage (Lesher and Collier 1973) during growth, and maturation, and the reverse relationship indicated above, the importance of a particular fat/lean ratio, on estrogen secretion and metabolism remain to be elucidated.

Adipose tissue itself may be a determinant of menarche and mature reproductive ability through: (1) the conversion of androgens to estrogen (Frisch, Canick, and Tulchinsky 1980b); Nimrod and Ryan 1975; Perel and Killinger 1979), a critical amount of estrogen may be necessary to prime the ovary (McArthur et al. 1976); (2) Body weight, hence fatness, influences the direction of estrogen metabolism to the most potent or least potent forms (Fishman, Boyar, and Hellman 1975). Extreme leanness may be related to the production of anti-estrogens, the catechol estrogens (Fishman 1976); (3) Changes in body-fat composition are correlated with changes in sex-hormone binding globulin thus regulating the availability of estradiol to the brain and other target tissues (Nisker, Hammond, and Siiteri 1980).

Clinically, the minimal weight for height findings have been found useful in cases of nutritional amenorrhea (Fries and Nillius 1973). Knuth, Hill, and Jacobs (1977) point out that "dietary treatment of patients with amenorrhea and loss of weight may replace gonadotropin therapy for induction of ovulation in a significant proportion of patients with anovulatory infertility.''

With the ever-increasing number of serious women athletes and dancers, clinicians must now add to the long list of possible causes of delayed menarche and amenorrhea, regular, intense, exercise (Dale, Gerlach, and Wilhite 1979; Frisch et al. 1981), which may be accompanied by bizarre food intakes (Frisch, Wyshak, and Vincent 1980c). These effects of undernutrition and exercise on menarche and the menstrual cycle are apparently reversible (McArthur et al. 1976; Frisch et al. 1980c; Warren 1980). In some subjects a one or two kilogram weight change will turn cycles on and off (Frisch 1977a; Frisch et al. 1981). However, nothing is known as yet about the mechanisms involved, or about the long-term effects on fertility.

References

Boyar, R.M., Katz, J., Finkelstein, J.W., Kapen, S., Weiner, E.D., and Hellman, L. 1974. Anorexia nervosa: Immaturity of the 24-Hour luteinizing hormone secretory pattern. *New England Journal of Medicine* 291:861-865.

Bulmer, M.G. 1970. *The biology of twinning in man*. Oxford, Eng.: Oxford University Press.

Coop, I.E. 1966. Effect of flushing on reproductive performance of lives. *Journal of Agricultural Science Cambridge* 67:305-323.

Dale, E., Gerlach, D.H., and Wilhite, A.L. 1979. Menstrual dysfunction in distance runners. *Obstetrics and Gynecology* 54:47-53.

Fishman, J. The catechol estrogens. 1976. *Neuroendocrinology* 22:363-374.

Fishman, J., Boyar, R.M., and Hellman, L. 1975. Influence of body weight on estradiol metabolism in young women. *Journal of Clinical Endocrinology and Metabolism* 41:989-991.

Fries, H., and Nillius, S.J. 1973. Dieting, anorexia nervosa, and amenorrhea after oral contraceptive treatment. *Acta Psychiatrica Scandinavia* 49:669-679.

Friis-Hansen, B.J. 1956. Changes in body-water compartments during growth. *Acta Paediatrica (Stockholm)* 110:1-67.

Frisch, R.E. 1972. Weight at menarche: Similarity for well-nourished and under-nourished girls at differing ages, and evidence for historical constancy. *Pediatrics* 50:445-450.

_____. 1975a. Demographic implications of the biological determinants of female fecundity. *Social Biology* 22:19-22.

_____. 1976. Fatness of girls from menarche to age 18 years, with a nomogram. *Human Biology* 48:353-359.

———. 1977a. Food intake, fatness and reproductive ability. In R. Vigersky, ed., *Anorexia nervosa.* New York: Raven Press, pp. 149-161.

———. 1978 Population, food intake, and fertility. *Science* 199:22-30.

———. 1980a. Pubertal adipose tissue: Is it necessary for normal sexual maturation? Evidence from the rat and human female. *Federal Proceedings* 39:2395-2400.

———. 1981. What's below the surface? *New England Journal of Medicine* 305:1019-1020.

Frisch, R.E., Canick, J.A., and Tulchinsky, D. 1980b. Human fatty marrow aromatizes androgen to estrogen. *Journal of Clinical Endocrinology and Metabolism* 51:394-396.

Frisch, R.E., Hegsted, D.M., and Yoshinaga, K. 1975b. Body weight and food intake at early estrus of rats on a high-fat diet. *Proceedings of the National Academy of Science* 72:4172-4176.

———. 1977b. Carcass components at first estrus of rats on high-fat and low-fat diets; body water, protein, and fat. *Proceedings of the National Academy of Science, USA* 74:379-383.

Frisch, R.E., and McArthur, J.W. 1974. Menstrual cycles: Fatness as a determinant of minimum weight for height necessary for their maintenance or onset. *Science* 185:149-151.

Frisch, R.E., and Revelle, R. 1971. Height and weight at menarche and a hypothesis of menarche. *Archives of Diseases of Childhood* 46:695-701.

Frisch, R.E., Welbergen, A., McArthur, J.W., Albright, T., Witschi, J., Bullen, B., Birnholz, J., Reed, R., and Hermann, H. 1981. Delayed menarche, irregular cycles, and amenorrhea of college athletes in relation to age of onset of training. Abstract #147, Endocrine Society Program, Cincinnati, (June):119, and *Journal of The American Medical Association* 246:1559-1563.

Frisch, R.E., Wyshak, G., and Vincent, L. 1980c. Delayed menarche and amenorrhea of ballet dancers. *New England Journal of Medicine* 303: 17-19.

———. 1980d. More on fatness and reproduction. *New England Journal of Medicine* 303:1125-1126.

Hammond, J., Ed., 1955. *Progress in the physiology of farm animals* vol. 2. London: Butterworths.

Harris, R.P. 1871. Early puberty. *American Journal of Obstetrics* 3:611-613.

Kennedy, G.C. 1969. Interactions between feeding behavior and hormones during growth. *Annals of the New York Academy of Science* 157: 1049-1061.

Kennedy, G.C., and Mitra, J. 1963. Body weight and food intake as initiation factors for puberty in the rat. *Journal of Physiology* 166:408-418.

Keys, A. et al. 1959. The biology of human starvation, vol. 1. Minneapolis: University of Minnesota.

Knuth, U.A., Hill, M.G.R., and Jacobs, H.S. 1977. Amenorrhea and loss of weight. *British Journal of Obstetrics and Gynecology* 84:801-807.

Lesher, A.I., and Collier, G. 1973. The effects of gonadectomy on the sex differences in dietary self-selection patterns and carcass compositions of rats. *Physiological Behavior* 11:671-676.

Marshall, J.C., and Frasier, T.R. 1971. Amenorrhea in anorexia nervosa: Assessment and treatment with clomiphene citrate. *British Medical Journal* 4:590-592.

McArthur, J.W., O'Loughlin, K.M., Beitins, I.Z., Johnson, L., Hourihan, J., and Alonso, C. 1976. Endocrine studies during the refeeding of young women with nutritional amenorrhea and infertility. *Mayo Clinic Proceedings* 51:607-615.

Mellits, E.D., and Cheek, D. 1970. The assessment of body water and fatness from infancy to adulthood. In Brozek, J., ed., *Physical growth and body composition*. Monogr Soc Res Child Dev. 35:12-26.

Nimrod, A., and Ryan, K.J. 1975. Aromatization of androgens by human abdominal and breast fat tissue. *Journal of Clinical Endocrinology and Metabolism* 40:367-372.

Nisker, J.A., Hammond, G.L., and Siiteri, P.K. 1980. More on fatness and reproduction. *New England Journal of Medicine* 303:1124.

Palmer, R.L., Crisp, A.H., MacKinnon, P.C.B., Franklin, M., Bonner, J., and Wheeler, M. 1975. Pituitary sensitivity to 50 Hg LH/FSH-RH in subjects with anorexia nervosa in acute and recovery stages. *British Medical Journal* 1:179-182.

Perel, E., and Killinger, D.W. 1979. The interconversion and aromatization of androgens by human adipose tissue. *Journal of Steroid Biochemistry* 10:623-626.

Tanner, J.M. 1962. *Growth at adolescence*. Oxford, Engl: Blackwell.

Vigersky, R.A., Andersen, A.E., Thomson, R.H., and Loriaux, D.L. 1977. Hypothalamic dysfunction in secondary amenorrhea associated with simple weight loss. *New England Journal of Medicine* 297:1141-1145.

Wade, G.N. 1975. Some effects of ovarian hormones on food intake and body weight in female rats. *Journal of Comparative Physiological Psychology* 88:183-193.

Wahren, J. 1979. Glucose turnover during exercise in health man and in patients with diabetes mellitus. *Diabetes Supplement 1* 28:82-89.

Wakeling, A., and Russell, G.F.M. 1970. Disturbances in the regulation of body temperature in anorexia nervosa. *Psychological Medicine* 1:30-39.

Warren, M.P. 1980. The effects of exercise on pubertal progression and reproductive function in girls. *Journal of Clinical Endocrinology and Metabolism* 51:1150-1157.

Warren, M.P., Jewelewicz, R., Dyrenfurth, I., Ans, R., Khalaf, S., and Vande Wiele, R.L. 1975. The significance of weight loss in the evaluation of pituitary response to LH-RH in women with secondary amenorrhea. *Journal of Clinical Endocrinology and Metabolism* 40:601-611.

Wyshak, G., and Frisch, R.E. 1982. Evidence for a secular trend in age of menarche. *New England Journal of Medicine* 306:1033-1035.

Zacharias, L., Rand, W.M., and Wurtman, R.J. 1976. A prospective study of sexual development and growth in American girls. *Obstetrics and Gynecology Survey* 31:325-337.

2 Endocrine Aspects of Menarche and Menopause— Milestones in the Woman's Life Cycle

Inge Dyrenfurth

Around two biological events, menarche and menopause, stands—unpronounced—the idea of the wholeness of a woman's life cycle. Its various phases are symbolically represented in Figure 2-1: childhood, adolescence, reproductive maturity, climacterium and seniority. It is a description of our somatic condition. This typical pattern is to a considerable degree under the control of our particular endocrine system, which we assume to be anchored in our genetic heritage, and is further modified into countless individual patterns by numerous environmental influences. The hormones secreted by the endocrine glands are active all through our lives. They interact in highly complex and continuously changing ways that we are far from comprehending. The endocrine system has been likened to an orchestra. As we hear the various instruments alternatively taking the lead during the performance of a symphony, so can we observe the various hormones dominating certain phases of our life cycle and at other times receding into the background. Thus we find growth hormone, thyroid and parathyroid hormones highly active in childhood when growth and skeletal development takes place. Adrenal and ovarian hormones enter into this interplay at puberty. The ovarian hormones powerfully dominate the years of reproductive maturity. With menopause, ovarian hormones disappear and we see a steady decline of the adrenal hormones as we move toward old age. Even the hormones of childhood lose their significance in the period of seniority.

Figure 2-2 indicates the position of the endocrine glands within our bodies. In the head we find the pineal and pituitary glands with the hypothalamus between them. In the neck region are the thyroid and parathyroids. In the chest is the thymus, a structure whose endocrine significance still eludes us, and in the abdomen are the pancreas, the adrenal glands, and the ovaries. Figure 2-2 also lists the hormones secreted by these glands. The endocrine events at puberty are not isolated processes. Rather, they are seen in this chapter as a sequel to the hormonal events of childhood and as preparation for those of maturity. They are also viewed in polarity to the endocrinology of the perimenopause. It is only in such context that adolescent physiology assumes a fuller meaning. In accordance with the

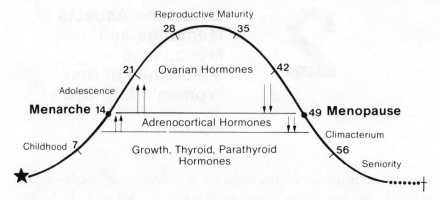

Figure 2-1. Symbolic Representation of the Woman's Life Cycle. Its Phases and Their Hormones

theme of this book the endocrine events of childhood and puberty will be dealt with most extensively while those of the mature menstrual cycle and of menopause and old age will be mentioned only briefly. They have been described in more detail in other publications (Dyrenfurth et al. 1974; Dyrenfurth 1982).

Childhood and Seniority

The physical growth and development of the child can be seen most clearly in longitudinal growth, changes in body proportions and in skeletal development. While the growth in the height of girls shows a linear progression until the age of fifteen and then begins to level out, the growth curves of individual organs and tissues present very diversified patterns (Figure 2-3). Relatively linear growth is seen for the pituitary and thyroid gland whereas pineal growth levels out at about nine years. Most interesting are the patterns for the adrenal glands and thymus. The weight of the latter is maximal at approximately age fourteen and then regresses, thus following the general growth pattern of lymphatic tissues. The adrenal glands are large at birth, then shrink and metamorphose over the first year of life. Thereafter begins a slow continuous growth that accelerates in early puberty, at eight to twelve years. Ovarian and uterine weights—not shown here—sharply increase in growth between ten and fifteen years (Scammon 1931). While these changes are not directly observable, the overall proportions of the child's body change markedly during its development, from the dominance of the head in the small child to a dominance of trunk and limbs

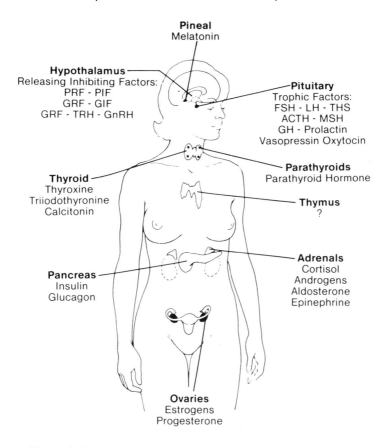

Figure 2-2. The Endocrine Glands and Their Hormones

in the adult. Particularly profound are the changes of the skeleton. In a newborn child only centers for shoulder and hipbones are present; wrists are even without centers. It is a long development to a fully calcified skeleton in the adult, which finds its conclusion when the epiphyses of the long bones are closed at puberty.

To point to the polarity of events as seen in the aged individual we note a distinct loss in height due to bending of the spine, reduction in intervertebral space, and maybe even crushfractures of the vertebrae. There is loss of calcium from the bone, resulting in brittleness and varying degrees of osteoporosis. Changes in numerous other tissues have been described generally in the direction of rigidification (Kohn 1978). Already such a sketchy description makes it clear that in addition to quantitative aspects we have to deal with changes in quality (form, texture, color). The endocrine

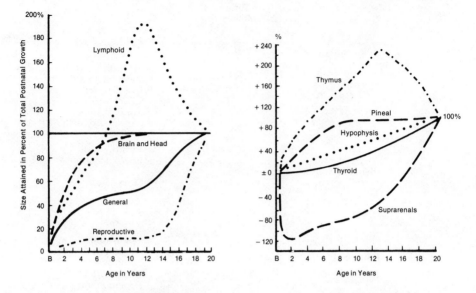

Source: Harris, J.A., Jackson, C.M., Peterson, D.G., and Scammon, R.E. *The measurements of man*. Minneapolis: University of Minnesota Press, © 1930, by the University of Minnesota. Reprinted with permission.

Figure 2-3. Growth Patterns of Some Tissues and of the Endocrine Glands

system, with the complex interrelationships of its various hormones and their continual state of flux, is an important factor contributing to these changes in form and function.

Growth Hormone (GH)

The secretion of this hormone is characterized by a peak at the onset of deep sleep (Parker et al. 1979). This was a startling discovery in the early 1970s when we were used to seeing plasma-cortisol levels rise in the early morning hours. The growth-hormone rhythm is established during the first three to six months of life and is fully developed when the child is one-year old (Vigneri and Agata 1971). Other observations in infants (Finkelstein et al. 1971) indicate that even at this early age there is a dual control of GH, its secretion being stimulated first by sleep and second by stress (crying). Sleep is the primary stimulus of GH in children. The role of GH for the longitudinal growth of a child can be seen from the growth curve of a girl whose pituitary had been removed for a craniopharyngioma and who was

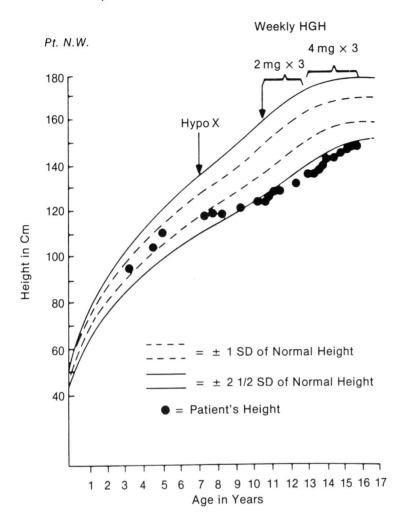

Source: Abrams, C.A.L., Grumbach, M.M., Dyrenfurth, I., and Vande Wiele, R.L. Ovarian stimulation with human menopausal and chorionic gonadotropins in a prepubertal hypophysectomized female. *Journal of Clinical Endocrinology and Metabolism*, 1967, 27:467-472. © 1967, The Endocrine Society. Reprinted with permission.

Figure 2-4. Growth Curve of a Child, before and after Hypophysectomy and following Treatment with Human Growth Hormone

subsequently treated with GH isolated from human pituitaries (see figure 2-4). Growth velocity—the centimeters grown per year—is very fast during the first two years, then becomes slower and more steady until around age 12 (in girls) when a renewed but transient acceleration occurs—the adoles-

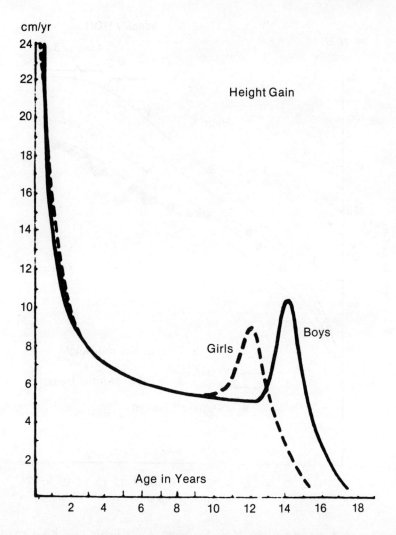

Source: Tanner, J.M., Whitehouse, R.H., and Takaishi, M. Standards from birth to maturity
for height, weight, height velocity, and weight velocity: British children. *Archives of Diseases
of Childhood*, 1966, 41:454-471, Figure on p. 466. Reprinted with permission.

Figure 2-5. Velocity Curves for Longitudinal Growth

cent growth spurt (see figure 2-5). During this growth spurt arginine and insulin (further stimuli for GH secretion) elicit heightened responses (Sperling, Kenny, and Drash 1970; Frasier, Hillborn, and Smith 1970). Also the
sleep-related peak is most pronounced at this age (see figure 2-6).

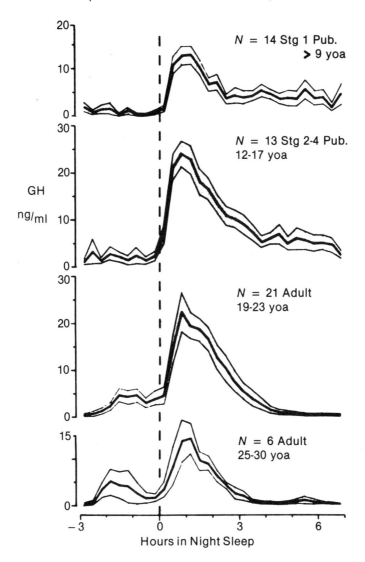

GH

ng/ml

Hours in Night Sleep

Source: Parker, D.C., Rossman, L.G., Kripke, D.F., Gibson, W., and Wilson, K. Rhythmicities in human growth hormone concentrations in human plasma. In D. Krieger (Ed.) *Endocrine rhythms.* New York: Raven Press, 1979. Figure on p. 163. Reprinted with permission.

Figure 2-6. Peak of Sleep-Related Serum Growth Hormone in Puberty as Compared to Childhood and Adulthood

The diminished role of GH in climacteric and aged women (absence of sleep-related peaks, reduced response to glucose, insulin, arginine) has been dealt with previously (Dyrenfurth 1982).

Thyroid Hormones: Thyroxine (T_4)
and Triiodothyronine (T_3)

Older measurements, using protein-bound iodine as an indicator for thyroid function, found this to be low during the years of puberty (Fisher 1967). This finding has been confirmed with newer methods (RIA) that show T_3 and T_4 plasma levels at age fourteen to sixteen years, presenting a minimum, but distinct, elevation of free T_3 and T_4 (the portion not bound to plasma thyroid-binding globulin—TBG). The free fraction of the thyroid hormones is generally thought of as the physiologically active form (see figure 2-7). Parallel with the increase in the free hormones goes an actual decline of TBG. These recent findings reconciled the hormone levels with another parameter of thyroid function—the basal metabolic rate (BMR), which is known to be elevated in puberty.

The aged thyroid secretes less T_3 and T_4 (Bermudez, Surks, and Oppenheimer 1975) and also loses responsiveness to its tropic hormone TSH and the releasing hormone TRH (Azizi et al. 1975).

Parathyroid Hormone (PTH) and Calcitonin (CT)

Bone and calcium metabolism is perhaps an area where genetics, endocrinology, and environmental influences (nutrition and light) are most closely interwoven. The two important hormones maintaining calcium homeostatis are PTH raising blood calcium, and CT lowering it. Together with other factors (such as vitamin D) they continually regulate absorption of calcium from the gut, deposition and resorption from bone, and excretion and reabsorption in the kidney. Estrogenic and androgenic hormones are further modifying influences acting upon these already highly complex processes. They assume particular importance in late puberty when they bring about the gradual closing of the epiphyses and eventual termination of longitudinal growth. Measurements of CT are relatively recent and those of PTH difficult because of the various molecular forms in which the hormone exists, so that our knowledge in the area is very much in flux. In children from six to thirteen years, blood levels of CT and PTH appear to take opposing courses with the CT/PTH ratio gradually declining, thus indicating a very active bone metabolism (Shaikin-Kerstenbaum et al. 1977). These

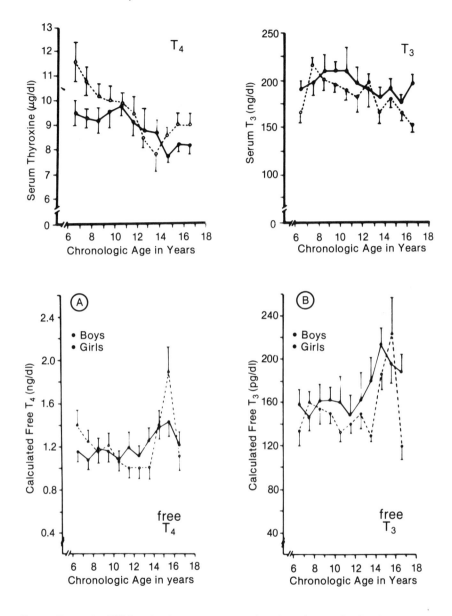

Source: Parra, A., Villalpando, S., Junco, F., Urguieta, B., Alatorre, S., Garcia-Bulnes, G. Thyroid function during childhood and adolescence. *Acta Endocrinologica*, 1980, 93:306. Reprinted with permission.

Figure 2-7. Total and Free Serum Thyroxine and Triiodothyronine in Children from Six to Seventeen Years of Age

observations were confirmed by an extensive study that found serum PTH in females high during childhood and adolescence, declining rapidly after the first two decades, reaching a minimum at the time of menopause and thereafter beginning to rise again (see figure 2-8). One may think of the early high levels as providing active calcium available for deposition in the bone matrix as opposed to the postmenopausal rise possibly reflecting the increased resorption from the bone, with resulting osteoporosis.

Measurement of CT from age twenty to eighty showed no significant changes (see figure 2-2) in basic levels while its capacity to respond to a calcium stimulus greatly diminishes in women from age sixty onward.

Adolescent and Menopausal Transition

The glucocorticoid and androgenic components of the adrenal secretion enter into the hormonal interpaly described so far, between the ages of eight to twelve. The result is an increase in muscle strength and the development of pubic and axillary hair (see figures 2-10 and 2-11).

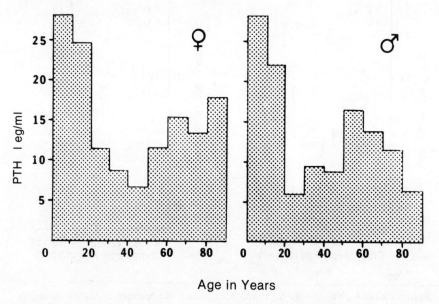

Source: Roof, B., Piel, C.F., Hansen, F., and Feudenberg, J. Serum PTH levels and serum calcium levels from birth to senescence. *Mechanisms of Ageing and Development*, 1976, 5:289-304. Reprinted with permission.

Figure 2-8. Serum-Parathyroid Hormone Concentrations through the Human Life Cycle

Generally somewhat later, (Grumbach, Grave, and Mayer 1974) between eleven and sixteen years of age, the breasts develop (see figure 2-12). Tanner (1978) has defined stages of these developments, where stage 1 represents the peripubertal and stage 5 the adult condition. In figure 2-13 the development of the rounded female proportions is indicated as these are brought about by fat depositions. Following menopause we may observe a shift in these fat deposits as well as a decline in muscle strength.

Adrenocortical Hormones: Cortisol,
Dehydroisoandrosterone, and Aldosterone

An acceleration in weight gain of the adrenal glands is seen in early puberty (see figure 2-3.) For a central European population this acceleration occurred at thirteen years (Dohm 1973). Plasma cortisol levels remain relatively unchanged throughout life but show a pronounced daily variation often with extremely low levels at night (9 P.M. to 2 or 3 A.M.) and highest levels

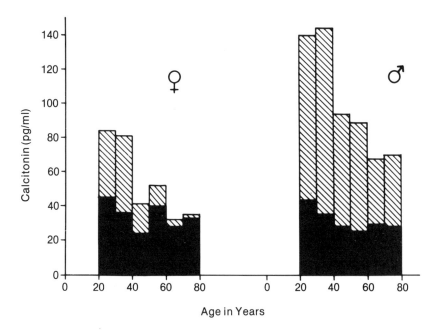

Source: Drawn from data from Deftos et al. (1979). *Conference on Endocrine Aspects of Aging* Bethesda, Maryland.

Note: Black bars, basal levels; shaded bars, response to calcium load.

Figure 2-9. Serum-Calcitonin Concentrations from Ages Twenty to Eighty

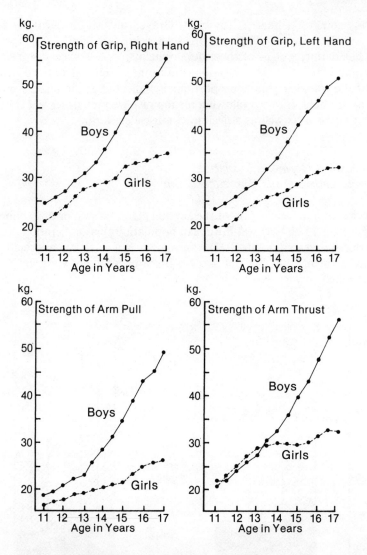

Source: Tanner, J.M. *Growth at adolescence*. 2nd ed. Oxford, Eng.: Blackwell Scientific
Publications, 1962 (based on data of Jones). Reprinted with permission.
Figure 2-10. Strength of Hands and Arms in Childhood and Adolescence

in the early morning hours (Blichert-Toft 1975). The daily production of
this hormone, however, as it comes to expression in the twenty-four-hour
urinary excretion of its metabolites (the 17-hydroxy-corticosteroids) is
markedly age dependent and shows curves with a steep rise and fall during
the adolescent and menopausal years (see figure 2-14). Maximal production
occurs from twenty to forty years. Similar curves have been obtained for the

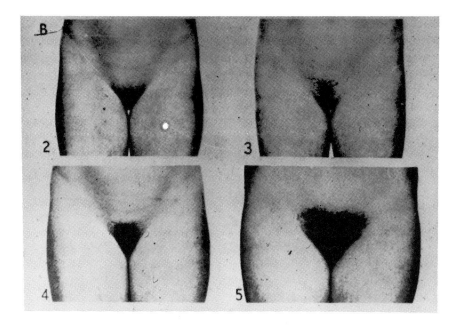

Source: Tanner, J.M. *Fetus into man*. Cambridge, Mass.: Harvard University Press, 1978. Figures on pp. 197, 199. © 1978, Harvard University Press. Reprinted with permission.

Figure 2-11. Pubic-Hair Stages in Female Adolescence

metabolites of the adrenal androgens, generally measured as 17 ketosteroids (Hamburger 1948). Such curves substantiate the generalized life chart presented in figure 2-1. One of the adrenal androgens is dehydroisoandrosterone, a substance exceeding in magnitude all other adrenocortical secretions, whose physiological function still remains a mystery. Its secretion over the life cycle follows closely that of the 17-ketosteroids (Smith et al. 1975) with serum concentrations showing a clear increase at age eight to twelve (Korth-Schütz, Levine, and New 1976). A third type of hormone secreted by the adrenal cortex is aldosterone, which is of significance in the regulation of water and electrolyte metabolism and shows an entirely different course over the life cycle; that is, a small gradual and steady decline from childhood to old age. But more significant, aldosterone is related to the decline in the capacity to respond to such stimuli as low sodium diet, upright posture, or high altitude (see figure 2-15). This curve is paralleled by the extracellular water of the body.

We may think of the basically fluid and succulent condition in childhood as favorable for all other structure-building hormones, while the drier basic conditions of age do not allow the hormones to exert their actions (repair) to the same extent.

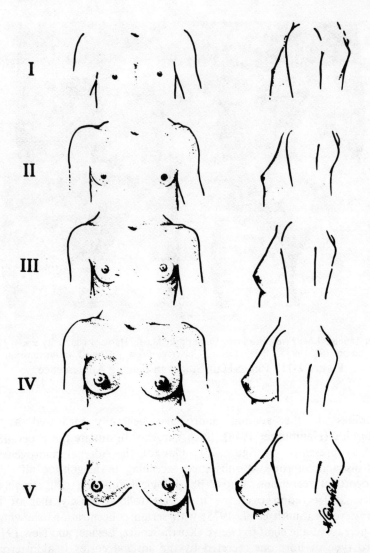

Source: Tanner, J.M. *Fetus into man*. Cambridge, Mass.: Harvard University Press, 1978.
Figures on pp. 197, 199. © 1978, Harvard University Press. Reprinted with permission.
Figure 2-12. Breast Stages in Female Adolescence

Ovarian Hormones (Estrogens and Progesterone)
and Pituitary Gonadotropins (FSH and LH).

While development of the secondary sex characteristics are observable
phenomena, maturation of the ovaries and uterus proceed unnoticed and

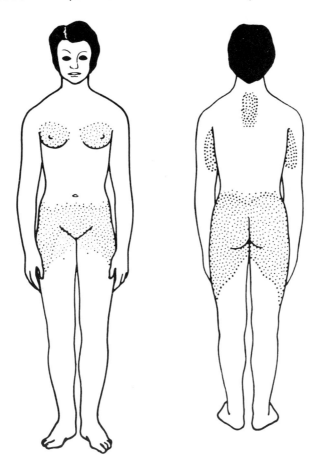

Source: Sinclair, D. *Human growth after birth*. 3rd ed. Oxford, Eng.: Oxford University Press, 1978. Figures on pp. 49, 107. 166. Reprinted with permission.

Figure 2-13. Sites of Fat Deposition in the Female Body at Puberty

only the first menstrual bleeding will indicate that the ovaries have assumed their regular function: the rhythmically changing secretion of estrogens, progesterone, and also some androgens. This process is set into motion by hypothalamic signals to the pituitary, which begins to secrete follicle-stimulating hormone (FSH) and luteinizing hormone (LH). Rises in the blood levels of both these gonadotropins are observed in early puberty, again mysteriously at night with the onset of sleep-like GH (see figure 2-16). Gradually FSH brings some of the ovarian follicles to development and LH stimulates estradiol secretion (Grumbach, Grave, and Mayer 1974). When estradiol levels are high enough they cause a sudden surge of LH

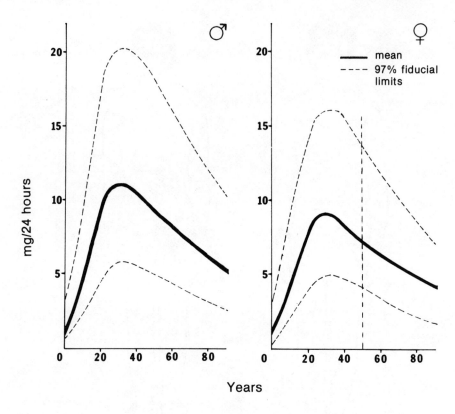

Source: Redrawn from Borth, Linder, and Riondel (1957). *Acta Endocrinologica* 25.

Figure 2-14. Daily Excretion of 17-Hydroxycorticosteroids as a Measure of Glucocorticoid Hormone Production

release from the pituitary—which in turn causes the first ovulation, corpus luteum formation, and fourteen days later the first menstruation, which we term *menarche.* Another hormone possibly supporting ovarian development is prolactin, which in adolescent girls appears to be secreted in elevated amounts (Ekara, Yen, and Siler 1975).

Menarche follows the adolescent growth spurt by one or two years (see figure 2-17). This sequence of events means that a certain stage of nonsexual development—weight, height, bone—is prerequisite to the onset of ovarian function, an observation that is being studied extensively in connection with anorexia nervosa. Much literature is available both on this topic and also on the shift of menarche to younger years.

A child does not always establish typical and regular cycles immediately. As a rule a transition period, which may last up to seven years, precedes full sexual maturity (Treloar et al. 1967). This period is characterized by en-

Aldosterone Excretion

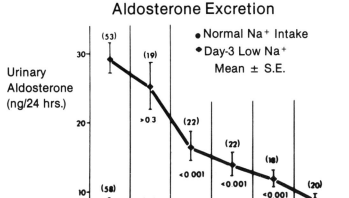

Urinary Aldosterone (ng/24 hrs.)

Age in Years

Extracellular Body Water

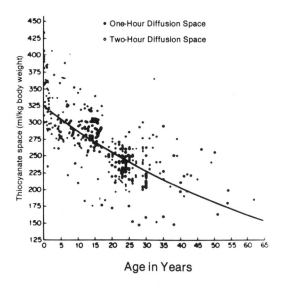

Age in Years

Source: Crane, M., and Genest, J. Essential hypertension: New concepts about mechanisms. *Annals of Internal Medicine*, 1973, 79:411-424. Reprinted with permission.

Source: Dittmer, D. (Ed.) *Blood and other body fluids*. Bethesda, Md.: Federation of American Societies for Experimental Biology, 1961 © 1961, by Federation of American Socieites for Experimental Biology. Reprinted with permission.

Figure 2-15. Urinary Aldoesterone and Extracellular Body Water with Age

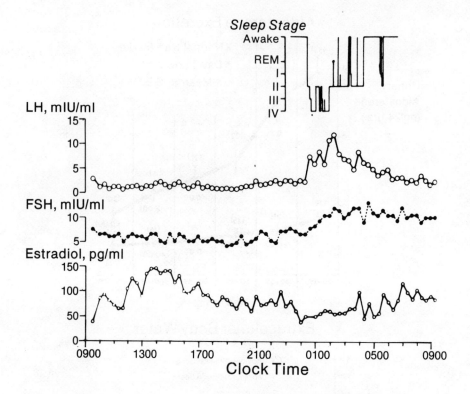

Source: Boyar, R.M., Wu, R.H.K., Roffward, H., Kapen, S., Weitzman, E.D., Hellman, L., and Finkelstein, J.W. Human puberty: 24 hour estradiol patterns in pubertal girls. *Journal of Clinical Endocrinology and Metabolism*, 1976, 43:1418-1420. © 1976, The Endocrine Society. Reprinted with permission.

Figure 2-16. Twenty-Four-Hour Pattern of Serum Gonadotropins (FSH and LH) and Estradiol in a Girl in Stage 3 of Pubertal Development

docrinologically incomplete cycles of varying length, interspersed with the occasional fertile cycle.

One example of an hormonally incomplete cycle is shown in figure 2-18. There is a typical peak of estradiol, followed by a likewise typical LH and FSH peak. But this peak occurs relatively late, twenty days following a menstruation. Then no progesterone is produced, indicating that no ovulation had taken place and no corpus luteum was formed. Accordingly bleeding followed not fourteen but five days after the gonadotropin peak.

A similar transition period leads up to the *menopause*, the last menstrual bleeding in a woman's life. The menopausal transition, too, is characterized by irregular—mostly prolonged —cycles often hormonally incomplete. Estrogen levels become lower until eventually they no longer can

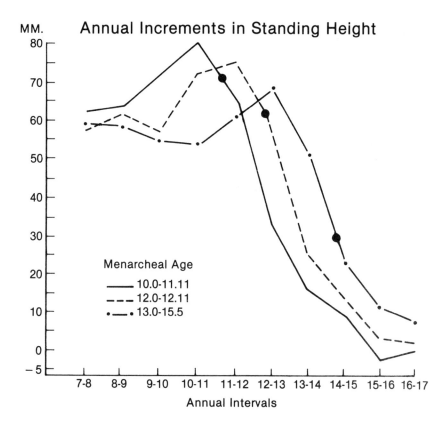

MM.   **Annual Increments in Standing Height**

Menarcheal Age

——— 10.0-11.11

- - - 12.0-12.11

•—• 13.0-15.5

Annual Intervals

Source: Sinclair, D. *Human growth after birth*. 3rd ed. Oxford, Eng.: Oxford University Press, 1978. Figures on pp. 49, 107, 166. Reprinted with permission.

Note: The rings indicate menarche.

Figure 2-17. Onset of Menarche in Relation to Adolescent Growth Spurt

provide either positive or negative feedback to the pituitary and FSH and LH increase dramatically and establish the woman's postmenopausal state (Wiede et al. 1973). Prolactin however, keeps declining in the postmenopausal years (Vekemans and Robyn, 1975). Excellent statistics about cycle length and regularity of both transition periods are available and date the mature period for reproduction from twenty to forty years (Presser 1974).

The Reproductive Years

The teenager gradually establishes regular, fertile cycles of twenty-six to thirty-days duration with typical hormonal function. Figure 2-19 shows daily

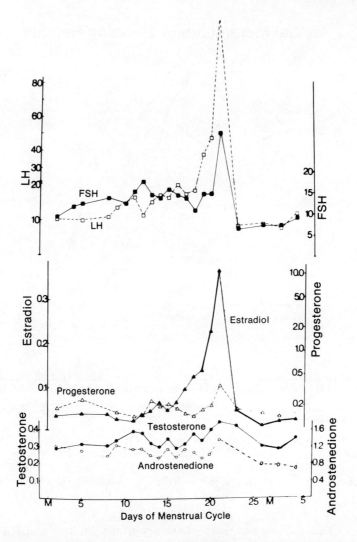

Source: Apter, D., Vinikka, L., and Vikho, R. Hormonal patterns in adolescent menstrual cycles. *Journal of Clinical Endocrinology and Metabolism,* 1978, 47:944-954. © 1978, The Endocrine Society. Reprinted with permission.

Figure 2-18. Example of a Hormonally Incomplete Menstrual Cycle during the Period of Adolescent Transition

measurements of plasma levels of the pituitary gonadotropins and ovarian estrogens and progesterone in forty-two normal, mature cycles.

Menses must be thought of as occurring at the beginning and end of the curves around day fourteen. At midcycle (day zero) a sharp peak in LH and

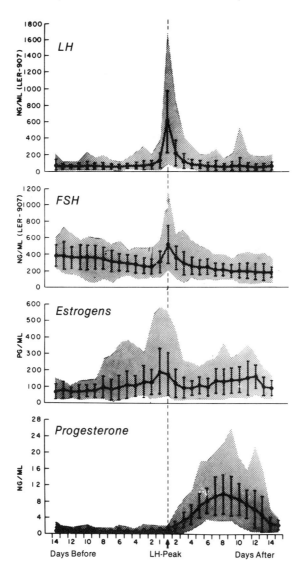

Source: Dyrenfurth, I., Jewelewicz, R., Warren, M., Ferin, M., and Vande Wiele, R.L. Temporal relationships of hormonal variables in the menstrual cycle. In M. Ferin, F. Halberg, R.M. Richart, and R.L. Vande Wiele (Eds.) *Biorhythms and human reproduction*. New York: John Wiley and Sons, 1974. Copyright © 1974 John Wiley & Sons. Reprinted by permission of John Wiley & Sons, Inc.

Note: The shaded area shows the entire range of measurements; the solid line means ± SD.

Figure 2-19. Hormonal Patterns of Forty-Two Menstrual Cycles in Healthy Women Aged Twenty to Thirty

FSH is seen, which is known to trigger ovulation. Leading up to it is a steep rise in estrogens while progesterone during this follicular phase remains at baseline levels. It rises and falls only during the two weeks following ovulation—the luteal phase. It does so in parallel with a renewed rise and fall of estrogens. In figure 2-20 the simultaneous anatomical events in ovary and uterus are indicated.

Under the influence of elevated levels of FSH at the onset of each cycle, a cohort of follicles begin to grow layers of granulosa and theca cells, which in the second week begin to secrete estrogens and to form an antral fluid-filled cavity. All but one of these follicles become atretic and regress while the one, named the Graafian follicle, will reach maturity and under the influence of the LH-surge will rupture and release a fertilizable ovum. The cells of the ruptured follicle luteinize and metamorphose into a new organ, the corpus luteum, which in turn produces progesterone in addition to estrogens. The ovarian hormones in their rhythmic sequence influence the structure of the uterine endometrium as symbolized in the lower panel of figure 2-20. Every month this endometrium is vascularized, become secretory, and, if no pregnancy occurs, is broken down again and the tissue expelled with the monthly bleeding. Many other physiological and even psychologic rhythms are known to occur in parallel with the four weekly rhythms of the female gonadal and pituitary function—to name but a few: rise and fall of basal body temperature with changing progesterone, increased

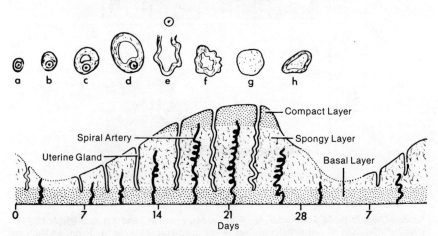

Source: Sinclair, D. *Human growth after birth*. 3rd ed. Oxford, Eng.: Oxford University Press, 1978. Figures on pp. 49, 107, 166. Reprinted with permission.

Note: Upper panel (ovary): follicle development, follicle rupture, and corpus-luteum formation and regression. Lower panel (uterus): endometrial build-up and regression.

Figure 2-20. Anatomical Changes in Ovary and Uterus during the Menstrual Cycle

and decreased production of cervical mucus with changing estrogen levels, and cyclic changes in vaginal cytology.

Summary and Conclusion

This chapter followed the development of the child to the young woman through the immensely important phase of puberty and adolescence from the endocrinologic view point. It also reflected on the polarity between the hormonal events in childhood and puberty and those in menopause and aging.

We saw the diurnal rhythms in the secretion of GH (maximal at onset of sleep) and cortisol (maximal in the early morning hours), which continue all through life, but are more pronounced in childhood and of lesser amplitude or even absent in age. We further saw the two ovarian hormones, estradiol and progesterone beginning their four-weekly rhythms at menarche and ending them at menopause. The picture of a life cycle evolved and is seen most clearly in the rise of glucocorticoid and androgen production from early puberty to a maximum at twenty to forty or 45 years with a decline following. We also saw the opposite form of curve in the case of PTH where there is a trough in the middle years with higher levels in the earlier and later decades. The course of aldosterone and particularly its responsiveness to stimuli revealed a different shape of curve, one characterized by a maximum at birth and a steady decline to old age. Most astonishing, the gonadotropins, especially FSH, remain at or below baseline all through childhood, showing rhythmically repeating peaks starting with puberty and then reaching their maximum levels in the years of climacterium and seniority.

Thus we have seen the maturation, regression, and rhythms that characterize the endocrinology of the female life cycle.

References

Abrams. C.A.L., Grumbach, M.M., Dyrenfurth, I., and Vande Wiele, R.L. 1967. Ovarian stimulation with human menopausal and chorionic gonadotropins in a prepubertal hypophysectomized female. *Journal of Clinical Endocrinology and Metabolism* 27:467-472.

Apter, D., Vinikka, L., and Vikho, R. 1978. Hormonal patterns in adolescent menstrual cycles. *Journal of Clinical Endocrinology and Metabolism* 47:944-954.

Azizi, F., Vagenakis, A.G., Portnay, G.I., Rapaport, B., Ingbar, S.H., and Braverman, L.E. 1975. Pituitary thyroid responsiveness to intramuscular thyrotropin releasing hormone based on analyses of serum thyroxine, triodothyronine and thyrotropin concentrations. *New England Journal of Medicine* 292:273-277.

Bermudez, F., Surks, M.I., and Oppenheimer, J.H. 1975. High incidence of decreased serum triiodothyronine concentrations with nonthyroidal disease. *Journal of Clinical Endocrinology and Metabolism* 41:27-40.

Blichert-Toft, M. 1975. Secretion of corticotrophin and somatotropin by the adenohypophysis in man. *Acta Endocrinologica Supplement 195,* 78.

Borth, R., Linder, A., and Riondel, A. 1957. Urinary excretion of 17-hydroxycorticoids and 17-ketosteroids in healthy subjects in relation to sex, age, body weight, and height. *Acta Endocrinologica* 25:33-47.

Boyar, R.M., Wu, R.H.K., Roffwarg, H., Kapen, S., Weitzman, E.D., Hellman, L., and Finkelstein, J.W. 1976. Human puberty: 24 hour estradiol patterns in pubertal girls. *Journal of Clinical Endocrinology and Metabolism* 43:1418-1820.

Crane, M., and Genest, J. 1973. Essential hypertension: New concepts about mechanisms. *Annals of Internal Medicine* 79:411-424.

Deftos, L.J., Weisman, M.H., Williams, G.H., Karpf, B.B., Frumar, A.M., Davidson, H.H., Parthemore, J.G., and Judd, H.L. 1979. Age and sex-related changes of calcitonin secretion in humans. *Conference on Endocrine Aspects of Aging.* (October) Bethesda, Maryland. (S. Korenman).

Dittmer, D., ed. 1961. Blood and other body fluids. Bethesda, Maryland: Federation of American Societies for Experimental Biology.

Dohm, G. 1973. The prepuberal and puberal growth of the adrenal (Adrenarche). *Beiträge Pathology* 150:337-362.

Dyrenfurth, I. 1982. Endocrine functions in the woman's second half of life. In A.M. Voda, M. Dinnerstein, and S.R. O'Donnell, eds. *Changing perpsectives on menopause.* Austin: University of Texas Press.

Dyrenfurth, I., Jewelewicz, R., Warren, M., Ferin, M., and Vande Wiele, R.L. 1974. Temporal relationships of hormonal variables in the menstrual cycle. In M. Ferin, F. Halberg, R.M. Richart, and R.L. Vande Wiele, eds. *Biorhythms and human reproduction.* New York: John Wiley and Sons.

Ekara, Y., Yen, S.S.C., and Siler, T.M. 1975. Serum prolactin levels during puberty. *American Journal of Obstetrics and Gynecology* 121:995-997.

Finkelstein, J.W., Anders, T.F., Sachar, E.J., Roffwang, H.P., and Hellman, L. 1971. Behavioral state, sleep stage and growth hormone levels in human infants. *Journal of Clinical Endocrinology and Metabolism* 32:368-371.

Fisher, O. 1967. Protein-bound iodine levels in childhood and adolescence. *Journal of Clinical Endocrinology and Metabolism* 27:89-92.

Frasier, S.D., Hillburn, J.M., and Smith, F.G. 1970. Effect of adolescence on the serum growth-hormone response to hypoglycemia. *Journal of Pediatrics* 77:465-467.

Grumbach, M.M., Grave, G.D., and Mayer, F.E. 1974. *The control of the onset of puberty.* New York: John Wiley and Sons.

Hamburger, C. 1948. Normal urinary excretion of neutral 17-ketosteroids with special reference to age and sex variations. *Acta Endocrinologica* 1:19-37.

Harris, J.A., Jackson, C.M., Peterson, D.G., and Scammon, R.E. 1930. *The measurements of man.* Minneapolis: University of Minnesota Press.

Jones, H.E. 1949. Motor performance and growth. A developmental study of static dynamomometric strength. Berkely: University of California Press.

Kohn, R.R. 1978. *Principles of mammalian aging,* 2nd ed. Englewood Cliffs, N.J.: Prentice Hall.

Korth-Schütz, S., Levine, L.S., and New, M.J. 1976. Dehydroepiandrosterone sulfate (DS) levels, a rapid test for abnormal adrenal androgen secretion. *Journal of Clinical Endocrinology and Metabolism* 42:1005-1013.

Parker, D.C., Rossman, L.G., Kripke, D.F., Gibson, W., and Wilson, K. 1979. Rhythmicities in human growth-hormone concentrations in human plasma. In D. Krieger, ed. *Endocrine rhythms.* New York: Raven Press.

Parra, A., Villalpando, S., Junco, E., Urguieta, B., Alatorre, S., and Garcia-Bulnes, G. 1980. Thyroid function during childhood and adolescence. *Acta Endocrinologica* 93:306.

Presser, H.B. 1974. Temporal data relating to the human menstrual cycle. In Ferin, M., Halberg, F., Richart, R.M., and Vande Wiele, R.L., eds. *Biorhythms and human reproduction.* New York: John Wiley and Sons.

Roof, B., Piel, C.F., Hansen, F., and Feudenberg, J. 1976. Serum PTH levels and serum calcium levels from birth to senescence. *Mechanisms of aging development* 5:289-304.

Scammon, R.E. 1965. Cited in Donovan, B.T., and Vander Werf ten Bosch, J.J. *Physiology of puberty.* London: Edward Arnold Publishers.

Shaikin-Kerstenbaum, R., Funkenstein, B., Conforti, A., Shani, S., and Berlyne, G.M. 1977. Serum calcitonin and blood mineral inter-relationships in normal children ages six to twelve years. *Pediatric Research* 11:112-116.

Sinclair, D. 1978. *Human growth after birth,* 3rd ed. Oxford, Eng.: Oxford University Press.

Smith, M.R., Rudd, B.T., Shirley, A., Rayner, P.H.W., Williams, J.W., Duignan, N.H., and Bertrand, P.V. 1975. A radioimmunoassay for the estimation of serum dehydroepiandrosterone sulphate in normal and pathological sera. *Clinical Chimical Acta* 65:5-13

Sperling, M.A., Kenny, F.M., and Drash, A.L. 1970. Arginine induced growth-hormone responses in children: Effect of age and puberty. *Journal of Pediatrics* 77:462-465.

Tanner, J.M. 1962. *Growth at adolescence.* 2nd ed. Oxford, Eng.: Blackwell.
_____ . 1978. *Fetus into man.* Cambridge, Mass. Harvard University Press.

Tanner, J.M., Whitehouse, R.H., and Takaishi, M. 1966. Standards from birth to maturity for height, weight, height velocity, and weight velocity. British children 1965. *Archives of Diseases of Childhood* 41:454-471.

Treloar, A.E., Boynton, R.E., Behn, G.G., and Brown, B.W. 1967. Variation of the human menstrual cycle through reproductive life. *International Journal of Fertility* 12:77-126.

Vekemans, M., and Robyn, C. 1975. Influence of age on serum prolactin levels in women and men. *British Medical Journal* 4:738-739.

Vigneri, R., and Agata, R. 1971. Growth hormone release during the first year of life in relation to sleep-wake periods. *Journal of Clinical Endocrinology* 33:561-563.

Wiede, L., Nillius, S.J., Gemzell, C., and Roos, P. 1973. Radioimmunoassay of FSH and LH in serum and urine of men and women. *Acta Endocrinologica Supplement* 174:41-58.

3

Age at Menarche and Year of Birth in Relation to Adult Height and Weight among Caucasian, Japanese, and Chinese Women Living in Hawaii

Madeleine J. Goodman, John S. Grove, and *Fred I. Gilbert, Jr.*

The secular trend toward earlier sexual maturation has been observed in the decline in age at menarche over the past century in many populations throughout the world. (See for example, Tanner 1962; Kumar 1975; Eveleth and Tanner 1976; Van Wieringen 1978; and Farid-Coupal Contreras de Castellano 1981.) While the upper limits from which this trend originated may not be as high as was once believed (Bullough 1981) and the lower limits of the trend may have been reached in some groups (Roberts and Dann 1975), the reality and general contours of the trend seem firmly established, although diverse populations may represent different phases of the same patterns of change. The investigation of that pattern from data cross-culturally is especially important in view of the wide variation in reported mean age at menarche among diverse populations (Hiernaux 1968). Are the recorded differences in mean age at menarche between women from the New Guinea Bundi group (18.8 years) and from Cuba (12.7 years) for example, merely indicative of the nutritional and other environmental differences historically associated with secular trends in Western populations (see Eveleth and Tanner 1976) or are there additional genetic differences in age at menarche between ethnic groups as Rona and Pereira (1974) suggest? The secular trend in age at menarche has been speculatively ascribed to a number of putative causes (Johnston 1974) including increased genetic intermixture (and resulting increases in heterozygosity), changes in climate, urbanization, and economic status.

The effects of variation in age at menarche on the completion of the growth process and on the pattern of fertility have been even less thoroughly explored. Age at menarche has not been found to be a good predictor of age at first pregnancy (Presser 1978; Goodman, Grove, and Gilbert 1980). And while menarche has long been associated with the tempo of female growth, the few existing prior studies have not yielded consistent results about the relationship between age at menarche and adult height. Dreizen, Spirakis, and Stone (1967) and Onat (1975) reported a trend toward increased adult stature with earlier menarche. Clegg (1980), after adjusting for year of birth, found later menarche to be associated with increased adult stature. Studies of the relationship between age at menarche and adult weight generally have been limited to special populations such as ballet dancers and athletes, who show late menarche and less weight-for-height than nonathletic women (Frisch 1980; Malina et al. 1978).

Yet, adult height is one of the best-established instances of a secular trend in human biometric data. Secular trends toward increased stature have been reported in many, but not all, populations around the world (Tanner 1978). Again, there is a question about upper limits, since some populations appear to have reached a plateau (Clegg 1980; Damon 1968). But wherever pronounced improvements in environmental conditions, such as health care and nutrition, are underway, this secular trend in height has been clearly observed.

It may be that the confounding effects of the two secular trends make the actual relationship of age at menarche to adult height difficult to compare from one population to the next. To tease out the complex effects of secular trends, adjustment must be made for the direct and indirect effects of year of birth on age at menarche, and on adult height and weight. The methodology of Path Analysis, after Li (1975) provides one approach for describing the web of the linear relationships among the variables. One of the strengths of this method is that it provides a means of comparing statistical relationships between age at menarche and adult height and weight among ethnic groups where secular trends differ.

The present chapter investigates the relationship of age at menarche to adult height and weight among Caucasian, Japanese, and Chinese women of comparable socioeconomic status (Goodman et al. 1982) living in the common microenvironment of Hawaii. It also describes the secular trends affecting these three variables.

Method

The population was drawn from 10,030 women who participated in a statewide breast-cancer-screening demonstration project run by the Pacific Health Research Institute in Honolulu between 1974 and 1980. As described previously (Goodman, Grove, and Gilbert 1980, Goodman et al. 1982), all data were collected by trained medical personnel using a standard medical-history form. Heights and weights were obtained concurrently with reproductive history for 3,205 parous women drawn randomly from the total population. These 1,291 Caucasian, 1,519 Japanese, and 395 Chinese women form the present study sample. The subject population included women of comparable socioeconomic level born between 1900 and 1940. Age at menarche was ascertained by oral interview conducted by specially trained interviewers and based on subjects' recollection.

The models developed were a set of interrelated linear equations that were fit by least-squares regression using the Statistical Package for the Social Sciences (SPSS) program package. Tests for lack of fit of the models were constructed by adding quadratic and cubic terms of the variables and their cross-products. The cross-product of an ethnic-group design variable with another variable measures the interaction of ethnic group with that variable (see Draper and Smith 1966).

Since the error degrees of freedom were always well over 300, for practical purposes we have assumed infinite degrees of freedom for significance testing. To simplify notation, all F test values were transformed to corresponding X^2 tests by simply multiplying each F value by its numerator degrees of freedom. Thus $F_{1,\infty} = X_1^2$; $3 \cdot F_{3,\infty} = X_3^2$, and so forth.

Results

The set of equations relating age at menarche and year of birth with adult height, adult weight, and other study variables was calculated separately for Caucasians, Japanese, and Chinese ethnic groups. The general linear model describing the network of relationships among the variables studied is presented in figure 3-1. The direction and sequence of effects specified in the equations can be seen. Each variable in the figure is presumed to be caused, at least indirectly, by those variables with path arrows leading to it. Means and standard deviations for variables studied in the path analysis are given in table 3-1.

Table 3-2 presents the analysis of variance summarizing the large hierarchical series of regression equations describing the linear, nonlinear, and interactive statistical relationships of each variable in the path diagram to its presumptive causal factors. It also gives tests of ethnic-group heterogeneity for the various statistical relationships between independent variables and the dependent variable in each model. In examining the complex web of relationships we will proceed according to the direction of the relationships among variables presented in figure 3-1: the model for age at menarche, followed by adult height, and, finally, the model for adult weight.

The Age-at-Menarche Model

The mean age at menarche in our study population did not vary significantly among ethnic groups $(X_2^2 = 3.24, p > .05)$ however the secular trend

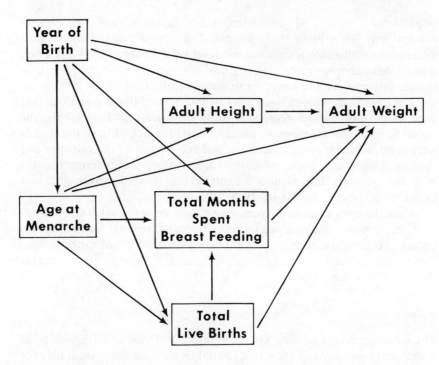

Figure 3-1. Path Diagram Illustrating the Relationship of Year of Birth
and Age at Menarche to Adult Height and Weight

toward earlier age at menarche appears to have been more rapid among
Orientals than Caucasians ($X_1^2 = 30.49$, $p < .001$). The average decline for
pooled Orientals is $-.051$ years at age at menarche per year of birth. In
Caucasians the average decline in age at menarche was only $-.019$ years per
year of birth. Chinese and Japanese did not differ significantly in their rates
of decline in age at menarche ($X_1^2 = 0.97$) and there was no evidence of a
highly significant nonlinear effect of year of birth on age at menarche in any
ethnic group ($X_6^2 = 9.22$, $p > .1$).

The Adult-Height Model

The relationship between age at menarche and adult height was studied in
each ethnic group separately and for all ethnic groups pooled. As observed
in table 3-1, mean adult height varied markedly among ethnic groups in our
sample ($X_2^2 = 1841.44$, $p < .001$). In the full model, given in table 3-2, it
was found that, overall, the regression coefficients for year of birth and age

Table 3-1
Means of Variables in Path Analysis by Ethnic Group

Variable	Caucasian N:1291		Japanese N:1519		Chinese N:395	
	Mean	Standard Deviation	Mean	Standard Deviation	Mean	Standard Deviation
Year of birth (1900-1940)	23.5724	9.6878	24.8308	8.0901	22.4354	8.7604
Age at menarche	12.8342	1.4829	12.8729	1.4723	12.9823	1.4661
Weight in pounds	135.5438	22.5791	118.4062	17.1932	120.5519	16.9292
Height in inches	64.3989	2.4418	61.0250	1.9427	61.8608	1.8670
Total number of live births	2.0209	1.5932	2.3443	1.5186	2.6532	1.5959
Total months breast-fed	4.5988	8.6286	8.3450	14.6281	6.0608	10.3848

at menarche, as well as for their squared terms did not differ significantly among ethnic groups ($X_8^2 = 12.66$, $p > .1$), although the effect of year of birth on adult height did differ marginally between Japanese and Chinese groups ($X_1^2 = 6.22$, $p < .05$). In the pooled data, the variables, year of birth and age at menarche, were found to exert not only independent positive linear effects on adult height ($X_2^2 = 137.10$, $p < .001$) but also independent positive quadratic effects ($X_2^2 = 17.04$, $p < .01$).

The Adult-Weight Model

As expected, mean adult weights varied among ethnic groups ($X_2^2 = 667.5$, $p < .001$). The linear model, as shown in table 3-2, was highly significant after adjustment was made for ethnic group ($X_5^2 = 550.95$, $p < .001$). Year of birth, age at menarche, height, and total live births, but not total months breastfed, made independent significant contributions to the determination of adult weight. The R^2 value for the total linear model was .27.

For every additional birth there was, on the average, a gain of approximately 1.5 pounds. For every extra inch in height there was an average gain of 3.2 pounds. There also was a modest secular trend toward increasing thinness ($X_1^2 = 230.79$, $p < .01$). The more recently a woman was born the less she was likely to weigh. The decrease was roughly 1.8 pounds per decade. A considerably stronger trend toward lower weight was found in the effect of later menarche ($X_1^2 = 82.22$, $p < .001$). For every year that menarche is delayed, a woman's predicted adult weight declines by 2.0 pounds, on the average. This rate of change was similar in all three ethnic groups.

The relationship between the independent variables and adult weight was found to be nonlinear ($X_{60}^2 = 80.2$, $p < .05$). As shown in table 3-2 (g)

Table 3-2
Analysis of Variance and Tests of Heterogeneity among Ethnic Groups

Source	Degrees of Freedom	X^2
I. Age at Menarche:		
(a) Ethnic group	2	3.24
(b) Year of birth	1	153.62[c]
(c) Oriental versus Caucasian × year of birth	1	30.49[b]
(d) Japanese versus Chinese × year of birth	1	.97
(e) Year of birth^2	1	2.74
(f) Oriental versus Caucasian × year of birth^2	1	1.17
(g) Japanese versus Chinese × year of birth^2	1	2.09
(h) Total heterogeneity among ethnic groups	4	34.70[c]
(i) Residual	3196 $MS = 2.06$ $R^2 = .06$	
II. Height:		
(a) Ethnic group	2	1841.44[c]
(b) Year of birth, age at menarche	2	137.10[c]
(c) Oriental versus Caucasian × year of birth	1	.54
(d) Oriental versus Caucasian × age at menarche	1	1.19
(e) Japanese versus Chinese × year of birth	1	6.22[a]
(f) Japanese versus Chinese × age at menarche	1	.002
(g) Year of birth^2, age at menarche^2	2	17.04[b]
(h) Oriental versus Caucasian × year of birth^2	1	2.46
(i) Oriental versus Caucasian × age at menarche^2	1	1.62
(j) Japanese versus Chinese × year of birth^2	1	.47
(k) Japanese versus Chinese × age at menarche^2	1	.16
(l) Total heterogeneity among ethnic groups	8	12.66
(m) Residual	3190 $MS = 4.41$ $R^2 = .38$	
III. Weight:		
(a) Ethnic group	2	667.5[c]
(b) Height, age at menarche, year of birth, total live births, total months breast-fed	5	550.95[c]
(c) Oriental versus Caucasian × (height, year of birth, total live births, total months breast-fed)	4	5.36
(d) Oriental versus Caucasian × age at menarche	1	4.81[a]
(e) Japanese versus Chinese × (height, year of birth, total live births, total months breast-fed)	4	4.16
(f) Japanese versus Chinese × age at menarche	1	.55

(g) Year of birth^2, height^2, births^2, menarche^2,   5   21.40[c]
     breast-fed^2

(h) Oriental versus Caucasian × (height^2, year   4   .64
     of birth^2, total live births^2, total months
     breast-fed^2)

(g) Year of birth^2, height^2, births^2, menarche^2, breast-fed^2	5	21.40[c]
(h) Oriental versus Caucasian × (height^2, year of birth^2, total live births^2, total months breast-fed^2)	4	.64
(i) Oriental versus Caucasian × age at menarche^2	1	1.04
(j) Japanese versus Chinese × (height^2, year of birth^2, total live births^2, total months breast-fed^2)	4	1.28
(k) Japanese versus Chinese × age at menarche^2	1	.03
(l) Total heterogeneity among ethnic groups	20	18.02
(m) Residual	3184	$MS = 324.08$ R^2 .28

IV. Total number of live births:

(a) Ethnic group	2	62.42[c]
(b) Year of birth, age at menarche	2	5.08
(c) Oriental × year of birth	1	64.30[c]
(d) Oriental × age at menarche	1	.80
(e) Japanese versus Chinese × year of birth	1	13.36[b]
(f) Japanese versus Chinese × age at menarche	1	.004
(g) Year of birth^2, menarche^2	2	4.58
(h) Oriental × year of birth^2	1	47.36[c]
(i) Oriental × age at menarche^2	1	.87
(j) Japanese versus Chinese × year of birth^2	1	11.27[b]
(k) Japanese versus Chinese × age at menarche^2	1	.009
(l) Total heterogeneity among ethnic groups	8	137.97[c]
(m) Residual	3190	$MS = 2.33$ $R^2 = .06$

V. Total months spent breast-feeding

(a) Ethnic group	2	107.44[c]
(b) Menarche, year of birth, births	3	1335.52[c]
(c) Oriental × year of birth, births	2	203.14[c]
(d) Oriental × age at menarche	1	9.77[a]
(e) Japanese versus Chinese × year of birth, births	2	69.26[b]
(f) Japanese versus Chinese × age at menarche	1	.07
(g) Year of birth^2, births^2, age at menarche^2	3	152.37[c]
(h) Oriental × (year of birth^2, births^2)	2	28.74[c]
(i) Oriental × age at menarche^2	1	1.92
(j) Japanese versus Chinese × year^2, births^2	2	18.72[c]
(k) Japanese versus Chinese × age at menarche^2	1	3.03
(l) Total heterogeneity among races	12	334.65[c]
(m) Residual	3184	$MS = 92.18$ $R^2 = .38$

[a] $p < 0.05$
[b] $p < 0.01$
[c] $p < 0.001$

the quadratic effects of the variables in the main model were highly significant ($X_5^2 = 21.40$, $p < .001$). In particular, age at menarche and height had strongly negative effects on adult weight. As in the case of height, however, no evidence was found for heterogeneity among ethnic groups ($X_{20}^2 = 18.02$). It thus appears that weight is predicted similarly, in parallel curves, by the variables considered in the model for all three ethnic groups. The only significant ethnic-group interaction, the interaction of being Oriental (as compared to Caucasian) with age at menarche on adult weight, was of borderline significance. A Type I error, in this isolated case, could not be ruled out.

The variable, total number of live births, which made an independent positive linear contribution to adult weight, was itself, subject to considerable ethnic-group heterogeneity ($X_8^2 = 137.97$, $p < .001$). Orientals, as compared with Caucasians, varied in their secular trends in childbearing, both in the linear effect of year of birth ($X_1^2 = 64.30$, $p < .001$) and in the quadratic effect of year of birth ($X_1^2 = 47.36$, $p < .001$). Similarly, Japanese exhibited significantly different secular trends from Chinese in total number of live births. The effects of the secular trend operated in linear ($X_1^2 = 13.36$, $p < .01$) and nonlinear fashion ($X_1^2 = 11.27$, $p < .01$) here too. It may be noted that age at menarche, which logically prefigured total live births in the path diagram, did not have a significant effect on the total number of live births.

While not significantly related to adult weight in the pooled model, total months spent breastfeeding also appeared to be a highly complex variable with substantial ethnic heterogeneity ($X_{12}^2 = 334.65$, $p < .001$). Year of birth and age at menarche exerted independent linear and nonlinear effects on total months spent breastfeeding as well as interactive effects with ethnic group, as shown in table 3-2.

Discussion

The secular trend towards earlier menarche, among Caucasians living in Hawaii, appears to conform with the projection of Tanner (1962) and Eveleth and Tanner (1976). We found among Caucasians in our sample a rate of decline in age at menarche of .2 years per decade, slightly slower than the Tanner projection of .3 years per decade. The secular trends towards earlier menarche among Japanese and Chinese in Hawaii, however, were more than twice as rapid (.5 years per decade) and were similar in both Oriental groups. Secular trends towards earlier menarche that exceed the rate of decline in European populations have also been recently reported in Latin American populations (Farid-Coupal, Contreras, and Castellano, et al. 1981). While current socioeconomic status is comparable among the three groups and the climatic effects would be held constant for women brought up in Hawaii, past nutritional differences and other, perhaps more subtle, cultural factors may well be implicated in defining the different secular trends toward earlier menarche among Oriental and Caucasian women in Hawaii. Perhaps because the most recent-born women in our sample were born in 1940, we have not detected any plateau or reversal in the decline in age at menarche reported in the literature (Roberts & Dann 1975; Roberts 1977).

Unlike Dann and Roberts (1969) and Clegg (1980) we found ample evidence for similar secular trends toward increased stature in all three ethnic groups. The rate of increase in height among Caucasians in our sample (.5 inches per decade) marginally exceeded reports by Tanner (1978).

It was apparent from the analysis of our data that even among the non-athletic women in our sample, later age at menarche was significantly associated with lower adult weight. It was also discovered that though the relationship between age at menarche and year of birth and adult weight was not a simple linear one, it did not differ appreciably among ethnic groups. (See table 3-2 III (l).) By comparison, total months spent breast feeding showed considerable ethnic heterogeneity in relation to age at menarche, and both total months spent breastfeeding and total live births were ethnically heterogeneous in their secular trends. (Age at menarche appeared not to be associated with total live births in our data.) Greater racial heterogeneity is thus found rather more in secular trends affecting variables connected with individual preferences and cultural differences than with the more strictly biological parameters. With respect to the more biological factors in sexual maturation, race seems not to have made a significant difference. It is possible that our population was not differentiated along ethnic lines by the relationship of height or weight to age at menarche because these relationships express pan-human biological phenomena. The similarity in secular trends among the ethnic groups for height and weight may reflect changes in environmental factors that affected all three ethnic groups in similar fashion.

In spite of the overall similarity of the regressions on height for the three ethnic groups in our sample, there was one significant subtest—the effect of year of birth on height differed between Chinese and Japanese ethnic groups. In view of this, and because of differing patterns of nonlinearity in the three ethnic groups, we felt it was safer to examine the three ethnic groups separately.

In Japanese, the secular trend toward increased height appeared to be virtually linear among women born between 1900 and 1930 but leveled off in women born between 1930 and 1940. Using women born between 1900 and 1930, the relationships between year of birth, age at menarche, and adult height can be adequately described linearly by the following diagram:

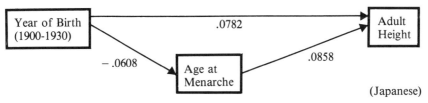

Among these Japanese women, the direct effect of year of birth on adult height was .0782 inches per year, and the indirect effect of the secular trend operating through age at menarche was $(-.0608) \times (.0858)$, or $-.00522$ inches per year. The total effect, the sum of the positive direct linear effect and the negative indirect effect was .0730 inches. Or, to express this differently, for every increase in the year of birth up to 1930, there was an increase in adult height of .073 inches, which effect can be broken down into two components, a direct time trend and an indirect effect through age at menarche.

The comparable calculations for Chinese are summarized as follows:

Direct effect of year of birth on height	.0256
Indirect effect of year of birth through age at menarche $(-.0437) \times (.0800)$	$-.0035$
Total direct and indirect effects	.0221

In Caucasians:

Direct effect of year of birth on height	.0474
Indirect effect of year of birth through age at menarche $(-.0192) \times (.132)$	$-.0025$
Total direct and indirect effects	.0449

Finally, because women with later years of birth were found to have earlier ages at menarche, on the average, as well as being slightly taller than earlier-born women, it is important to correct for year of birth when examining the relationship between age at menarche and adult height. If there is no control by matching or covariance adjustment, the estimate of the regression of adult height on age at menarche will be seriously biased toward zero and there may appear to be little or no effect of age at menarche. For the three ethnic groups in these data, for example, the regression coefficients for height on age at menarche both without adjustment and with adjustment (by linear regression) are given in table 3-3.

Table 3-3
Regression of Height on Age at Menarche

Ethnic Group	No Correction for Year of Birth	Correction for Year of Birth made
Japanese	$-.019 \pm .034$	$.077 \pm .034*$
Chinese	$.040 \pm .064$	$.080 \pm .066$
Caucasians	$.094 \pm .046*$	$.132 \pm .045**$

$*p > .05$ $**p < .01$

For Caucasians and for Japanese the corrected regression coefficients shown above become significant and positive, a striking change and further evidence for Johnston's plea (1974) that researchers studying menarche apply sufficient sophistication in design to disentangle the various factors that operate to create its variability, and we might add, that may mask its effect.

References

Bullough, V. 1981. Age at menarche: A misunderstanding. *Science* 213: 365-366.

Clegg, E.J. 1980. Secular changes in age at menarche and adult stature in Hebridean women. *Journal of Biosocial Science* 12:83-91.

Damon, A. 1968. Secular trend in height and weight within old American families at Harvard 1870-1965. *American Journal of Physical Anthropology* 29:45-50.

Dann, T.C., and Roberts, D.F. 1969. Physique and family environment in girls entering a Welsh college. *British Journal of Preventive and Social Medicine* 23:65-71.

Dreizen, S., Spirakis, C.N., and Stone, R.E. 1967. A comparison of skeletal growth and maturation in undernourished and well-nourished girls before and after menarche. *Journal of Pediatrics* 70:256.

Draper, N.R., and Smith, H. 1966. *Applied regression analysis.* New York: John Wiley and Sons.

Eveleth, P.B., and Tanner, J.M. 1976. *Worldwide variation in human growth. International Biological Programme 8.* Cambridge, Eng.: Cambridge University Press.

Farid-Coupal, N., Contreras, M.L., and Castellano, H.M. 1981. The age at menarche in Carabobo, Venezuela, with a note on the secular trend. *Annals of Human Biology* 8:283-288.

Frisch, R.E., Wyshak, G., and Vincent, L. 1980. Delayed menarche and amenorrhea in ballet dancers. *New England Journal of Medicine,* 303:17-19.

Goodman, M.J., Grove, J.S., and Gilbert, F. 1980. Age at first pregnancy in relation to age at menarche and year of birth in Caucasian, Japanese, Chinese, and part-Hawaiian women living in Hawaii. *Annals of Human Biology* 7:29-33.

Goodman, M.J., Gilbert, F.I., Mi, M.P., Grove, J.S. Catts, A., and Low, G., in press. Breast cancer screening in Hawaii 1974-1980: Results of a six-year program. *Hawaii Medical Journal.*

Hiernaux, J. 1968. Ethnic differences in growth and development. *Eugenics Quarterly* 15:12-21.

Johnston, F.E. 1974. Control of age at menarche. *Human Biology* 46:159-171.

Kumar, J. 1975. The recent level of age at menarche and the effect of nutrition level and socio-economic status on menarche: A comparative study. *Eastern Anthropologist* 28:99-132.

Li, C.C. 1975. *Path analysis.* Pacific Grove, Cal.: Boxwood Press.

Malina, R.M., Spirduso, W.W., Tate, C., and Baylor, A.M. 1978. Age at menarche and selected menstrual characteristics in athletes at different competitive levels and in different sports. *Medicine and Science in Sports* 10:218-222.

Onat, T. 1975. Prediction of adult height of girls based on the percentage of adult height at onset of secondary sexual characteristics, at chronological age and skeletal age. *Human Biology* 47:117-130.

Presser, H.B. 1978. Age at menarche, socio-sexual behavior and fertility. *Social Biology* 25:94-101.

Roberts, D.F. 1977. The changing pattern of menarcheal age. *Symposia Biologica Hungarica* 20:167.

Roberts. D.F., and Dann, T.C. 1975. A 12-year study of menarcheal age. *British Journal of Preventive and Social Medicine* 29:31-39.

Rona, R., and Pereira, G. 1974. Factors that influence age of menarche in girls in Santiago, Chile. *Human Biology* 46:33-42.

Tanner, J.M. 1962. *Growth at adolescence,* 2nd ed. Oxford, Eng.: Blackwell.

_____ . *Foetus into man: Physical growth from conception to maturity.* London: Open Books Publishing Ltd.

Van Wieringen, J.C. 1978. Secular growth changes. In F. Falkner and J.M. Tanner, eds. *Human growth, 2 postnatal growth.* New York: Plenum.

**Part II
Psychological Aspects
of Menarche**

Introduction to Part II

Despite the interest that adolescent behavior has held for scientists and philosophers since the time of Aristotle (Conger 1973), remarkably little attention has been given to the psychological aspects of menarche. One possible explanation for the dearth of research in this area is the difficulty inherent in doing it. Anne Petersen, in describing her work, discusses some of the problems she confronted in studying girls around the time of puberty; that is, getting endocrine measures, Tanner ratings, or anthropometric measures. Nevertheless, Petersen worked directly with a large sample of sixth- and seventh-grade boys and girls, asking if they had noticed any pubertal changes, noting the relationship between menarche and other measures of pubertal change, and assessing feelings about these pubertal changes both directly and indirectly. Petersen found that girls were both happy and frightened about menstruation. And she also noted some interesting discrepancies between reports from mothers and their daughters, with inaccurate reporting of menarche apparently related to the difficulty girls had with the experience. Petersen also found that unlike boys, girls want to mature at the same time as their peers. The initial reactions of early maturing girls were primarily negative: they experienced more stress after menarche, whereas the late maturers suffered until menarche.

Many theorists have suggested that menarche is a significant, organizing event in a woman's psychosexual development (Whisnant and Zegans 1975). Elissa Koff explored this in a study of the effect of menarche on normal girls. Koff hypothesized that with menarche there would be a dramatic shift in girls' self-perception and expression. She asked seventh-grade girls for two sets of figure drawings, six months apart. The results were dramatic. Postmenarcheal girls produced more sexually differentiated drawings and indicated greater awareness of sexual differentiation. Moreover, the girls who changed menarcheal status during the six-month interval also showed an increase in sexual differentiation in their drawings. A sentence-completion task suggested that the girls expected immediate bodily change to be associated with their first menstrual periods. Koff concludes that menarche is a powerful organizing force resulting in girls experiencing themselves as more feminine and more sexually mature.

Roberta Danza looked at the changes in family relations resulting from a change in menarcheal status. She found that regardless of age, postmenarcheal girls were more likely to wear make-up or date; they functioned more independently; and they reported less closeness and more conflict with their parents. In addition to having intrapersonal meaning, menarche seems to be a marker signaling a change in relationships between girls and their parents.

Some researchers have suggested that negative menarcheal experiences have a long-standing influence on women's lives. For example, Shainess (1961) found that women who had negative recollections of menarche also experienced premenstrual tension. Nancy Woods and her colleagues have done a careful study of the relationship between recollections of menarche and current attitudes and symptoms. Woods found ambivalent recollections of menarche among this adult sample; they described a mixture of happy and proud with embarrassed and scared feelings. Woods also found those with a later menarcheal age to have more positive recollections of the experience, thus confirming Petersen's observation that early onset is more disturbing. However, age at menarche and negative recollections of it were not found to be related to current attitudes or symptoms. Rather, current attitudes were related to current symptoms, leaving unanswered the question of which causes which.

One of the common beliefs regarding menstruation is that a woman looks different, presumably less attractive, when she is menstruating. In one study (Golub 1981), 67 percent of the college women sampled responded that they believed this idea to be true. Rhoda Unger and her coauthors hypothesized that both men and women would associate low attractiveness with menstruation. In a clever study using photographs of women labeled as menstruating or nonmenstruating, she found no significant difference in the attractiveness ratings assigned to the two conditions. However, people with colds were judged to be less attractive than those without colds. Unger suggests that menstruation may be becoming less of a social stigma.

References

Conger, J.J. 1973. *Adolescence and youth.* New York: Harper and Row.

Golub, S. 1981. Sex Differences in attitudes and beliefs regarding menstruation. In P. Komnenich, M. McSweeney, J.A. Noack, and Sr. N. Elder, eds., *The menstrual cycle: Research and implications for women's health.* vol. 2. New York: Springer.

Shainess, N. 1961. A reevaluation of some aspects of femininity through a study of menstruation. *Comparative Psychiatry* 2:20-26.

Whisnant, L., and Zegans, L. 1975. A study of attitudes toward menarche in white middle-class American adolescent girls. *American Journal of Psychiatry* 132:809-814.

4

Menarche: Meaning of Measures and Measuring Meaning

Anne C. Petersen

Menarche is a fascinating topic to study. For those of us interested in bio-psychosocial development, it provides a specific focus for the study of the various interactions among biological, social-cultural, and psychological processes. It is a biological event, embedded within the longer biological process of puberty with internal-systemic and external-evolutionary implications (Petersen and Taylor 1980). It is also a social-cultural event in most societies (Paige and Paige 1981). The biological and social-cultural significance of menarche is integrated within the person of each girl through perceptual, attributional, attitudinal, and emotional processes. Through menarche, we can examine the reciprocal influences among these various factors. For example, in the usual course of development, menarche is followed by, or "causes," changes in self-perception (for example, Brooks-Gunn and Ruble in press; Koff, Rierdan, and Silverstone 1978; Rierdan and Koff 1980). In many societies it signals the onset of womanhood. But, perhaps because of its social-cultural significance to girls who perceive this event as threatening to their selves, the process of menarche can be delayed or reversed, as in anorexia nervosa. Other examples of reciprocal relations could be cited. Thus, menarche is important to understand not just for its inherent qualities but also because it is an ideal focus for understanding the complex relations among biological, psychological, and social factors.

Pubertal change and its relation to other aspects of development are among the issues addressed in our longitudinal study of biopsychosocial development at early adolescence. The broader study focuses on the development of sex differences in self-image and cognitive performance. Though little research has been done with early adolescents, the existing information suggests that this stage of life is particularly difficult, especially for girls (Hamburg 1974; Lipsitz 1977). Pubertal change, and especially menarche in girls, are factors often thought to be stressful. There are strong stereotypes about the ill effects of both "raging pubertal hormones" and "raging menstrual hormones." Given the prevalent belief that puberty and menarche create difficulties for young adolescents, it is surprising to see how little research exists on this topic. The fact that so little research exists is itself notable. What the paucity means, however, is unclear. Several research groups have begun to explore the psychological significance of menarche and puberty (for example, Brooks-Gunn and Ruble in press; Rierdan and Koff 1980). The specific issues that will be addressed in this chapter are twofold: (a) How can pubertal change be measured? and (b) What do these measurements mean in terms of the subjective experience of and reactions to pubertal change? We have been working hard on both issues, and while we have improved the specific measurement of pubertal change and subjective meanings, we find that the "errors" of measurement are not random and provide important information about each aspect.

The Early-Adolescent Study

Before I describe the results of our studies thus far, let me first describe the overall research program of which the study of menarche and puberty is a part.

Our theoretical framework for this reseach utilizes a biopsychosocial model for development assuming that a transaction occurs over time among biological, psychological, and social factors (Petersen 1980). Figure 4-1 shows the basic model. We are testing models that propose specific linkages between biological change and psychosocial factors. One of two specific models described earlier (Petersen and Taylor 1980) is relevant to the topic of this chapter (see figure 4-2); it depicts unidirectional influences of biological change on psychosocial factors. As indicated earlier, it is assumed that these two aspects interact reciprocally. The present chapter focuses on the *reporting* of information, rather than actual changes, and on how psychosocial factors can influence the reports of biological change.

The study focuses on development from sixth through eighth grades, utilizing a cohort-sequential design with a second cohort to replicate the first. This design is shown in table 4-1. The sampling design involved 200 subjects per cohort from two suburban school districts, both predominantly middle to upper-middle class and white. One school district is smaller than we had anticipated, and both are declining in enrollment, a fact reflected in our actual sample sizes of 188 for Cohort I and 139 for Cohort II. The present chapter is based upon available data from both cohorts.

Our study focuses on information obtained from the children four times annually, in two individual interviews and two group sessions that take place each fall and spring. Parents are interviewed when their children are in sixth and eighth grades. The total assessment design is shown in table 4-2. Interviewers remain blind to other sources of information except that the young adolescent has a single interviewer over the course of the study. We have just completed three years of assessment on Cohort I. There is only one sixth-grade assessment in Cohort I with most measures, due to a delay in funding, together with a special situation in one school district that prompted us to proceed with data collection despite the lost data point.

Table 4-1
Cohort-Sequential Longitudinal Design for the Early-Adolescent Study

| | | | Grade | | |
			6	7	8
Cohort	I	(1967)	1979	1980	1981
Year of birth	II	(1968)	1980	1981	1982

The Measurement of Pubertal Change

We consider menarche within the context of other pubertal changes that are occurring. Although menarche is the easiest measure of puberty in girls, it actually occurs relatively late in a process that takes about four years if the focus is on observable changes, longer if the focus is on hormonal changes (Petersen and Taylor, 1980). Menarche generally occurs after the peak spurt in height, usually between Tanner's last two stages (4 and 5) of pubic-hair development and around stage 4 of breast development (Marshall and Tanner 1969, 1970; Tanner 1962).

The best way to measure pubertal change, now that x-rays of bone growth are known to be risky, is to obtain objective ratings using Tanner's Sexual Maturity Scale of pubic-hair development for both boys and girls, breast development for girls, and penis development for boys. Ratings of whole body photographs taken at three views can be used although some levels of pubertal status can be difficult to rate reliably, particularly if the photographs are black and white rather than color (Petersen 1973).

The ideal set of pubertal-change measures would also include anthropometric measurements, at least height and weight. Height is especially useful for assessing the rate of change as well as for determining the age at peak growth (Bock, et al. 1973; Thissen et al. 1976). Endocrine measures, such as testosterone and estradiol, can also be used to monitor pubertal growth and may be essential depending on the research questions (Petersen and Taylor 1980). They also, however, pose both methodological and ethical problems, the methodological problems becoming serious, though very interesting, with girls around the time of and after menarche (Petersen 1979; Warren in press).[1]

Unfortunately, we do not have *any* of these measures in our study. The proposed endocrine measures were deleted early in the funding process, due to the current state of endocrine methodology. The Tanner ratings and anthropometric measures were deleted by the school districts. In one school district, this aspect of the study was refused at the outset, though they did offer (and we accepted) their annual height and weight data. In the second school district, we spent a year negotiating but finally withdrew the puberty

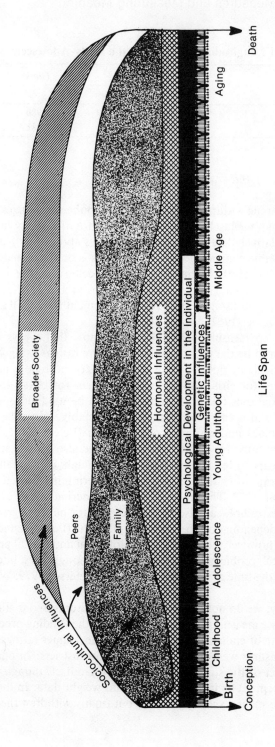

Source: Petersen, A.C. Biopsychosocial processes in the development of sex-related differences. In J.E. Parsons (Ed.) *The psychobiology of sex differences and sex roles.* Washington, D.C.: Hemisphere Publishing Company, 1980. Reprinted with permission.

Figure 4-1. Biopsychosocial Development over the Life Span

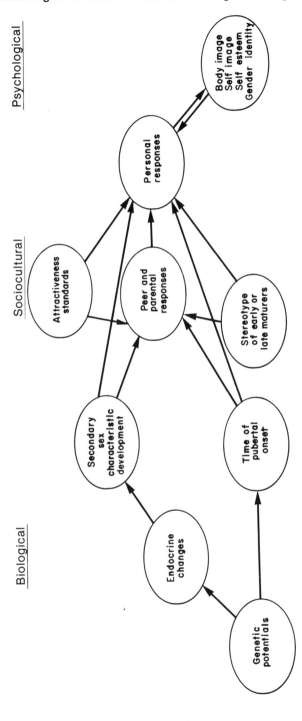

Source: Petersen, A.C., and Taylor, B. The biological approach to adolescence: Biological change and psychological adaptation. In J. Adelson (Ed.) *Handbook of adolescent psychology.* New York: John Wiley & Sons, 1980. Copyright © John Wiley & Sons. Reprinted by permission of John Wiley & Sons, Inc.

Figure 4-2. Hypothetically Important Paths from Pubertal Change to Psychological Responses

Table 4-2
Assessment Design for the Early-Adolescent Study

Assessments	Descriptions	Frequency
	For Adolescents	
Interview	Semistructured; focuses on school, friends, family, and self	Twice annually
Self-Image Questionnaire for Young Adolescents	Nine scales and total score of adjustment	Annually
Cognitive measures	Formal operations (Linn, Peel); spacial ability (PMA); fluent production (DAT); field independence (Water Level, GEFT)	Annually
Sentence completion test (Loevinger)	Measures stage of ego development	Annually
Sex-role inventories	Bem Sex Role Inventory; Attitudes toward Women Scale for Adolescents (Petersen)	Annually
Lowman Inventory of Family Feelings	Measures feelings about family members	Sixth, Eighth grades
Teacher ratings	Ratings of classroom behavior	Sixth, Eighth grades
School achievement	Average GPA, standardized-test ranking	Obtained once for all three grades
	For Parents	
Interview	Parallels child interview plus	Sixth, Eighth grades
Self-Image Questionnaire for Young Adolescents (parent form)	Parent report of child's self-image	Sixth, Eighth grades
Lowman Inventory of Family Feelings	Measures feelings about family members	Sixth, Eighth grades

component rather than risk losing the entire study. After our initial despair, we began instead to ask the young people to self-report their stage of growth on the various indices. We felt that the use of self-report responses to nude pictures such as proposed by others (Duke, Litt, and Gross 1980; Morris and Udry 1980) would meet with equivalent or perhaps greater disapproval than the use of pediatricians to perform the ratings. Fortunately, our scales show the predicted sequences of pubertal changes when analyzed as Guttman scales and form scales with the desired psychometric properties.

If nothing else, our research shows that a sensitive subject like puberty can be measured in a large school-based study. In our discussions with other researchers, we have found that many have had experiences like ours, especially if they are beginning the study during early adolescence rather than earlier in life. We have pondered some over why the study of early adolescents was so difficult an issue. Among other factors, it seemed that the parents equate puberty with sex, reflecting, we suspect, societal taboos. While there is an obvious link between the two, we were *not* interested in sexual behavior.

Results of Pubertal-Status Assessment

The across-item consistency, as measured by the alpha coefficient, demonstrated that the pubertal items do form a scale. The alphas increased over time and cohort from .42 and .45 for boys and girls, respectively, for the first interview with Cohort I, to .68 and .78 (boys and girls, respectively) one year later, and .65 and .77 (boys and girls, respectively at the same time for the spring sixth-grade interview for Cohort II. These results support our sense that we had become more proficient at asking these questions each time. We were quite cautious at first (spring of sixth grade with Cohort I) and only tentatively asked each child whether he or she had noticed any pubertal changes (after first defining puberty); if the answer was yes, we asked what changes had occurred. Since this procedure seemed to elicit plausible responses and produced no complaints that we heard,[2] we felt comfortable asking the questions more directly. We now ask whether growth has not begun, barely begun, is definitely underway, or ceased, on eight developmental indicators: growth in height, foot growth (included since the data reported here), body hair, skin change, facial hair growth and voice change (boys only), breast development and menarche (girls only). The most recent scales produced alpha coefficients in respectable ranges for both boys and girls, and slightly higher for girls. Not all of the measures are equally good and they vary in power across time, as would be expected. Skin change (that is, pimples) is less good, for example, because factors other than pubertal development influence its emergence. The variation in relevance to the scale across time occurs because the timing of the events varies. The improvement in our measures makes this variation over time more difficult to detect in the table. Our entire series, once we have it, will reveal this change more adequately.

Menarche shows lower correlations with the scale. This effect is due in part to the fact that menarche is a dichotomous variable. Thus, for most of the early changes in other measures, menarche remains at zero.

We have also had the interviewer assess pubertal stage using a four-point scale: prepubertal, barely pubertal, quite pubertal, and postpubertal, with specific descriptions of each level used to make the rating more reliable. The addition of the interviewer ratings to the scale increases the scale consistency even more, to .82 for girls at the most recent assessments for each cohort and to .73 and .69 for Cohort I and II boys, respectively.

Therefore, even crude self-report measures of pubertal change can have psychometric properties that are desirable. The levels of the most recent alpha coefficients are higher than those attained with some standard psychological measures.

Table 4-3 shows the correlations between menarche and other measures of pubertal change. Recall that our scales in early interviews were less reliable, a factor that will decrease the correlations. Focusing on the most recent times, it appears that breast development is the best correlate at both ages, with body hair and pimples declining in importance from sixth to seventh grade. This result is comparable to that obtained before using more rigorous measures of physical growth (Petersen 1979). The interviewer rating is highly correlated with menarche, probably because that development is necessary for a postpubertal rating.

The Meaning of Puberty and Menarche

We have been interested in the psychological significance of puberty since the beginning of this study. At first, I thought—naively—that we could obtain this information by simply asking these young adolescents. While a few young people could articulate their feelings about the changes in their bodies, most could not. Some of this inability to discuss pubertal change surely relates to cognitive development and the fact that most sixth graders still think concretely, in Piagetian terms (Inhelder and Piaget 1958). We doubt, however, that cognitive development is the complete explanation for the discomfort and inarticulateness of some children. Since our first attempts to assess feelings about pubertal change, we have added some less open-ended questions to the interview and some projective measures as well.

One projective measure uses the beginnings of stories based on passages from Judy Blume's book *Are You There God? It's Me Margaret,* a book that

Table 4-3
Correlations between Menarche and Other Variables by Cohort and Time

	Cohort I			Cohort II	
	Spring Sixth	Fall Seventh	Spring Seventh	Fall Sixth	Spring Sixth
Body hair	.34	.15	.26	.22	.53
Breast development	.04	.20	.42	.22	.48
Skin change	.14	.10	.25	.09	.43
Growth	.02	.21	.32	.34	.39
Interviewer rating	—	.74	.69	.62	.69

—Data not obtained.

is popular with pubertal girls and focuses on puberty. We administered two versions of this assessment to the girls in Cohort I in the spring of seventh grade. In version 1, the responses to the questions were open ended and in version 2, the girls were asked to rank order four alternative responses. The story about menarche is:

> "Mom—hey, Mom—come quick!" When Nancy's mother got to the bathroom she said: "What is it? What's the matter?" "I got it," Nancy told her. "Got what?" said her mother.

In the open-ended version, the first question was *What happened next?* Of the forty-three girls completing this version, 37 percent gave responses like, "She told her mom that she had gotten her period." Another 42 percent did not mention menstruation but gave responses about mom explaining, helping, or praising. The next question was *How did Nancy feel?* While 33 percent of the girls gave negative or fearful responses, 49 percent were positive or pleased with maturing, and another 5 percent were both, or ambivalent.

In the close-ended version, the responses to the question, *What did Nancy say?* were *I got the measles, I caught a spider, I got my period,* and *It. You know. It.* The third response (*period*) was ranked first by 63 percent of the thirty-eight girls while the *it* response was ranked first by an additional 32 percent. These responses were the most frequent second choices as well. The next question, *"How did Nancy feel?"* had responses, *happy scared, sad,* and *nothing.* Half of the girls ranked *scared* first, while 39 percent selected *happy* first, and no girl ranked *sad* first. *Happy* and *scared* were also the most popular second choices. *Nothing* was the winner for fourth ranking (53 percent).

These results are summarized in table 4-4. They suggest that girls are both happy and frightened about menstruation. When it is possible to express ambivalence in the responses, some girls do. Other results of ours suggest that ambivalence might be more prevalent than these data suggest.

Table 4-4
Seventh-Grade Girls' Projective Responses to Menarche

Response	Form 1[a] (n = 43)	Form 2 (n = 38)
Negative, scared	33%	50%
Positive, happy	49%	39%
Ambivalent	5%	—[b]

[a]Form 1: open responses, Form 2: first ranking of four alternatives.
[b]Not possible.

More direct evidence about difficulties with menarche, especially among early maturers comes from examination of the convergence (or its lack) of reports from mothers, fathers, and girls regarding menarche. We initially pursued the issue of convergence as a way of establishing reliability of the reports of the girls. Of the girls in Cohort I with both parents at sixth grade (n = 87), 77 percent agreed with both parents about their menarcheal status, 6 percent stating that menarche had occurred and 71 percent saying that it had not yet occurred. In another 12 percent of the cases, the fathers didn't know but the mothers and daughters agreed, 9 percent no and 3 percent yes. In the remaining 10 percent of the cases, there was a discrepancy between the daughter's report and that of the mother and father. Of these nine girls, three were cases where the parents both said that menarche had not occurred while the daughter either refused to respond or said that she didn't know if any pubertal change had occurred. Because the discrepancy in report could be real—for example, the parents interviewed later than the girl, with menarche occurring in between, or an initial period of spotting with a "real period" occurring up to a year later, we carefully checked all available information to insure reliability.

The six who denied menarche when it had in fact occurred are most interesting. Six is not many girls but it is 43 percent of all postmenarcheal girls at that point! (The percentage estimate can be replicated with our second cohort when these data are ready.) In the overall sample of menarcheal girls, only 2 mothers said that their daughters felt positive about their development. It should be noted that the daughter in one of these cases reports quite a different story. The second positive response reported by a mother was by the mother of one of the girls who *denied* having menstruated. Over 70 percent of the mothers report that the experience was very difficult for their daughters. Over 83 percent of the girls (five of six) who denied menarche had mothers who reported the negative aspects of the experience for them. These mothers provided the most negative reports of all mothers of menarcheal girls. One of these mothers said, "When she got her first period, I found her pants. She was 11½ [early in sixth grade]. She wouldn't tell me—she denied it the first two times. I saw it as denying her femininity. She would hide her pants. I finally told her she had to use the stuff or she couldn't go on a ski trip." The daughter denied menstruating at sixth grade and said she had "no particular feelings" about pubertal change. In the fall of seventh grade, she again denied menstruating and said that her feelings about pubertal change were neutral: "It doesn't bother me."

In response to the card in the Thematic Apperception Test (Murray 1943) that shows a middle-aged woman with a girl holding a doll, she said:

> There is a little girl with . . . holding her doll. And she was . . . she asked her mom . . . she was . . . now what is it? When am I going to have you know, the (unclear). And, you know, her mom explained to her, you

know, about having her (unclear) and everything. And then she was scared, you know, about how it is, you know. I guess what she was, the mother was rather scared of telling her daughter. Because she was thinking her girls are growing up and the daughter was a little scared herself of growing up. (*Hm*) That's all. (*Um hm. What happens?*) What? (*What's the end of the story?*) The end of the story? Oh, she grows up. (laugh) And she has a baby. (*Um hm. How does she feel about it?*) And she's happy that her mom told her. (*Uh huh*) That's all I guess. (*Okay*)[3]

  She first acknowledged menarche in the fall of eighth grade, saying that she had started in June of seventh grade. Another mother of a girl who followed a similar pattern said of her sixth grader, "I thought she would need a psychiatrist!" At sixth grade, we had no cases of a girl reporting menarche when the parents did not. We think we have had such cases in eighth grade and await the parent data to corroborate our hunches.

  While the initial reactions to menarche of early maturers appear to be primarily negative, most of the girls accommodate to the change eventually. Later on they describe how difficult it had been. We are just beginning to hear these reports in eighth grade so it appears that it takes the early maturers some time to adjust. Later maturers appear not to have difficulties of such intensity or duration. These data are just now going into computer-data sets so we can soon test the hypotheses that we have generated from our impressions in the interviews.

  From other analyses and papers (for example, Tobin-Richards, Boxer, and Petersen in press; Wilen and Petersen 1980), we have concluded that girls, unlike boys, would prefer to mature at the same time as everyone else. For boys, earlier maturation is related significantly to more positive self-esteem, more positive body image, and more positive feelings about the timing of their development. For girls, all of these factors are related in a curvilinear way to timing, with average timing always being best. Even though being late is almost as negative for girls as being early, we expect that, unlike early maturers who suffer after menarche, late maturers suffer *until* menarche. This is another hypothesis that we plan to test with the later maturers in our eighth-grade data.

  We also have found that postmenarcheal girls are more likely than their premenarcheal age-mates to report being overweight and to be dissatisfied with their weight (Tobin-Richards, Boxer, and Petersen in press). Postmenarcheal girls at seventh grade are more likely to report that they are maturing faster than other girls their age. These results help validate our measures.

Summary

This chapter has focused on two issues in the study of menarche. First, how can this aspect and other aspects of puberty be measured, particularly in a large school-based study? Second, how reliable is self-reported information about menarche and pubertal change and how do the reports of these changes relate to the girls' subjective experiences of changes?

We find that self-reports of pubertal changes appear to be reliable and valid for most girls. The changes occur in the order that they should and they form a consistent scale. Inaccurate reporting of menarche, when it occurs, appears to be related systematically to the difficulty of the experience. Girls who deny menarche when it has in fact occurred seem to be having particular difficulty with accepting this change. We expect that late maturers may be more likely to report menarche when it has not yet occurred.

Girls, unlike boys, prefer that their pubertal changes occur at the same time as everyone else. Boys would rather be early maturers. The greater concern for conformity among girls may place particular stress on early maturing girls. This finding is consistent with that of Roberta Simmons and her colleagues in which they find that girls who are pubertal, have changed to junior high school, and are dating are more likely to have lower self-esteem, lower school achievement, and more behavior problems than boys and non-pubertal, nondating girls in K-8 schools (Simmons et al. 1979).

Most girls, however, especially if they begin menstruation at about the same time as others in their grade, accept pubertal change with some amount of comfort. There do seem to be some good books and pamphlets available although school programs seem weak apart from such materials. At the same time, school remains the most prevalent source (66 percent in our data) for such information, with only 21 percent of the girls citing books or other media sources. Now that we are beginning to understand what information to provide and who needs it most, we need to see that young girls are well-informed. Early maturers would seem to be a particularly vulnerable group.

Notes

1. Since the development of a mature menstrual cycle, like puberty itself, is a process rather than an event, it is very difficult to know what stage in the process any single measurement represents. The only solution to this dilemma is frequent, repeated measurements, a solution not very feasible until a method less intrusive than relatively large plasma samples is available.

2. A few children are quite uncomfortable about these questions as evidenced by direct comments (or in a few cases by refusal to answer these questions) or by citing these questions as ones on which some children might not be totally honest.

3. The interviewer's statements are italicized.

References

Bock, R.D., Wainer, H., Petersen, A.C., Thissen, D., Murray, J., and Roche, A. 1973. A parameterization for human growth curves. *Human Biology* 45:63-80.

Brooks-Gunn, J., and Ruble, D.N. In press. The experience of menarche from a developmental perspective. In J. Brooks-Gunn and A.C. Petersen, eds. *Girls at puberty: Biological, psychological, and social perspectives.* New York: Plenum.

Duke, P.M., Litt, I.F., and Gross, R.T. 1980. Adolescents' self-assessment of sexual maturation. *Pediatrics* 66:918-920.

Hamburg, B. 1974. Early adolescence: A specific and stressful stage of the life cycle. In G. Coelho, D.A. Hamburg, and J.E. Adams, eds, *Coping and adaption.* New York: Basic Books.

Koff, E., Rierdan, J., and Silverstone, E. 1978. Changes in representation of body image as a function of menarcheal status. *Developmental Psychology* 14: 635-642.

Inhelder, B. and Piaget, J. 1958. The growth of logical thinking from childhood to adolescence, New York: Basic Books.

Lipsitz, J. 1977. *Growing up forgotten.* Lexington, Mass.: Lexington Books.

Marshall, W.A., and Tanner, J.M. 1969. Variations in the pattern of pubertal changes in girls. *Archives of Disease in Childhood* 44:291-303.

_____ . 1970. Variations in the pattern of pubertal changes in boys. *Archives of Disease in Childhood* 45:13-23.

Morris, N.M., and Udry, J.R. 1980. Validation of a self-administered instrument to assess stage of adolescent development. *Journal of Youth and Adolescence* 9:271-280.

Murray, H.A. 1943. *Thematic Apperception Test.* Cambridge, Mass.: Harvard University Press.

Paige, K.E., and Paige, J.M. 1981. *The politics of reproductive ritual.* Berkeley: University of California Press.

Petersen, A.C. 1973. *The relationship of androgenicity in males and females to spatial ability and fluent production.* Unpublished doctoral dissertation, University of Chicago.

_____ . 1979. Female pubertal development. In M. Sugar, ed., *Female adolescent development.* New York: Brunner/Mazel.

_____ . 1980. Biopsychosocial processes in the development of sex-related differences. In J.E. Parsons, ed., *The psychobiology of sex differences and sex roles.* Washington, D.C.: Hemisphere Publishing Company.

Petersen, A.C., and Taylor, B. 1980. The biological approach to adolescence: Biological change and psychological adaptation. In J. Adelson ed., *Handbook of adolescent psychology.* New York: John Wiley and Sons.

Rierdan, J., and Koff, E. 1980. The psychological impact of menarche: Integrative versus disruptive changes. *Journal of Youth and Adolescence* 9:49-58.

Simmons, R.G., Blyuth, D.A., Van Cleave, E.F., and Bush, D.M. 1979. Entry into early adolescence: The impact of school structure, puberty, and early dating on self-esteem. *American Sociological Review* 44:948-967.

Tanner, J.M. 1962. *Growth at adolescence.* Springfield, Ill.: Thomas.

Thissen, D., Bock, R.D., Wainer, H., and Roche, A.F. 1976. individual growth in stature: A comparison of four growth studies in the USA. *Annals of Human Biology* 3:529-542.

Tobin-Richards, M., Boxer, A., and Petersen, A.C. In press. The psychological impact of pubertal change: Sex differences in perceptions of self during early adolescence. In J. Brooks-Gunn and A.C. Petersen, eds., *Girls at puberty: Biological, psychological, and social perspectives.* New York: Plenum.

Warren, M. In press. Hormonal aspects of puberty. In J. Brooks-Gunn and A.C. Petersen, eds., *Girls at puberty: Biological, psychological, and social perspectives.* New York: Plenum.

Wilen, J.B., and Petersen, A.C. 1980. Young adolescents responses to the timing of pubertal changes. Unpublished manuscript, Laboratory for the Study of Adolescence, Michael Reese Hospital and Medical Center, Chicago.

5 Through the Looking Glass of Menarche: What the Adolescent Girl Sees

Elissa Koff

Helene Deutsch (1944), struck by the variety and numerosity of psychological responses to menarche, or the first menstruation, was moved to recommend the "psychology of menstruation" as a specific problem area demanding empirical investigation. She, like Judith Kestenberg (1961, 1967), ascribed special significance to menarche; both writers conceptualize menarche as the critical turning point in the adolescent girl's development and suggest that her reaction to this event has far-reaching consequences for her subsequent adult behavior.

Deutsch's proposal, for the most part, appears to have gone unheeded. While the physical changes associated with menarche have been described in some detail (Frisch and Revelle 1970; Tanner 1978), there are in fact relatively few systematic studies concerned with the psychological correlates of the event. Theoretical speculations, emerging primarily from clinical case material of girls and women in psychotherapy or psychoanalysis, have yet to be complemented by a body of empirical data collected from nonclinical samples around the time the girls are experiencing menarche. The studies discussed in this chapter are an attempt to provide empirical support for some of the clinically derived speculations about the impact of menarche upon body image and sexual identification.

Several writers (Blos 1962; Hart and Sarnoff 1971; Kestenberg 1967; Koff, Rierdan, and Silverstone 1978) have observed a salutary effect of menarche upon body image and sexual identification. This position is perhaps best articulated in the writings of Kestenberg (1961, 1967). Drawing mainly from clinical materials, Kestenberg characterizes the premenarcheal state as one of confusion and disequilibrium, during which the girl experiences difficulty in organizing and communicating her thoughts. The onset of menstruation is associated with a dramatic shift; the postmenarcheal girl is seen to express herself more clearly and to be better able to organize her thoughts. One concomitant of this apparent reorganization is that premenarcheal confusion about body image and sexual identity typically is succeeded by postmenarcheal acceptance of womanhood, along with a corresponding reorganization and articulation of body image (Hart and Sarnoff 1971; Kestenberg 1961).

Interviews with a nonclinical sample of pre- and postadolescent girls (Whisnant and Zegans 1975b) have corroborated Kestenberg's clinical impressions. Postmenarcheal girls identified several personal changes following the first menstruation. They experienced themselves as more womanly and noted that they had begun to reflect upon their future reproductive roles. They also described greater definition and acceptance of their bodies as feminine and clarification and recognition of the self as female. Other evidence suggests that a greater general awareness and differentiation of female and male bodies (Haworth and Normington 1961) also is associated with such personal changes.

Menarche is experienced by the average U.S. girl at about thirteen years of age (Zacharias, Rand, and Wurtman 1976), and occurs relatively late in the sequence of physical changes associated with adolescence. It can succeed the period of maximum growth spurt and the emergence of secondary sex characteristics by as long as two-and-one-half years (Tanner 1978). Thus, while the actual feminizing changes associated with puberty commence long before, and continue long after menarche, it appears that the onset of menstruation—a sharply defined biological event—serves as a nodal event around which the psychological and biological changes occurring more or less continuously throughout adolescence are organized and assimilated. The girls who were interviewed by Whisnant and Zegans reported (1975b) that menarche provided "proof" that they really were women; not until this time do adolescent girls appear able to accept or integrate the feminizing changes of puberty.

Deutsch (1944) also has described more negative affective responses such as anxiety, shame, anger, and depression as the aftermath of the onset of menstruation. From this vantage, because the young girl's fantasies about the event and, in particular, her expectations of auspicious personal and environmental changes cannot be fulfilled, menarche must inevitably bring some degree of disappointment and distress in its wake.

As noted above, ideas about the young adolescent girl's fantasies and expectations concerning the personal and interpersonal consequences of menarche have been derived principally from the clinical literature and in the main from retrospective accounts of the experience. Surprisingly little direct evidence from girls in the throes of the experience is available. As part of a series of studies concerned with the psychosocial impact of menarche, questions concerning these expectations have been posed, indirectly and directly, to young adolescent girls at about the time of their menarche. Following is a discussion of two converging lines of data, gathered from two different groups of girls, which address the expectations girls harbor regarding changes in their bodies associated with the onset of menstruation.

In one study (Koff, Rierdan, and Silverstone 1978), longitudinal data collected from girls at two points in time suggested that significant changes in body image, reflected in human-figure drawings, accompanied the first menstruation. Drawings from a comparable group of girls, who had not yet experienced menarche but who had experienced the same passage of time, did not reflect this dramatic shift toward maturity. Struck by these findings, we became curious about the extent to which adolescent girls concurred in this belief. Toward this end, we conducted a second study using a projective sentence-completion task that presented a series of sentence stems concerned with a variety of feelings, responses, and circumstances related to menarche, including several concerned with bodily changes (Koff, Rierdan, and Jacobson 1981).

Method and Results

In the first study (Koff, Rierdan, and Silverstone 1978), seventh-grade girls produced drawings of male and female human figures on two occasions approximately six months apart. From eighty-seven girls sampled, three groups were discriminated: thirty-four who were premenarcheal on both test occasions, twenty-three who were postmenarcheal on both test occasions, and thirty whose menarcheal status changed between the two test occasions.

The main dependent measure was a sexual differentiation score, derived by scoring the subjects' male- and female-figure drawings according to criteria provided by Haworth and Normington (1961) for a four-level sexual-differentiation scale. This measure was chosen because of data suggesting the progressive awareness of sexual differentiation and greater acceptance of one's sex role would be reflected in the degree to which human-figure drawings are rendered as sexually differentiated. It was expected that menarche would be associated with greater awareness of sexual differentiation and greater acceptance of one's sex role. A second dependent measure was sex of the first drawn figure, a popular index of sex-role identification.

To summarize the results briefly, postmenarcheal girls, as a group, produced drawings that were significantly more sexually differentiated than those of their premenarcheal peers. Among those girls whose menarcheal status changed during the course of the study, there was a significant increase in the sexual differentiation of their drawings from the first to the second test occasion. Further, a greater percentage of postmenarcheal girls than premenarcheal girls drew their own sex first, and for those girls whose menarcheal status changed, all but one who had drawn a boy first on initial testing drew a girl first on the second test occasion.

The difference between pre- and postmenarcheal girls can be seen in the drawings themselves, some of which are reproduced here. While these drawings are indeed representative of the larger whole, they have been selected with an eye toward their particularly dramatic character. While I am presenting only the female drawings, it should be borne in mind that the sexual differentiation score entails the comparison of male- and female-figure drawings. The drawings in figures 5-1a and 5-1b were produced by a girl who was premenarcheal on both test occasions, and those in figures 5-2a and 5-2b by a girl who was postmenarcheal when the study began. The drawings in figures 5-3a and 5-3b are those of a girl whose menarcheal status changed over the course of the study.

The data suggested that the onset of menstruation was associated with a better articulated and defined body image and a clearer sexual identification, and the drawings provided strikingly graphic visual representations of bodily changes perceived to be associated with the onset of menstruation. Prior to menarche, drawings were relatively undifferentiated with regard to sexual features, while after menarche, they were significantly more highly differentiated. It was *as if* the concrete event of menarche somehow resulted in a magical and almost instantaneous transformation from young girl to sexually mature woman. Drawings from girls who had not yet experienced menarche, but who had experienced the same passage of time, did not reflect this dramatic shift toward maturity.

Given these striking data, we were curious about the extent to which young adolescent girls actually subscribed to the belief that menarche would determine this rather sudden and momentous transformation. Toward this

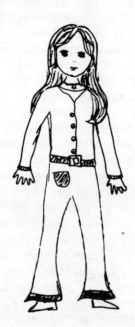

Figure 5-1a. Drawing of a Premenarcheal Girl, Time 1

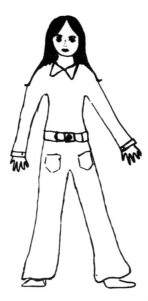

Figure 5-1b. Drawing of a Premenarcheal Girl, Time 2

end, we administered the sentence-completion task (Koff, Rierdan, and Jacobson 1981) structured around themes suggested by our data, other empirical studies, and clinical observations and theory. Descriptions of changes associated with menarche, including reorganization of body image and sexual identification, were generated from the responses of thirty-four seventh- and eighth-grade girls (sixteen premenarcheal, eighteen postmenarcheal) to open-ended sentences referring to the cue sentence, "Ann just got her period for the first time." The descriptions of bodily changes, embodying primarily a fantasy of instant metamorphosis from child to adult woman, accorded well with what had been seen in the human-figure drawings.

The data from the interview study by Whisnant and Zegans (1975b) and from our human-figure drawings suggested the expectation of immediate bodily changes attendant upon the first period. This sentiment was echoed by the majority of girls in this study, in such statements as, "she saw herself in a different way," "she thought she had changed," "she felt very grown up," "she felt mature," "she thought she looked older." Variations on this theme were the predominant responses of both pre- and postmenarcheal girls as they completed the sentence stem, "When Ann looked at herself in the mirror that night . . . "

A second item concerned with perception of the body ("Ann regarded her body as . . . ") discriminated the pre- from the postmenarcheal girls

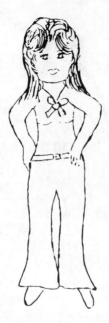

Figure 5-2a. Drawing of a Postmenarcheal Girl, Time 1

somewhat more. A greater number of premenarcheal girls described an altered body image—Ann's body was "more mature than it was," "a woman's body," "grown up," "different," "pretty much the same, but older,"—than did girls who had begun to menstruate. Several of these girls reported no change—for example, Ann regarded her body as "she did before" or "the same as yesterday"—a possibility not mentioned by any of the premenarcheal girls.

Discussion

What is most compelling about these two data sets is the degree of correspondence between the human-figure drawings and the statements generated in the sentence-completion task. The changes that are apparent in the drawings of the girls whose menarcheal status changed over the six-month period are captured so vividly in the sentence completions—for example, "When Ann looked in the mirror that night, it seemed to her she had grown and looked more like an adult."

It is interesting to speculate about these responses. It certainly is possible that these expectations are mere facsimile of what girls are told by their mothers or of what they read in the materials prepared and distributed by

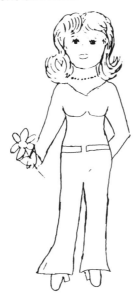

Figure 5-2b. Drawing of a Postmenarcheal Girl, Time 2

the manufacturers of sanitary products (Whisnant, Brett, and Zegans 1975a). These commercial materials, proclaiming to the young girl that on the day of her first period, she is a woman (!), certainly do nothing to dispel a fantasy of instant metamorphosis. The powerful media representation then could certainly account for the development of such an expectation, especially among the premenarcheal girls. However, the responses of the postmenarcheal girls are not so easily dismissed, for these girls, having actually experienced menarche, and not possibly having experienced this promised overnight attainment of adulthood, appear to be subscribing to the same belief. Such behavior suggests that menarche is indeed both anticipated to be, and experienced as, a powerful organizing force. Girls appear subjectively to experience this event as a "turning point in [their] maturity" (to quote one of our subjects), and the actual configurational changes that occur for most girls at too continuous a rate to be perceptible, are less important than the physical-psychological change that occurs with menarche.

It appears that regardless of the actual physical changes that are taking place, the girl at menarche anticipates and experiences a reorganization of her body image in the direction of greater sexual maturity and feminine differentiation. Such an interpretation accords with observations that the degree of feminine identification women experience is independent of the way they actually may appear. The "boyish" looking woman may feel every

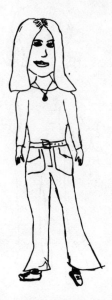

Figure 5-3a. Drawing of a Girl Whose Menarcheal Status Changed over Course of Study—Premenarcheal, Time 1

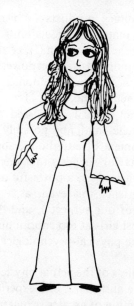

Figure 5-3b. Drawing of a Girl Whose Menarcheal Status Changed over Course of Study—Postmenarcheal, Time 2

bit as "feminine" as the most stereotypically feminine-looking woman, while the latter may lack clear sexual identification despite all outward appearances.

A similar process may be in effect for the adolescent girl. It is not how she looks, but how she feels, that the data are reflecting. Menarche does appear to provide a critical impetus, which results in the girls's subjective experience of herself as more feminine and sexually mature. This experience is then manifested in the human-figure drawings in the most appropriate way: inner feelings about the sexual parts of the body are reflected in the external representational mode of a drawing.

References

Blos, P. 1962. *On adolescence.* New York: Free Press.

Deutsch, H. 1944. *The psychology of women*, vol. 1. New York: Grune and Stratton.

Frisch, R.E., and Revelle, R. 1970. Height and weight at menarche and a hypothesis of critical body weights and adolescent events. *Science* 169:397-399.

Hart, M., and Sarnoff, C.A. 1971. The impact of the menarche: A study of two stages of organization. *Journal of the American Academy of Child Psychiatry* 10:257-271.

Haworth, M.R., and Normington, C.J. 1961. A sexual differentiation scale for the D-A-P Test. *Journal of Projective Techniques* 25:441-450.

Kestenberg, J.S. 1961. Menarche. In S. Lorand and H.I. Schneer, Eds., *Adolescents: Psychoanalytic approach to problems and therapy.* New York: Paul B. Hoeber, Inc.

_____ . 1967. Phases of adolescence, Parts I and II. *Journal of the American Academy of Child Psychiatry* 6:426-463, 577-611.

Koff, E., Rierdan, J., and Jacobson, S. 1981. The personal and interpersonal significance of menarche. *Journal of the American Academy of Child Psychiatry* 20:148-158.

Koff, E., Rierdan, J., and Silverstone, E. 1978. Changes in representation of body image as a function of menarcheal status. *Developmental Psychology*, 14:635-642.

Tanner, J.M. 1978. *Fetus into man: Physical growth from conception to maturity*, Cambridge, Mass.: Harvard University Press.

Whisnant, L., Brett, E., and Zegans, L. 1975a. Implicit messages concerning menstruation in commercial educational materials prepared for young adolescent girls. *American Journal of Psychiatry* 132:815-820.

Whisnant, L., and Zegans, L. 1975. A study of attitudes toward menarche in white middle-class American adolescent girls. *American Journal of Psychiatry* 132:809-814.

Zacharias, L., Rand, W.M., and Wurtman, R.J. 1976. A prospective study of sexual development and growth in American girls: The statistics of menarche. *Obstetrical and Gynecological Survey* 31:325-337.

Recollections of Menarche, Current Menstrual Attitudes, and Perimenstrual Symptoms

Nancy Fugate Woods,
Gretchen Kramer Dery,
and *Ada Most*

Beliefs about menstruations are acquired at an early age, and these beliefs usually reflect the general cultural stereotypes about menstruation as a negative and symptom-laden phenomenon. When adolescent females are asked to describe their reactions to their first menstrual period, their feelings are typically negative. Indeed, they used terms such as "scared," "upset" or "ashamed" (Whisnant and Zegans 1975). Studies of adult women's recollections of menarche often confirm these negative feelings (Shainess, 1961). Clarke and Ruble (1978) found that even premenarcheal girls and boys of the same age, as well as girls who have experienced menarche, believe that many symptoms are associated with the menstrual cycle. When asked about their beliefs concerning the effects of menstruation on activities and mood, both the boys in the study and premenarcheal and postmenarcheal girls described these effects as negative or neutral. More postmenarcheal than premenarcheal girls demonstrated a dislike of menstruation.

In a subsequent study of 350 girls from fifth to twelfth grade, Ruble and Brooks[1] examined the influence of grade and menarcheal status on symptoms that girls anticipated as well as those that they experienced. Older girls reported greater cycle-phase differences in symptoms, but when age was held constant there was little difference between what premenarcheal girls expected to experience and what postmenarcheal girls reported they did experience. This same sample evaluated menstruation as quite negative although they agreed it was part of becoming a woman.

In contrast, Brooks, Ruble, and Clarke (1977) found that college women at a private university accepted menstruation rather routinely and

This research was funded by a grant from Sigma Theta Tau and BRSG SO7 RR05758 awarded by the Biomedical Research Support Grant Program, Division of Research Resources, National Institutes of Health. Presented at the Menarche: An Interdisciplinary Research Conference, New Rochelle, New York, 12-13 June 1981. Portions of this research were reported in *Psychosomatic Medicine* 44 (1982):285-293 and are reprinted by permission of the publisher. Copyright 1982 by The American Psychosomatic Society, Inc.

did not find it overly disruptive. They also found that current attitudes toward menstruation were related to the cycle-phase differences in symptoms that women expected to experience. The attitudes reflected five dimensions: menstruation as a debilitating event, as a natural or positive event, as a bothersome event, as an event that can be anticipated, and as an event that should not influence one's behavior (denial). When these women responded to the Moos Menstrual Distress Questionnaire (MDG) as if they were premenstrual or intermenstrual, their scores on the debilitation and anticipation dimensions of the menstrual attitude scales were positively associated with cycle-phase differences in most of the MDQ scales. When they reported actual physical and psychological distress they experienced with menstruation, women with higher levels of distress were more likely to believe that menstruation is debilitating and can be anticipated and less likely to deny that it affected one's behavior.

A subsequent study of women from private and state-supported universities, (Brooks-Gunn and Ruble 1980) confirmed that certain menstrual attitudes were related to menstrual symptoms women experienced as well as to those they anticipate experiencing or would expect women, in general, to experience. Seeing menstruation as debilitating and predictable was again associated with greater cyclic changes in symptom experiences and expectations, whereas denial of the effect of menstruation was negatively associated with actual or expected cycle-phase changes.

These studies, taken together, show that young girls' feelings about menarche tend to be negative and that even premenarcheal girls and similar-aged boys have expectations about menstrual symptoms. Yet studies of college-aged women show that they generally find menstruation minimally disruptive. Their current menstrual attitudes, however, are related to both those symptoms they anticipate experiencing and those they actually experience. To date, however, there has been no study to explore the influence of menarcheal experiences on subsequent menstrual attitudes and symptoms in a free-living population of adult women.

If negative menarcheal experiences have important effects on women's future menstrual experiences, then we would anticipate a strong association between women's recollections of menarche and their current menstrual attitudes. If perimenstrual symptoms are, indeed, partly a product of menarcheal experience, then one would also anticipate a strong association between negative recollections of first menstruation and perimenstrual symptoms. If recollections of first menstruation do not establish a self-fulfilling prophecy, then negative responses to menarche should exist independently of current negative menstrual attitudes or perimenstrual symptoms. The purpose of this chapter is to assess the associations between recollections of menarche, current menstrual attitudes, and perimenstrual symptoms in adult women.

Method

Sample

We chose a population of women residing in five neighborhoods of varying racial composition and socioeconomic status of a large southeastern city as the sampling frame. We identified all households in each neighborhood from a census listing for the city, and then randomly selected households from this listing. Trained interviewers contacted each household by telephone or in person and determined whether or not one of the household residents met the criteria for inclusion in the study.

The inclusion criteria were that participants be female, eighteen to thirty-five years of age, and not pregnant at the time of the telephone contact, to optimize the likelihood of interviewing women who were currently menstruating. Only one woman per household was studied. Of 650 randomly selected households contacted, 255 potential participants were available, and 193 (77 percent) actually agreed to participate in the study.

Measures

Perimenstrual Symptoms. We used an adaptation of the Moos Menstrual Distress Questionnaire (MDQ) (Moos 1968)[2] to measure perimenstrual symptoms (PMS). Our previous work had revealed that of the forty-seven symptoms on the MDQ, only sixteen varied significantly and substantially across menstrual cycle phase (Woods, Most, and Dery).[3] These symptoms included: weight gain, crying, lowered performance, taking naps or staying in bed, headache, skin disorders, cramps, anxiety, backache, fatigue, painful or tender breasts, swelling, irritability, mood swings, depression, and tension. We used factor analysis, with a varimax rotation, to identify four factors for each cycle phase: pain, water retention, negative affect, and impaired performance for the premenstrual and menstrual phases. The scales were found to be internally consistent (Cronbach's alpha from .64 to .88). On the MDQ, women are asked to report their perceptions of each of the symptoms for (1) their most recent flow; (2) the week before their most recent flow; and (3) the remainder of the cycle. They were asked to use a rating scale in which responses range from 1 for "no experience of the symptom" to 6 for "acute or partially disabling." *Cycle phase* was defined in the same manner as the MDQ required, such that the premenstruum included the week prior to the last menstruation, the menstruum included time during the most recent flow, and the remainder of the cycle included all residual days after accounting for the premenstruum and menstruum.

Current Menstrual Attitudes. We used the Menstrual Attitudes Questionnaire (MAQ) to describe women's attitudes toward menstruation (Brooks-

Gunn and Ruble 1980). This instrument consists of thirty-three items designed to tap five dimensions of menstrual attitudes: menstruation as a debilitating event, a bothersome event, or a natural event, and anticipation and prediction of the onset of menstruation and denial of any effect of menstruation. An example of an item reflecting menstruation as a debilitating event is: "Women are more tired than usual when they are menstruating." Menstruation as a natural event is reflected in items such as "Menstruation is a recurring affirmation of womanhood." Women rate each item on a 7-point scale such that 1 = disagree strongly and 7 = strongly agree. Scale homogeneity is high (Cronbach's alpha = .80 to .93) in our sample.

Recollections of First Menstruation (RFM). We used the Recollections of First Menstruation (RFM) items (Brooks-Gunn)[4] to reflect the women's initial experiences with menstruation. These eight adjectives describe how the woman felt the first time she got her period; for example, happy, embarrassed. Women respond to a Likert-type scale where responses range from 1 = not at all to 4 = a lot. Four items constitute a negative scale (upset, embarrassed, angry, scared), and three a positive scale (happy, proud, excited). An additional item asks whether the woman felt surprised at menarche.

We also considered the woman's self-reports of menstrual-cycle length, days of flow, estimation of amount of blood lost, ability to predict the next menstruation, pregnancy history, use of oral contraceptives or intrauterine devices, and the woman's age.

Procedure

Interviewers initially contacted the women by phone and arranged a mutually convenient time for interviewing the women in their homes. The interviewer obtained informed consent prior to conducting the interview, and the interviews were completed in about one hour. During the interview we administered the MDQ and obtained demographic information and data about recollections of menarche and current menstrual attitudes. The interviews were conducted between March and July of 1979.

Results

Participants

The 193 participants ranged in age from 18 to 35 years with a mean age of 27.7 years (*SD* = 4.6). One hundred-six (54.9 percent) of the women were married; 57 (29.5 percent), single; 11 (5.7 percent) remarried; 9 (4.7 percent) divorced, 7 (3.6 percent) separated, 2 living with a partner (1 percent), and 1 (0.5 percent widowed. Thirty-three percent of the sample was black, and 67 percent was white. The income of the study sample ranged from less than $2,000 to more than $40,000 annually, with a median of about $6,700. The women had attained educational levels ranging from completion of the eleventh grade to doctoral preparation. The women in the sample also represented a variety of religious denominations: 128 were Protestant, 20 Catholic, 4 Jewish, 13 other denominations, and 28 claimed no religion. Seventy-eight of the women in the sample had one or more children, with the mean number of children in these families being 1.7.

One-hundred fifty-six or 80.8 percent of the women were currently employed, and 37 or 19.2 percent were not employed. Twenty (51.3 percent) of the latter described themselves as students, with the remainder being homemakers. The employed women reported working five to sixty hours per week, with the mode being forty hours. Their occupations varied widely with some women employed in areas employing only 1 percent women and some in occupations in which women constituted 65 percent or more of the labor force. The social status of the women's occupations also varied widely.

Fourteen of the women interviewed had had a hysterectomy and did not complete the MDQ. Forty-three of the women were using oral contraceptives, and twenty-two had an IUD in place.

Because we were concerned with the relationship of recollections of menarche, current menstrual attitudes, and perimenstrual symptoms, it was important to determine whether use of oral contraceptives (OC) or an intruterine device (IUD) might confound these relationships. To ascertain the effect of OC or IUD use, we inspected the correlations between OC and IUD with the recollections of first menstruation, MAQ, and PMS scale scores. We found that IUD use is not correlated with any of these variables. Use of oral contraceptives is weakly correlated with negative feelings about menarche (rho = .174, p < .011), denying the effects of menstruation (rho = .164, p < .015), and with a low tendency to see menstruation as a natural phenomenon (rho = $-.207, p$ < .004). Because neither IUD use nor OC use was strongly correlated with recollections of first menstruation and symptoms, and OC only weakly correlated with two of the five menstrual-attitude scales, women who used both forms of contraception are included in these analyses.

Characteristics of Menarche

Recollections of first menstruation reflected women's ambivalence. Most women reported being happy (58 percent) proud (65 percent), or excited (75 percent) at menarche, but most women also recalled negative responses. Sixty-seven percent reported feeling upset, 82 percent embarrassed, 29 percent angry, and 74 percent scared. Eighty percent were surprised. Age at menarche ranged from 9 to 16 with a mean age of 12.3 ± 1.4 years, and a median of 12.25 years. This finding is consistent with the expected age at menarche for this age cohort of women in the United States where the mean is approximately 12.5 years (Zacharias, Wurlman & Schatzoff 1970).

Current Menstrual Attitudes

In general, the women slightly disagreed that menstruation is debilitating ($M = 3.75 \pm 1.45$), or that it has no effect ($M = 3.51 \pm 1.56$), but slightly agreed that it is bothersome ($M = 4.64 \pm 1.35$), a natural event ($M = 4.92 \pm 1.23$), and that their next menstruation could be anticipated or predicted ($M = 5.24 \pm 1.13$).

Perimenstrual Symptoms

Mean scores for the perimenstrual symptom scales are given in table 6-1. In general, the average severity on each scale ranges from 2 to 3, consistent with descriptions of these symptoms as "barely noticeable" to "mild." The difference in symptom severity across cycle phase is minimal.

Relationships between Characteristics of Menarche and Current Menstrual Attitudes

Age at menarche was not related to any of the current menstrual attitudes. Women who experienced menarche at a later age had slightly more positive recollections (rho = .130, $p < .04$). In general, characteristics of men-

Table 6-1
Scores on Perimenstrual-Symptom Scales
(N = 179) (Mean ± S.D.)

| | Perimenstrual Symptom Scales | | | |
	Pain	Water Retention	Negative Affect	Impaired Performance
Premenstrual	1.988 ± .941	2.333 ± 1.015	2.238 ± .873	2.100 ± .852
Menstrual	2.199 ± .933	2.062 ± .925	2.070 ± .828	2.123 ± .871

arche have little relationship to current menstrual attitudes. Women with more positive feelings about menarche were more able to anticipate and predict their next menstruation (rho = .219, $p < .05$). Surprise at menarche and negative recollections of menarche were not related to current menstrual attitudes.

Relationship between Characteristics of Menarche and Current Perimenstrual Symptoms

Characteristics of menarche are only slightly related to perimenstrual symptoms (see table 6-2). Women who have positive recollections of menarche have more severe premenstrual and menstrual negative affect and impaired-performance symptoms. Women who felt surprise at menarche are likely to have menstrual-pain symptoms. Negative recollections of menarche are not significantly associated with any of the symptoms, although there is a small and nonsignificant correlation between negative recollections and menstrual pain. Women who began menarche later are slightly less likely to have premenstrual pain, but this relationship is not statistically significant. Age at menarche is unrelated to other symptoms.

Table 6-2
Correlations (Spearman's rho) between Characteristics of Menarche and Current Perimenstrual Symptoms
(N = 179)

Characteristics of Menarche	Pain	Water Retention	Negative Affect	Impaired Performance
		Premenstrual Symptoms		
Recollections of First Menstruation				
Positive recollections	.187	.173	.337*	.257*
Negative recollections	.044	.066	.067	− .036
Surprise	− .182	.008	− .085	− .042
Age at menarche	− .143	− .022	.045	.050
		Menstrual Symptoms		
Recollections of First Menstruation				
Positive recollections	.106	.155	.278*	.268*
Negative recollections	.182	.034	− .020	.012
Surprise	.261*	.163	.121	.104
Age at menarche	.081	.011	.031	− .076

Source: Dunn and Clark (1974). *Applied statistics: analysis of variance and regression,* New York: John Wiley and Sons.
*$p < .05$ adjusted for number of tests.

Relationship between Current Menstrual Attitudes
and Perimenstrual Symptoms

As seen in table 6-3, there is a positive and statistically significant relationship between seeing menstruation as debilitating and each of the perimenstrual-symptom scales except premenstrual water retention. Likewise, anticipation of menstruation is positively correlated with each of the PMS scales. Denial of effects of menstruation is negatively related to each of the symptom scales except menstrual water retention. Neither seeing menstruation as bothersome nor seeing it as a natural event is related to PMS.

Discussion

Characteristics of menarche appear to have only a weak relationship to current menstrual attitudes, with women who have positive recollections of menarche being more able to anticipate their next menstruation. Age at menarche has no effect on current menstrual attitudes and is only weakly associated with having less premenstrual pain. Surprisingly, women who have the most positive recollections of their first menstruation have more

Table 6-3
Correlations between Current Menstrual Attitudes and Perimenstrual Symptoms
(Spearman's rho: N = 179)

| | Premenstrual Symptoms | | | |
	Pain	Water Retention	Negative Affect	Impaired Performance
Debilitating	.248*	.209	.351*	.404*
Bothersome	.005	−.028	−.113	−.098
Natural	.057	.098	−.034	.014
Anticipation	.378	.324*	.294*	.314*
Denial	−.269*	−.220*	−.403*	−.334*
	Menstrual Symptoms			
Debilitating	.263*	.252*	.449*	.523*
Bothersome	.046	.026	−.001	−.096
Natural	.011	.082	.065	.063
Anticipation	.414*	.259*	.282*	.354*
Denial	−.283*	−.155	−.307*	−347*

Source: Method of analysis from Dunn and Clark (1974). *Applied statistics: analysis of variance and regression,* New York: John Wiley and Sons.
*$p < .05$ adjusted for number of tests.

symptoms of premenstrual and menstrual negative affect and impaired performance. Women who were more surprised at menarche have more
menstrual pain. Women who currently see menstruation as debilitating and
anticipate their next period have higher scores on all PMS scales, whereas
women who deny the effects of menstruation have lower PMS scale scores.

Although Shainess (1961) in her study of one hundred women, some of
whom were her psychotherapy patients, found that women who had negative menarcheal experiences also had premenstrual tension, and Deutsch
(1944) cautions that "in the course of a woman's lifetime the subjective
events connected with the first menstruation have a tendency to recur at
every other menstruation, but normally in a very weakened form" (p. 186)
these results lend little support to the theory that negative recollections of
the first menstrual experience have an important effect on subsequent
attitudes toward menstruation and symptom experience. Thus, the self-
fulfilling prophecy that might have been set in motion by negative menarcheal experiences seems more a myth than reality. This lack of confirmation,
however, may be a function of the population studied—primarily well
women living in the community instead of women seeking treatment for
symptoms about whom the self-fulfilling prophecy theory was generated
(Deutsch 1944; Shainess, 1961).

The fact that current menstrual attitudes and symptoms seem independent of recollections of menarche may also be attributable to the design
employed in the study. Because data about menarcheal experiences were
gathered retrospectively, these women had considerable opportunity to
reconstruct their feelings at menarche. If subjects were reconstructing their
feelings, however, one would expect to see much more consistency between
their recollections of menarche and current attitudes and, perhaps, less ambivalence about menarche.

It is likely that women's feelings about menstruation changed as a consequence of the changing sociocultural milieu in which the stereotypes
about menstruation and women in general have recently been challenged.
This age cohort of women began menstruating during the early to midsix-
ties, the reference point used for the items about recollections of menarche.
They reported their current menstrual attitudes in 1979 after nearly a decade
of change had occurred in women's roles (U.S. Department of Labor 1975)
and in the sex-role norms about women (Thornton & Freedman 1979). Thus
it is possible that as girls, these women had quite negative feelings about
menarche, but by the time of this study, their attitudes toward menstruation
had become more positive.

Although women's attitudes toward menstruation may have changed in
response to sociocultural change, they also reflect their current experiences
with menstrual symptoms. That is, women who have severe menstrual
symptoms may come to see menstruation as debilitating and something to

anticipate inasmuch as it disrupts their lives—if only for a short time. These women also would probably find it most difficult to deny that menstruation has negative effects. Thus the causal path is probably not a unidirectional one, and changes in either attitudes or symptoms are probably reflected in the other variable.

Finally, while menarche marks a major transition in the lives of adolescents, menstruation represents continuity in the lives of adult women, and thus evokes a different response. While young girls respond to a single and dramatic event, menarche, adult women's attitudes probably are a function of their ongoing symptom experience.

In sum, recollections of menarche seemingly have little influence on subsequent menstrual attitudes or symptoms in adult women. Women's current menstrual attitudes, however, are moderately associated with, and probably influenced by, the symptoms they experience.

Notes

1. Ruble, D., and Brooks, J. "Adolescents' attitudes about menstruation." Unpublished manuscript, 1977.

2. Moos, R.H. *Menstrual distress questionnaire.* Preliminary manual. Palo Alto, Cal., Department of Psychiatry, Stanford University and Veterans Association Hospital, 1977.

3. Woods, N., Most, A. and Dery, G.K. Toward a construct of perimenstrual distress. Submitted for publication.

4. Brooks-Gunn, J. Personal communication, 1981.

References

Brooks, J., Ruble, D., and Clarke, A. 1977. College women's attitudes and expectations concerning menstrual-related changes. *Psychosomatic Medicine* 39:288-298.

Brooks-Gunn, J., and Ruble, D. 1980. The menstrual attitude questionnaire. *Psychosomatic Medicine* 42:503-512.

Clarke, A., and Ruble, D. 1978. Young adolescents' beliefs concerning menstruation. *Child Development* 49:231-234.

Deutsch, H. 1944. *The psychology of women.* New York: Grune and Stratton.

Dunn, O., and Clark, V. 1974. *Applied statistics: Analysis of variance and regression.* New York: John Wiley and Sons.

Moos, R.H. 1968. The development of a menstrual distress questionnaire. *Psychosomatic Medicine* 30:853-867.

Shainess, N. 1961. A re-evaluation of some aspects of femininity through a study of menstruation. *Comparative Psychiatry* 2:20-26.

Thornton, A., and Freedman, D. 1979. Changes in the sex role attitudes of women, 1962-1977:Evidence from a panel study. *American Sociological Review* 44:831-842.

U.S. Department of Labor. 1975. *Handbook on women workers,* U.S. Department of Labor Employment Standards Administration, Women's Bureau.

Whisnant, L., and Zegans, L. 1975. A study of attitudes toward menarche in white middle-class American girls. *American Journal of Psychiatry* 132:809-814.

Zacharias, L., Wurlman, R., and Schatzoff, M. 1970. Sexual maturation in contemporary American girls. *American Journal of Obstetrics and Gynecology* 108:833.

7

Menarche: Its Effects on Mother-Daughter and Father-Daughter Interactions

Roberta Danza

Many researchers on family development identify significant events and transitional crises during the life of the family as agents of major change in the family organization (Duvall 1967; Solomon 1973). Adolescence is one such event that precipitates a normative crisis in family-life development (Blos 1963; Erikson 1959), and is a time of major reorganization within the family (Ravenscroft 1974).

For the female adolescent, the onset of the first menses, is a "sharply defined biological event" (Koff, Rierdan, and Silverstone 1978, p. 638) that provides a focal point of investigation. Significant changes between pre-and postmenarcheal girls in cognition (Kestenberg 1961; Koff, Rierdan, and Silverstone 1978), thought organization (Kestenberg 1961; Koff, Rierdan, and Silverstone 1978; Whisnant and Zegans 1975), maturity in attitudes and interests (Davis 1977; Stone and Barker 1939), as well as acceptance of feminity and sexuality (Koff, Rierdan, and Silverstone 1978; Lambert et al. 1972) have been documented.

In addition, menarche has the rare characteristic among developmental events of containing a long and vital historical, cultural, and emotional heritage (Delaney, Lupton, and Toth 1976) that I predicted inevitably must affect relationships between the newly menarcheal girl and her mother and father. The purpose of this chapter is to explore the way in which female maturation, specifically menarche, affects mother-daughter and father-daughter relationships.

The following areas were investigated:

1. The differences that exist between pre- and postmenarcheal girls in the extent of: (a) limits that are set and the person(s) setting them; (b) responsibility given and by whom; (c) closeness or distance to/from each parent; and (d) amount of conflict with each parent.
2. The effects that parental attitudes toward menstruation have on parental interaction with the daughter, with particular emphasis on: (a) limits set for the daughter; (b) amount of responsibility given to the daughter; (c) closeness or distance between parent and daughter; and (d) amount of conflict occurring between parent and daughter.

Method

The subject of this chapter is a study that was designed to survey family units comprised of adolescent daughters, their mothers, and their fathers. A convenience sample was obtained. Forty-eight sixth- and seventh-grade female students, aged 11 to 14 years, were recruited on a voluntary basis from a privately financed middle school ($N = 12$; $\overline{X}$ age $= 11.9$) and a public junior-high school ($N = 36$; $\overline{X}$ age $= 12.8$). The sample consisted of twenty-four premenarcheal girls ($\overline{X}$ age $= 12.47$) and twenty-four postmenarcheal girls ($\overline{X}$ age $= 12.68$). There was no significant difference in age between the pre- and postmenarcheal girls. The sample came from families that were predominantly white (85 percent), Christian (40 percent Catholic, 35 percent Protestant), and of middle income (mothers, \$10-15,000; fathers, \$20-25,000). The mothers' ($N = 24$) mean age was 39.7 years and they had had an average of 13.6 years of schooling. The fathers' ($N = 16$) mean age was 42.1 and they had an average of 14.2 years of schooling. Twenty mothers were married, two divorced, and one widowed.

The students were recruited by the investigator who told the subjects that she was interested in learning about the kinds of changes that occur in the families of young adolescent girls. Parental participation was not required for the daughter's participation, and no attempt was made to determine the subject's age or menstrual status in advance.

A questionnaire comprised of more than 175 questions was given to the girls in a group setting in their schools and to the parents in their homes.

Major dependent variables were defined as follows:

1. *Limit Setting* included both the person(s) who determined the control and direction of the subject's behavior, and the extent of the limits set. The extent of limits set was measured on two scales: *Developmental Tasks* and limits set around *Times* (see appendix 7A).

2. *Responsibility*, defined as an increase or decrease in the tasks expected of the daughter (care of younger siblings, meal preparation, chores of greater difficulty, outside employment, allowance, and the amount of participation the daughter had in deciding her own limits and privileges).

3. *Closeness/Distance*, defined by the frequency of discussion of emotionally charged topics by the daughter and each parent (see appendix 7A) and the degree of discomfort experienced in these discussions; also, comfort with separation and whether the daughter perceived a change in closeness to each parent.

4. *Conflict and the Emotional Tone* of interaction with mother and father, specifically the nature of any change in closeness or distance experienced and in the frequency of arguments (see appendix 7A).

5. *Menstrual Attitudes.* Positive or negative feelings about menstruation in the mother and father. These included the openness with which

menstruation was discussed among family members and friends, and each family member's knowledge and involvement in the menarcheal event of the female subject. In addition, mothers were asked to rate their physical comfort during menses, past and present; and to identify the emotions they experienced on first learning of menstruation, at their own menarche, and presently when menstruating.

The instrument was hand-scored, computer-card punched, and the data analyzed using the Datatext program with matched t-tests, analysis of variance, and Pearson product-moment correlations as appropriate.

Results

Significant differences were found between pre- and postmenarcheal girls on all four axes. Moreover, the differences were related to menarcheal status and not to age.

Postmenarcheal girls as compared with premenarcheal girls:

1. Experienced a greater number of the developmental tasks (were more likely to wear make-up, a bra, to date, and such) ($t = 2.930$, $p < .006$),
2. Did more limit setting on their own ($t = 3.063$, $p < .004$),
3. Slept less on school nights ($t = 4.093$, $p < .001$),
4. Had more liberal time limits ($t = 2.413$, $p < .02$),
5. Experienced less comfort in emotionally charged discussions with their mothers ($t = 2.00$, $p < .05$),
6. Were significantly less comfortable in discussions with their fathers than with their mothers ($t = 2.70$, $p < .01$),
7. Reported more conflict with their parents (t $= 2.030$, $p < .05$),
8. Evaluated their parents as getting along less well ($t = 2.20$, $p < .03$).

The premenarcheal girls reported more emotional interaction (see appendix 7A) with their fathers than did the postmenarcheal girls ($t = 2.639$, $p < .01$).

Correlations between parental attitudes toward menstruation and the variables reflecting parent-child relationships were also done. (Because of the limited number of fathers responding, only the mothers' responses were analyzed). When the mothers' menstrual attitudes were distributed on a scale from positive to negative a number of significant correlations were found. However, the small number of subjects, particularly at the negative end of the scale, made interpretation somewhat tentative. These findings, then, are considered *suggestive* of interactions between maternal menstrual attitudes and family dynamics.

Preliminary indications are that when the mothers' menstrual attitudes are negative: there is more distance between mother and daughter; the daughter is closer to her father and more discussions take place between them; the father tends to be the primary limit setter and imposes stricter limits; there is more conflict in the triad; the daughter is less comfortable with her parents going out together; and she tends to maintain the more "child-like" nine-hour daily sleep pattern.

While the previously cited statistical constraints still pertain, this picture nevertheless appears to contrast markedly with those families in which the mother reports more positive attitudes toward menstruation. In these instances there appears to be greater closeness between the mother and daughter; more likelihood that the mother is the primary limit setter and that the limits are more liberal (for example, the daughter experiences more developmental tasks and later time limits); less conflict in the triad; the daughter reports greater comfort with her parents going out together; and her sleep pattern takes on the more "adult-like" eight-hour cycle.

The contrasts between the models described are provocative and suggest that further investigation with larger populations might be rewarding.

Discussion

This chapter suggests that it is menarche, not age or peer norms, that differentiates the extent of limits, roles, and responsibilities given to and assumed by the early-adolescent female. There is a definite change in the interaction between the postmenarcheal girl and her parents. This change is reflected in her increased reluctance to discuss so called charged topics with her parents and her changed perception of her parents' relationship. Whether their relationship is, in fact, more in conflict at this nodal point of change in their daughter or the daughter perceives them in a less idealized manner is not known.

The findings suggest that the postmenarcheal girl both experiences herself and also is perceived by her parents as more mature. Behaviors and expectations are adjusted accordingly. There is even a change in a simple biological dimension: postmenarcheal girls get by on an hour-less sleep each night than do their premenarcheal peers. Menarche appears to be a factor in producing a shift from the more child-like average of nine-plus hours of sleep each night to the more adult average of eight hours.

The relationship between mothers' menstrual attitudes and family interactions, while only suggestive on the basis of these data, also appears to be important. The daughter of a mother with negative menstrual attitudes seems less likely to identify with and become close to her mother. Instead, she becomes close to her father who sets stricter limits. Thus, the growth of the daughter away from the family appears to be curtailed. This impression is substantiated to some extent by the finding that these daughters maintain the child-like sleep patterns. The picture that emerges is one in which the girl's opportunity to leave the family in an age-appropriate way and direct sexual and aggressive drives outward is limited. Conflict within the family increases.

In contrast, when the mother's attitudes toward menstruation are positive, the daughter seems better able to achieve a closer identity with her mother as a mature female model; she feels comfortable about maturing and experiencing an increased number of activities with peers of both sexes and begins to negotiate the delicate balance between closeness to her parents and moving into a new life of her own.

It is important to be cautious in speculating about the meaning of the relationship between mother's attitudes toward menstruation and family dynamics. It is probable that the high degree of correlation is due in part to the influence of other factors, such as personality variables or degree of comfort with disclosure, which are also at play.

The final picture that emerges, then, is one in which menarche appears to have a significant impact on the family-life cycle. In this study, menarche affected the limits, responsibilities, closeness, distance, conflict and roles the daughter experienced, and it served as a nodal point for changing the mother's and father's relationship to their developing daughter.

The implications for clinical practice are many. Certainly those female adolescent patients identified as exhibiting problem behaviors and grappling with issues of control, independence, and sexuality can be helped through an understanding of family dynamics at and around the time of menarche. In addition, this chapter suggests that the Oedipal issues that emerge again in early adolescence are not merely an interesting theoretical construct or solely a helpful way of viewing family psychodynamics but can be seen in actual quantifiable behaviors. Family dynamics are not only understandable through anecdotal reporting and general psychodynamic impressions but can be determined by a rigorous statistical approach in which appropriate behaviors are counted and analyzed.

References

Blos, P. 1963. *On adolescence: A psychoanalytic interpretation.* New York: Free press.

Davis, B.L. 1977. Attitudes towards school among early and late maturing adolescent girls. *Journal of Genetic Psychology* 131:261-266.

Delaney, J., Lupton, M.J., and Toth, E. 1976. *The curse: A cultural history of menstruation.* New York: Mentor.

Duvall, E.M. 1967. *Family development*. Chicago: Lippincott.

Erikson, E.H. 1959. *Identity and the life cycle*. New York: International Universities Press.

Kestenberg, J. 1961. Menarche. In S. Lorand and H. Schneer, eds., *Adolescents, psychoanalytic approach to problems and therapy*. New York: Paul B. Hoeber, Inc.

Koff, E., Rierdan, H., and Silverstone, E. 1978. Changes in representation of body image as a function of menarcheal status. *Developmental Psychology* 14:635-642.

Lambert, G., Rothschild, B., Altand, R., and Greer, L. 1972. *Adolescence*. Monterey, Cal.: Brooks/Cole.

Ravenscroft, K. 1974. Normal crises in the family life cycle: Family structure and mental health. *Family Process* 2:68-80.

Solomon, M. 1973. A developmental conceptual premise for family therapy. *Family Process*. 12:179-188.

Stone, C.P., and Barker, R.G. 1939. The attitudes and interests of pre-menarcheal and post-menarcheal girls. *Journal of Genetic Psychology* 54:27-71.

Whisnant, L., and Zegans, L. 1975. A study of attitudes toward menarche in white middle-class American adolescent girls. *American Journal of Psychiatry* 132:809-814.

Appendix 7A:
Selected Sections from
the Questionnaire

A. Developmental Tasks:

At what age did you?	Age in Years and Month?	Who Decided?[a]
1. Wear make-up outside the home		
2. Shave your legs		
3. Wear a bra		
4. Choose your own clothes		
5. Date in groups		
6. Date with one boy		
7. Go to boy-girl parties		
8. Go driving alone with a boy		
9. See any movie you choose		

[a]The subjects were asked to place the letter(s) corresponding to those involved in making the decision (M-Mother, F-Father, D-Daughter, O-Other, and explain)

B. Times:

What time do you?	Time	Who Decided?
1. Usually awaken on school days		
2. Usually awaken on nonschool days		
3. Go to bed on school nights		
4. Go to bed on nonschool nights		
5. Stay out on school nights		
6. Stay out on nonschool nights		

C. Topics of Discussion:

Over the past year approximately how many meaningful discussions have occurred between you and your mother or father about:	Amount M	Amount F	Rate according to your comfort with the discussions: 1-2-3-4-5 1-Most comfortable 5-Most uncomfortable	Who initiated the discussions? M-mother D-daughter F-father Other
1. Physical changes of womanhood				
2. Pregnancy				
3. Sexuality				
4. Love				
5. Boyfriends				
6. Use of alcohol				
7. Use of drugs				
8. Requests for advice				

D. Conflict and Emotional Tone

In your relationships over the last year, has there been more (M), less (L), or the same (S) amount of: (compared to previous years)	Mother	Father	Rate your comfort with the changes that have occurred: 1-2-3-4-5 1-most comfortable 5-most uncomfortable	If more, who initiated this? M-mother F-father D-daughter O-other
1. Conflict (arguments)				
2. Humor				
3. Willingness				
4. Warmth				
5. Affection				
6. Trust				
7. Anger				

8

Physical Attractiveness and Physical Stigma: Menstruation and the Common Cold

Rhoda K. Unger,
Virginia H. Brown,
and *M. Victoria Larson*

A rapidly accumulating body of evidence suggests that perceptions of lower physical attractiveness are associated with negative social judgments for both females and males. The pioneer study in this area (Goldberg, Gottesdiener, and Abramson 1975) found that both male and female college students selected photos of less attractive women as perceived supporters of feminism. Less attractive males were also seen as more likely to be feminists (Johnson et al. 1978) as were individuals of both sexes who were considered active rather than passive supporters of the women's movement (Johnson, Holborn, and Turcotte 1979).

Recently, research has indicated that association between low physical attractiveness and negative evaluative judgments are not limited to feminism. Less attractive individuals of either sex are much more likely to be sorted into social categories representing various forms of minor behavioral deviance (Unger, Hilderbrand, and Madar in press). Both female and male college students selected photographs of less attractive individuals as more likely to be involved in a politically radical organization. Lesbians were also perceived as less attractive than heterosexual women although less attractive males were perceived as homosexuals only by female subjects. Both sexes perceived that less attractive males were more likely to be those men with stereotypically feminine occupational aspirations but did not penalize females with stereotypically masculine aspirations in a similar manner.

Association of decreased physical attractiveness with socially unpopular activities represents a subtle form of stereotyping. It is possible that such perceptions are mediated by the belief that the individuals so perceived have deliberately chosen their deviant behavior. This interpretation is consistent with the finding that both female and male subjects perceive that less attractive women *need* feminism (Jacobson and Koch 1978).

Physical unattractiveness, however, has been found to be associated with conditions not under the stimulus person's control. Thus, it has been found that less attractive individuals are more likely to be selected as showing

107

symptoms of psychopathology (Jones, Hansson, and Phillips 1978) and are even seen as more likely to have epilepsy (Hannson and Duffield 1976).

It has not yet been shown that perceptions of unattractiveness are associated with less serious forms of physical disorder. Because of the general stigma associated with menstruation in our culture (compare Unger 1979; Weideger 1975), this condition is a likely target for perceptions such as the ones discussed above. It was hypothesized, therefore, that when subjects were asked to sort stimulus photographs into groups on the basis that half the photographs had been taken when the subjects were menstruating and half when they were not, less attractive women would be selected as those who had posed when menstruating. Since negative evaluations of menstruation appear to be so global, it was also hypothesized that both male and female students would hold similar associations between menstruation and physical unattractiveness.

It is important to determine whether such associations are more common when females are the stimulus persons than when males are. Research using labels of behavioral deviance suggests that perceptions of unattractiveness affect both females and males although situational differences may exist. It is impossible, of course, to provide a plausible control condition using males and menstruation. We decided, therefore, to provide another condition—the common cold. This condition is roughly as common a phenomenon as menstruation and afflicts males and females equally. It has also been shown that people are less likely to be blamed for disagreeable behavior if they have a cold or are portrayed as premenstrual (Schilling and Jacobi).[1] Therefore, it was hypothesized that both males and females would select less attractive individuals of both sexes as those who had a cold when photographed. Comparison of the effects for the two physical labels—menstruation and the common cold—would indicate the strength and extent of negative social judgments associated with menstruation.

Methodology

Subjects

Subjects were 180 students (90 female and 90 male) randomly selected from the campus of a suburban New Jersey state college. All subjects were contacted by a female experimenter who asked if they would participate in a brief study involving photographs. Subjects were promised anonymity and no demographic information other than observed age (eighteen to twenty-five) was requested. No subject participated in more than one sorting condition.

Stimuli

Forty black-and-white photographs of college-age women and men were used in this study. All photographs were previously rated for physical attractiveness on a 5-point scale similar to that described by Goldberg, Gottes-diener, and Abramson (1975). An average rating for each photograph was calculated for the fifteen male and the fifteen female raters. Since the ratings obtained from each sex were highly correlated, all ratings for each photo were pooled yielding a single attractiveness rating. The mean rating for female stimulus photographs was 2.85 (range 1.90 to 3.98). The mean rating for male stimulus photographs was 2.60 (range 1.48 to 3.63).

Task

Two kinds of physical labels were used in this study. Subjects in all condi-tions (fifteen females and fifteen males) were individually presented with either the male or the female stimulus photographs in random order. They were informed that half the individuals in these photographs had had their photograph taken when the physical condition was present and half had had them taken when it was absent. The subjects were asked to sort the photographs into two equal groups: (1) menstruating versus nonmenstruat-ing and (2) cold versus no cold. In the cold condition, sex of subject and sex of stimulus person were varied resulting in a completely crossed factorial design. In the menstrual condition, of course, both male and female sub-jects viewed only female photographs. In all, six conditions were run: menstruation label—males sorting females and females sorting females; cold label—males sorting females, females sorting females, males sorting males, and females sorting males.

Results

Overall, female stimulus photographs were perceived as significantly more attractive than male stimulus photographs ($p < .0001$). This outcome was a result of the original attractiveness evaluations that were used as a depen-dent variable in the present study. Therefore, meaningful interactions with the sex of the stimulus could not be analyzed (such an analysis was also pro-blematic because of the empty cells with male stimuli in the menstrual-label condition). Therefore, the data were first analyzed using a two-way analysis of variance with sex of subject and physical label as the independent variables. Physical label proved to have a significant effect: $F = 35.63$; $p < .0001$. However, the sex of the subject had no significant effect nor did any interaction between sex of subject and physical label.

Data were then subjected to a post-hoc analysis using Duncan's multiple-range test for variable means. The average attractiveness labels of photos sorted into condition-present and condition-absent groups by male and female subjects combined were compared. It was found that subjects did not make any difference in sorting in terms of attractiveness using the menstruation/nonmenstruation label. The mean attractiveness of females sorted as menstruating was 2.81 versus 2.88 for photos sorted into the menstruation-absent condition. Perceptions of attractiveness, however, did play a role in the cold/no-cold evaluation. The mean attractiveness of females seen as having colds was 2.73 versus 2.96 for those seen as having no colds. The mean attractiveness of males seen as having colds was 2.56 versus 2.64 for those seen as not having a cold when photographed. All of these means were significantly different from each other as measured by the Duncan (alpha level = .05). There appears to be a greater magnitude of difference for female stimuli than for male, but since the photos were originally different in their base level of attractiveness it is difficult to determine what, if any, differential perceptions are present. These data suggest that menstruation has ceased to act as a social stigma, at least among college-educated individuals.

Conclusions

These data suggest that menstruation may have lost some of its negative social properties. Thus, they are in conflict with some of the more field-oriented measures such as those of Ernster (1975), which suggest that menstruation is the target of many pejorative labels. Data suggesting that there are no sex differences in perceptual behavior are consistent with previous studies cited, which showed little variation in terms of sex in the social perception of the sexes (Johnson et. al. 1978; Unger, Hilderbrand, and Madar in press).

Although it is difficult to discuss data that fail to reject the null hypothesis, it is noteworthy that the cold/no-cold sorting did produce differential perceptions about attractiveness using the same stimulus photographs and a comparable subject population. These findings suggest that lack of results was not due to the manipulations having no effect. In fact, requesting people to sort photographs into various categories provides a considerable source of information about the on-going social judgment processes of our society. The task may be particularly useful because subjects are largely unaware of the bases on which they are making their judgments. Nevertheless, few subjects refuse to participate because they cannot make judgments about physical or behavioral states on the basis of physical appearance.

These data suggest that judgments involving physical appearance extend beyond behavioral deviance to conditions involving minor levels of physical stigma. It is hopeful that in this study, at least, negative evaluations of the menstruating woman did not appear to exist. Physical-appearance variables, however, may be more important to females than males—not because they are indeed made differentially—but because physical appearance is seen as more salient to judgments of females than of males (Unger 1979). Concern with physical appearance is particularly important during adolescence. Beliefs about negative stigma may easily be incorporated into the self-image during this period. It is important, therefore, to determine whether stereotypic assumptions about menstruation and attractiveness continue to persist in younger and/or noncollege populations.

Notes

1. Schilling, K.M., and Jacobi, M. Attribution of menstrual distress. Paper presented at the meeting of the American Psychological Association, San Francisco, August 1977.

References

Ernster, V.L. 1975. American menstrual expressions. *Sex Roles* 1:3-13.

Goldberg, P.A., Gottesdiener, M., and Abramson, P.R. 1975. Another put-down of women? Perceived attractiveness as a function of support for the feminist movement. *Journal of Personality and Social Psychology* 32:113-115.

Hannson, R.C., and Duffield, B.J. 1976. Physical attractiveness and the attribution of epilepsy. *Journal of Social Psychology* 99:233-240.

Jacobson, M.B., and Koch, W. 1978. Attributed reasons for support of the feminist movement as a function of attractiveness. *Sex Roles* 4:169-174.

Johnson, R.W., Doiron, D., Brooks, G.P., and Dickinson, J. 1978. Perceived attractiveness as a function of support for the feminist movement: Not necessarily a put-down of women. *Canadian Journal of Behavioral Science* 10:214-221.

Johnson, R.W., Holborn, S.W., and Turcotte, S. 1979. Perceived attractiveness as a function of active versus passive support for the feminist movement. *Personality and Social Psychology Bulletin* 5:227-230.

Jones, W.H., Hansson, R.C., and Phillips, A.L. 1978. Physical attractiveness and judgments of psychopathology. *Journal of Social Psychology* 105:79-84.

Unger, R.K. 1979. *Female and male: Psychological perspectives.* New York: Harper and Row.

Unger, R.K., Hilderbrand, M., and Madar, T. In press. Physical attractiveness and assumptions about social deviance: Some sex-by-sex comparisons. *Personality and Social Psychology Bulletin.*

Weideger, P. 1975. *Menstruation and menopause.* New York: Knopf.

**Part III
Menstrual Education**

Introduction
to Part III

Menstrual education: Who needs it? What should be taught? And who is to do the teaching? In a cross-cultural study of ninety-five women from twenty-three nations, Logan (1980) found that mothers were the most common source of information prior to the onset of menstruation. Yet one-third of these girls were not told about menarche before its occurrence. For U.S. premenarcheal girls, female friends are an important source of information, as are the schools and commercial educational materials (Whisnant and Zegans 1975).

How adequate was the preparation these women received? Twenty-eight percent of the foreign women and 39 percent of a sample of U.S. women reported that their preparation for menarche was inadequate (Logan 1980; Weidegger 1976). The data also suggest that where one learns about menstruation seems to be less important than the tone of the interaction: free discussion, whether among friends and family or in school, fosters fewer reports of inadequate preparation.

Who needs menstrual education? In a recent study, Golub[1] found that 25 percent of a group of college women felt frightened when they discovered their first menstruation. Others have also found menarche to be an anxiety-producing or negative event (Koff, Rierdan, and Jacobson 1981; Whisnant and Zegans 1975); mixed feelings are common (Petersen 1982; Woods, Dery, and Most 1982). Some theorists have argued that menarche, because of its link with adult sexuality and childbirth, must of necessity be an anxiety-producing experience (Deutsch 1944). However, there may be a simpler explanation. Blood frightens most people. Usually, it means that something is wrong. Perhaps the fear that researchers have found among girls discovering their first menstruation is related to an atavistic fear of blood and a lack of understanding of what is happening, rather than to such future events as childbirth.

In the next chapter, Jill Rierdan discusses a study of college women in which she found that preparation for menstruation does indeed allay fear and anxiety. Girls who were adequately prepared were more likely to report a positive initial experience with menstruation. Rierdan's research was also aimed at determining what women think they need to know to be adequately prepared. She found that young women wanted information about menstrual physiology and menstrual hygiene as well as information about the experience "as a personal event." This desire for something more than just factual data would appear to mean that some recognition of the emotional impact of the menstrual experience is needed too.

Commercial educational materials have been found to be an important source of information about menstruation for young adolescent girls (Whisnant, Brett, and Zegans 1975). Vera Milow describes the educational program that has been developed by TAMPAX Incorporated over the past forty years. Based upon empirical experiences of educational consultants as well as research data, this program has broadened in scope from the presentation of anatomy and physiology and menstrual hygiene to the inclusion of new medical information and a responsiveness to questions regarding all aspects of menstruation. Moreover, in recent years the menstrual education program has been reaching girls at earlier ages. Milow notes the continued need for menstrual education demonstrated by *The TAMPAX Report*, a nationwide study of attitudes toward menstruation, which showed the persistence of menstrual taboos and misinformation. And she stresses the importance of educating mothers so that they too are able to participate in preparing their daughters for menstruation.

Edna Menke addresses the role of mothers by comparing the beliefs regarding menstruation and menstrual symptoms of a sample of mothers and their adolescent (twelve- to sixteen-year-old) daughters. Menke hypothesized that mothers are an important influence on their daughters' perception of menstruation. She found that mother's and daughter's attitudes were quite similar, thus emphasizing the importance of mothers' role in menstrual education.

Lenore Williams's research focused on the knowledge, beliefs, and attitudes of nine- to twelve-year-old girls. She found that among these premenarcheal girls attitudes toward menstruation were generally positive, with many relating menarche to growing up. Yet the girls did hold some of the common negative stereotypic beliefs about menstruation and were influenced by concealment taboos. Williams also identified a need for more information about internal reproductive anatomy in this group. Her chapter, and the others in this part, confirm the need for broadly based menstrual education programs that reach premenarcheal girls and their mothers.

Note

1. Golub, S. Recollections of menarche. Unpublished study.

References

Deutsch, H. 1944. *The psychology of women*, vol. 1. New York: Grune and Stratton.

Koff, E., Rierdan, J., and Jacobson, S. 1981. The personal and interpersonal significance of menarche. *Journal of the American Academy of Child Psychiatry* 20:148-158.

Logan, D.D. 1980. The menarche experience in twenty-three foreign countries. *Adolescence* 15:247-256.

Petersen, A. 1983. Menarche: Meaning of measures and measuring meaning. In S. Golub, ed., *Menarche*. Lexington, Mass.: Lexington Books, D.C. Heath and Company.

Weidegger, P. 1976. *Menstruation and menopause*. New York: Knopf.

Whisnant, L., and Zegans, L. 1975. A study of attitudes toward menarche in white middle-class American adolescent girls. *American Journal of Psychiatry* 132:809-814.

Whisnant, L., Brett, E., and Zegans, L. 1975. Implicit messages concerning menstruation in commercial educational materials prepared for young adolescent girls. *American Journal of Psychiatry* 132:815-820.

Woods, N.F., Dery, G.K., and Most, A. 1983. Recollections of menarche, current menstrual attitudes, and perimenstrual symptoms. In S. Golub, ed., *Menarche*. Lexington, Mass.: Lexington Books, D.C. Heath and Company.

9

Variations in the Experience of Menarche as a Function of Preparedness

Jill Rierdan

Recently,[1] investigators have stressed the dearth of research on female adolescent development (for example, Sugar 1979). Study of girls' psychological responses to puberty, in general, has been limited; systematic assessment of girls' responses to the onset of menstruation—menarche—has just begun.

The paucity of systematic empirical investigations of menarche is particularly surprising in light of clinicians' views that menarche is the single most-important event of puberty for girls. Kestenberg (1967) and Ritvo (1977), for example, have theorized that menarche presents a normative developmental crisis, with favorable resolution of this crisis entailing a more mature and integrated sense of self as female. Shainess (1961) reports that a girl's experience of menarche affects her subsequent adult adjustment. Similarly, Ritvo (1977) suggests that the body image of adolescent girls—found by Koff, Rierdan, and Silverstone (1978) and Rierdan and Koff (1980) to change significantly with the onset of menstruation—is crucial to women's adult sexuality.

Findings from the empirical investigations of menarche that have recently been undertaken support the view that menarche is an important developmental milestone. Adolescent girls assessed by Koff, Rierdan, and Jacobson (1981) and Whisnant and Zegans (1975) indicated that menarche was a highly focal event, experienced with intense ambivalence. On the one hand, menarche was experienced positively; it provided so-called proof of womanhood and, as such, was associated with maturity. On the other hand, menarche was experienced negatively as an anxiety-producing, embarrassing event, resulting in increased self-consciousness within the family and also with peers. The latter negative experiences of menarche have been thought to impede girls' subsequent development of a mature, positive female identity. Accordingly, the question has been raised as to whether the disruptive psychological impact of menarche might be minimized, thus leading to increased self-acceptance by adolescent girls and adult women.

Some have been pessimistic concerning the possibility of reducing the traumatic impact of menarche. Deutsch (1944) and Rosenbaum (1979), for

119

example, suggest that menarche is necessarily a disruptive and anxiety-producing experience and contend that such feelings are not mitigated by adequate preparation or intellectual knowledge of the biological mechanisms involved in menstruation.

Deutsch's reasoning derives from the psychoanalytic view that menarche arouses anxiety concerning castration, adult sexuality, and childbirth. Others, writing from a more social-psychological vantage point, share this basic pessimism, although perhaps to a lesser degree. Clarke and Ruble's (1978) study indicates that girls, before menarche, have a set of quite negative expectations and attitudes about menstruation. Since boys also appear to share this set of expectations (Brooks-Gunn and Ruble)[2] it has been suggested that there exist culturally determined beliefs about menstruation that countervail specific efforts to present menstruation in a more positive light. Further testimony to the existence of culturally shared negative attributions about menstruation comes from Ernster's (1975) review of euphemisms used in the United States for menstruation, which have primarily negative connotations.

To some degree, there is support for pessimism regarding the efficacy of preparing girls for menstruation. Girls questioned by Koff, Rierdan, and Jacobson (1981) and Whisnant and Zegans (1975) reported themselves to be well-prepared intellectually for menarche but nevertheless experienced, often to their surprise, considerable distress.

There is also some evidence, however, to suggest that certain types of preparation for menarche may reduce, if not eliminate, the negative impact. Brooks-Gunn and Ruble,[3] for example, noted a relationship between perceived adequacy of preparation for menarche and some aspects of subsequent menstrual distress.

The aim of this chapter is to explore some further psychological dimensions of girls' preparation for menstruation. The results of a large-scale retrospective study of college women's memories of menarche, conducted in collaboration with Elissa Koff, Karen Sheingold, and Jenny Flaherty,[4] will be reported. This age group was selected since these women were believed to be distanced enough from their menarche to be able to reflect thoughtfully and respond dispassionately to an inquiry, while being close enough to be able to reconstruct their experiences reliably. Women were asked to evaluate their own preparation, to report on their initial experience of menstruation, and to indicate, on the basis of their experience, what would be helpful in preparing a girl for menarche. The results of this investigation provide (a) an empirical assessment of the relationship between adequacy of preparation and experience of menstruation, and (b) a descriptive data base relevant to women's own views of what constitutes helpful preparation for menstruation.

Method

Subjects

Informants were ninety-seven college women (mean age, 19.20 years), who experienced menarche between 9.25 and 16.00 years, at a mean age of 13.00 years.

Materials and Procedure

Informants completed an eleven-page questionnaire concerning their menarche. Initial questions sought factual information about the onset of menstruation and were designed to provide an affectively neutral introduction for the survey. Subsequent questions dealt with preparation for menarche and with the subjective experience of menstruation, as recollected by the informants.

Preparation. Two dimensions of preparation were investigated. To assess *perceived adequacy* of preparation, informants were asked to rate the degree to which they felt prepared for menstruation on a scale ranging from 1 (completely unprepared) to 7 (completely prepared). To assess *prior knowledge* about menstruation, informants were asked to recall what they knew about six aspects of menstruation prior to their menarche. Specifically, they were asked to indicate what they knew about (a) the cause of bleeding, (b) the sensation of menstruation, (c) the frequency of menstruation, (d) the amount of bleeding per day, (e) the duration of menstruation, and (f) the mechanics of menstrual hygiene. Informants' answers were scored as correct or incorrect, with a score of 1 awarded for each correct response. Total scores for each informant could range from 0 to 6.

Experience. Informants were asked to rate their initial experience of menstruation on a scale ranging from 1 (completely positive) to 7 (completely negative), with the midpoint labeled "equally positive and negative."

Results and Discussion

Preparation and Menstrual Experience: Empirical Assessment

The following descriptive statistics may provide an initial glimpse of informants' preparation for and experience of menarche. In terms of perceived adequacy of preparation, informants gave the following ratings: 1; that is, completely unprepared (N = 7); 2 (N = 2); 3 (N = 8); 4 (N = 15); 5 (N = 20); 6 (N = 30); 7; that is, completely prepared (N = 15). For amount of prior knowledge, the distribution of scores was as follows: 0; that is, no accurate information (N = 5); 1 (N = 5); 2 (N = 9); 3 (N = 20); 4 (N = 32); 5 (N = 22); 6; that is, correct answers to all items (N = 4). Thus, according to both measures most subjects appear to have been relatively well prepared for menarche. In contrast, there was more heterogeneity in ratings of subjective experience of menarche, with the distribution of scores as follows: 1; that is, completely positive (N = 11); 2 (N = 10); 3 (N = 10); 4; that is, equally positive and negative (N = 24); 5 (N = 16); 6 (N = 16); 7; that is, completely negative (N = 10).

The two dimensions of preparation, perceived adequacy and prior information, were significantly correlated (r = .56, p < .001), as expected. Further, each was significantly correlated with the initial experience of menstruation. Girls who perceived their preparation as more adequate were more likely to report positive initial experiences (r = .48, p < .001), as were girls who recalled more accurate information prior to their first menstruation (r = $-$.19, p < .06).

Since data were available regarding girls' ages at menarche, the importance of preparation in the context of menarcheal age could be assessed. Not surprisingly, significant correlations were found between perceived adequacy of preparation and age (r = .41, p < .001) and between prior information and age (r = .33, p < .001), with early maturers less prepared for menarche than later maturers.

More surprising were the results of a final set of analyses directed toward differentiating the relative contributions of age and preparation to the experience of menarche. With age controlled, the correlation between perceived adequacy of preparation and initial experience was significant (r = $-$.44, p < .001). The more prepared a girl judged herself to have been prior to menarche, the more likely she was to rate her initial experience as positive, regardless of her age at menarche. In contrast, when perceived adequacy of preparation was controlled, no systematic relationship between age at menarche and initial experience of menarche (r = $-$.01) was found, indicating that preparedness is a more critical factor in influencing initial menstrual experience than age.

In summary, these analyses demonstrate empirically that adequacy of preparation does have an important impact on girls' initial experience of menarche. Further, the results indicate that the social-psychological/educational variable of preparation for menstruation is a more important determinant of first menstrual experience than is rate of biological development as such.

Adequacy of Preparation: Descriptive Data Base

Having an indication that more adequate preparation is an important determinant of girls' initial experiences of menstruation, it is appropriate to explore the meaning of the term *preparation*. What does it mean to be prepared for menarche? To answer this question the responses that informants provided as they offered suggestions for preparing girls for menstruation may be examined.

Two areas of knowledge deemed important by informants—information about the physiology of menstruation and information about menstrual hygiene—typically are included in most educational materials. The women in this study also emphasized the need for information about the concrete experience of menstruating; they indicated that abstract information about menstruation as a biological event is insufficient preparation for menstruation as a personal event.

In keeping with this focus on menstruation as a personal event, informants also emphasized the individuality and variability of menstrual experience. Further, women stressed the need to inform girls about the *normality* of menstruation. Their suggestion that menstruation needs to be distinguished from disease, injury, and uncleanliness indicates that such associations are very much a matter of awareness. That they are not often addressed directly may be attributable in part to taboos against discussing menstruation at all; as likely, however, may be well-meant, but ultimately unhelpful, attempts to comfort girls by telling them that they should not feel upset or distressed. The women in this study would reassure girls of the normality of menstruation and, in so doing, would acknowledge as normal the experience of fright and embarrassment at menarche. Women suggested that validation of a girl's negative experiences of menstruation, rather than denial of these experiences, may more successfully facilitate a girl's experience of the positive feelings of pride in herself as more mature and female, which can also be associated with menarche.

In this regard, informants advocated offering a balanced view of menstruation. While they would present it positively as a symbol of womanhood and as a uniquely female experience, they would also acknowledge that it can be alarming, messy, and embarrassing. In this sense, they suggest the need to help girls integrate the positive and negative aspects of menstruation, rather than to attempt to eliminate distress itself.

This end cannot be accomplished through educational materials alone. Many women emphasized a girl's need for support and reassurance at the time of menarche, and many referred specifically to the importance of an informed, understanding, accepting mother. Interviews with mothers of adolescent girls, however, indicate that most mothers are poorly prepared to act as informed, supportive models for their daughters (Bloch 1978).[5]

This fact suggests that efforts to prepare girls for menarche must include attention to the informational and emotional needs of mothers as well as daughters. The benefits of such attention to preparing girls and their mothers for menarche is clear from the demonstrated relationship between adequacy of preparation and more positive menstrual experiences.

Notes

1. Portions of this research are reported in Koff, Rierdan, and Sheingold (1982) and in Rierdan, Koff, Flaherty, and Sheingold.
2. Brooks-Gunn, J., and Ruble, D.N. The social and psychological meaning of menarche. Paper presented at the Society for Research in Child Development, San Francisco, March 1979.
3. Ibid.
4. Rierdan, J., Koff, E., Flaherty, J., and Sheingold, K. Guidelines for preparing girls for menstruation. Manuscript under review.
5. Bloch, D. Level and sources of sex knowledge of 12-year old girls. Paper presented at the American Public Health Association, Maternal and Child Health Section, New York, November 1979.

References

Bloch, D. 1978. Sex education practices of mothers. *Journal of Sex Education and Therapy* 4:7-12.

Clarke, A.E., and Ruble, D.N. 1978. Young adolescents' beliefs concerning menstruation. *Child Development* 49:231-234.

Deutsch, H. 1944. *The psychology of women*, vol. 1. New York: Grune and Stratton.

Ernster, V.L. 1975. American menstrual expressions. *Sex Roles* 1:3-13.

Kestenberg, J.S. 1967. Phases of adolescence, Parts I and II. *Journal of the American Academy of Child Psychiatry* 6:426-462, 577-611.

Koff, E., Rierdan, J., and Jacobson, S. 1981. The personal and interpersonal significance of menarche. *Journal of the American Academy of Child Psychiatry* 20:148-158.

Koff, E., Rierdan, J., and Sheingold, K. 1982. Memories of menarche: Age, preparation, and prior knowledge as determinants of initial menstrual experience. *Journal of Youth and Adolescence* 11:1-9.

Koff, E., Rierdan, J., and Silverstone, E. 1978. Changes in representation of body image as a function of menarcheal status. *Developmental Psychology* 14:635-642.

Rierdan, J., and Koff, E. 1980. The psychological impact of menarche. *Journal of Youth and Adolescence* 9:49-58.

Ritvo, S. 1977. Adolescent to woman. In H. P. Blum, ed., *Female psychology: Contemporary psychoanalytic views*. New York: International Universities Press.

Rosenbaum, M. 1979. The changing body image of the adolescent girl. In M. Sugar, ed., *Female adolescent development*. New York: Brunner/Mazel.

Shainess, N. 1961. A re-evaluation of some aspects of femininity through a study of menstruation: A preliminary report. *Comprehensive Psychiatry* 2:20-26.

Sugar, M. 1979. *Female adolescent development*. New York: Brunner/Mazel.

Whisnant, L., and Zegans, L. 1975. A study of attitudes toward menarche in white middle-class American adolescent girls. *American Journal of Psychiatry* 132:809-814.

10 Menstrual Education: Past, Present, and Future

Vera J. Milow

TAMPAX Incorporated initiated a consumer-education program in menstrual health forty years ago. Its initial aim was to teach consumers how to use tampons, a product introduced by TAMPAX in 1936, and to dispel widespread public ignorance about menstruation.

Early in the program it was evident that many people did not want to talk about this subject, and we learned that often people didn't know what we were talking about when we spoke of menstruation and the menstrual cycle. Expressions such as "the curse," "I'm sick," and "being unwell" were more commonly used to indicate menstruation. Our aim was to give women an awareness of this part of their lives and to teach that menstruation is a healthy, normal function of a woman's body.

Since the time we started our program, we have made major inroads in promoting menstrual health education. To make our education program a success we have had to confront three problems: (1) to identify what attitudes and information levels exist about menstruation among different groups; (2) to determine how to reach those groups, especially the young people, with correct information about menstruation before its onset; and (3) to overcome the onus of being a commercial company involved in the education process.

To better educate the public about the menstrual cycle, TAMPAX has a staff of educational consultants who regularly visit school and community groups throughout the United States and Canada to initiate programs in menstrual health. We conduct workshops and in-service programs with teachers and other professionals, and make presentations to students. We also contact and work with community health organizations, health teaching groups, clinics, physicians and nurses, and other allied groups.

Our basic lecture plan includes discussion of the anatomy and physiology of menstruation, from premenarcheal development through the normal menstrual cycle and its variations, ending with menopause. Also covered are health habits related to menstruation: exercise, posture, hygiene, diet, and menstrual protection. And, in response to the changing needs of students and teachers, existing myths and misconceptions are discussed and new medical information is given.

TAMPAX does not believe that all that needs to be taught can be conveyed in one easy lesson. For this reason, we offer free educational materials, including written brochures and visual aids to teachers and students for reference. Designed as supplementary material, they are not expected to replace classroom discussion. Moreover, we have learned that professional people will accept materials and counsel from a company only if the information is educationally sound—not developed for the purpose of advertising the product. For this reason, our materials are widely used.

TAMPAX Studies

Our experience with menstrual health education confirms the observations of others that much remains to be learned about young women, their understanding and experience of menarche, and their attitudes toward it (Whisnant and Zegans 1975). To identify educational needs, research was done. In the early 1950s and through the 1960s, tabulations were made of questions asked of the TAMPAX educational consultants addressing audiences in elementary and high schools, colleges, and occupational settings. An analysis of these sessions was done in 1953 by Martha Rogers of New York University (Rogers 1953) based on questions that arose in 232 talks across the United States. A second analysis was done by Edith Anderson (Anderson 1965) on the basis of questions asked in 343 lectures in the United States and Canada.

The subjects in these two studies were a random sample of the audiences addressed by our consultants during the 1950s and 1960s. In 1953, 47 percent of the lectures were given to college students and 36 percent were given to junior and senior high-school groups. In 1963, only 14.5 percent of our lectures were to college students, while 72 percent were to high-school students. However, we have always kept in touch with the college group, particularly in the area of teacher education.

Both sets of questions (those from the 1953 and 1963 studies) were categorized into major areas: anatomy and physiology of menstruation, menstrual discomfort, treatment of discomfort, sex, swimming, personal hygiene, folklore, embarrassment, education, and menopause. These studies helped us to determine general information levels and attitudes. Moreover, comparison of the two sets of questions gave us a perspective on the changes that occurred between 1953 and 1963.

Trends

Over the ten-year period our studies spanned, most of the questions (80 percent) asked by students were about menstruation, particularly dysmenorrhea. Questions related to the menses and water were the second most frequently asked, and 85 percent were from the younger age groups. Common misconceptions were illustrated by such questions as: "Does cold water cause cramps?" "Is it bad to bathe and take cold drinks during menstruation?" and "Can I really eat oranges and citrus fruit? I was told not to during menstruation." Questions about whether exercise was advisable during menstruation were asked by teachers as well as school-age girls.

In the 1960s new patterns emerged. Premenstrual tension became an area of major interest. In the first study, ten years earlier, the problem was not clearly identified. Young people also proved to be increasingly curious about sexual activities, and questions related to oral contraceptives, intercourse, fertility, and pregnancy were all common. The subject of menopause was raised by college groups in particular.

Another change occurred in the groups we were addressing. In the early sixties, high-school groups displayed more eagerness to discuss the subject of menstruation than did the college-age groups that had shown a great deal of interest in the early fifties. This change pointed out a growing sophistication among young people about the menstrual cycle. We also like to think it showed that we were getting through at the college and professional level and with those working with younger people.

Over the years, folklore and embarrassment continued to be stumbling blocks. Regional differences were often profound. Some of the old wives' tales we discovered were shocking, yet widespread. We had girls who asked: "Is it true that menstrual blood is bad blood?" and "Can menstruation wilt flowers?" We had young women in their early twenties who said; "I can't go to the school prom if I'm menstruating because the flowers that my date gives me will wilt." They also wanted to know if it were true that a hair permanent wouldn't take when they were menstruating. Or, they were told that if they had a tooth filled during menstruation it wouldn't take and would fall out.

The first time I was asked, "Why did mother slap me across the face when I started to menstruate?" I didn't know what to say. I had never heard that question before. We tried to find an answer, and I was given two, not very scientific, explanations. One answer was physiological in nature: to bring the blood back to her face; the other was sociological: the mother was now slapping her daughter because the daughter was of an age when she could be a threat to her. More recently I have heard the slap related to being a woman, a recognition of the girl as a sexual person.

Questions posed by teachers offered insight into sex and menstrual education. For example, it was a matter of debate as to whether coeducation was appropriate, and at what age; how "far" to go in answering questions by students; and how to answer "all those questions." With my twenty-nine years of experience I still don't know what all those questions are that can't be answered. Any question asked usually can be answered by referring back to scientific information already presented. If not, it is appropriate to say, "I don't know, but I'll try to find out for you," or to direct the inquirer to a professional source.

Our education consultants have continued to address many of the same questions in the fifteen years since our last study. Yet our society has undergone the so-called sexual revolution and the liberation of women. How these movements have influenced Americans' understanding of and attitudes toward menstruation is explored in depth in *The TAMPAX Report* (Research and Forecasts 1981).

The TAMPAX Report

The TAMPAX Report is based on a statistically valid, major study of the nations's attitudes toward menstruation done in 1981. A total of 1,034 men and women fourteen years and older (including an oversample of 154 teenagers aged fourteen to seventeen were interviewed.

The TAMPAX Report reveals that menstruation still may be one of our most controversial and misunderstood subjects. According to the report, most Americans believe that menstrual education should be taught in school, yet their attitudes toward menstruation are often negative, their understanding of it confused. Menstruation remains a taboo subject for many Americans. Two-thirds of our country believe menstruation should not be discussed in the office or socially. One-quarter think it an unacceptable topic even for the family at home.

How do people find out about menstruation if they can't talk about it? Sometimes they don't. Our experience in teaching is that many women did not even *know* about menstruation before they first experienced it and our studies confirm this fact. Indeed, *The TAMPAX Report* finds that about one-third of the women in this country were not prepared for menstruation. Furthermore, the study reveals that two-fifths of U.S. women claim that their first reaction to menstruation was negative. While younger women (under thirty-five) appear to be better educated about menstruation than older women, their attitudes are not very different.

The TAMPAX Report found that, in general, men's and women's beliefs about menstruation are similar. Most people think that menstruation does affect women physically and emotionally but that it does not impair a woman's ability to function normally at work. However, more than one-quarter of the U.S. public think women *cannot* function normally at work when they are menstruating.

There are a number of key questions regarding menstruation on which Americans are divided. Half of the country believe that women should not have sexual intercourse while menstruating; a third believe that menstruation affects a woman's ability to think; one-third believe that women should restrict their physical activities; and 22 percent believe that menstrual pain is strictly in women's heads.

Men and women share many attitudes about menstruation, but there are some pronounced differences. For instance, more women than men say that menstruation is painful (56 percent versus 39 percent). More women (81 percent) believe that they can function as well at work when menstruating (only 66 percent of men agree). And, oddly, more men believe that it is socially acceptable to discuss menstruation than do women (38 percent versus 27 percent).

Two groups have a particularly open view of menstruation: those who favor equal rights for women and professional and white-collar workers. People with a less open point of view are more likely to reside in the South, be less educated, less affluent, blue collar, black, highly moral or religious, and politically conservative.

In view of the persistence of myths about menstruation, it seems reasonable to ask where Americans learn about menstruation? Although most Americans (56 percent) learn a great deal about health-related matters from doctors and health professionals, only 1 percent claim they first learned about menstruation from these same sources. Mother is still the most common source of information about menstruation for young women. *The TAMPAX Report* found that young men learn from a wider variety of people, most often from friends. Outside of the home, schools are the main sources of information. Today, ten times as many teenagers aged (fourteen to seventeen) learn about it in schools as did people over fifty-five (33 percent versus 3 percent). Moreover, Americans overwhelmingly support menstrual education in the school—91 percent are in favor.

Future Directions

Despite what appears to be a greater sophistication among young people today, much of the information students have is superficial, and misconceptions are apparently as widespread as they were a decade ago. Given these findings, our goal should be to begin menstrual education at the elementary-school level. However, this goal is not always easy to achieve.

Though we know that there is a strong need for menstrual education and menstrual health programs have become part of the curriculum in many schools, they are absent from many others. TAMPAX Incorporated believes that it has a responsibility to contribute to efforts in the field of menstrual health education. We must work within the educational system, making contact with school boards and parent-teacher groups, and we will continue to work with teachers and other professionals to instruct students.

A new film by TAMPAX Incorporated, "Accent on You,"for young people (nine to fourteen years old) addresses today's more sophisticated, coeducational audience. It features a twelve-year-old boy and girl who discuss puberty, menstruation, and the male and female reproductive systems in a mature, comprehensive fashion. Spanish and French editions of the film will be available. Also being developed are *It's a Woman's World,* a new booklet for older students (fifteen years through college age), and a teaching guide offering comprehensive, updated information in answer to a wide range of questions regarding the female reproductive system, the menstrual cycle, medical concerns and new treatments, menstrual protection and hygiene, and healthy attitudes about being a woman.[1]

Note

1. Information regarding the TAMPAX educational program and materials offered may be obtained by writing to: TAMPAX Incorporated, Dept. MIV, P.O. Box 7001, Lake Success, New York 11042.

References

Anderson, E. 1965. Who wants to know what about menstrual health? *Nursing Outlook* 13:47-50.

Research and Forecasts. 1981. *The TAMPAX Report.*

Rogers, M.E. 1953. Responses to talks on menstrual health. *Nursing Outlook* 1:272-274.

Whisnant, L., and Zegans, L. 1975. A study of attitudes toward menarche in white middle-class American adolescent girls. *American Journal of Psychiatry* 132:809-814.

11 Menstrual Beliefs and Experiences of Mother-Daughter Dyads

Edna M. Menke

Menarche is an indication of sexual maturation that usually occurs between the ages of eleven and fifteen. At this time in their lives girls are adjusting to changes in their body size, height, and shape, as well as to their first and subsequent menstrual cycles (Sommer 1978). Information about the menstrual cycle is obtained from the girl's mother, friends, school, and culture. And since the menstrual cycle is surrounded by superstitions, taboos, and folklore, as well as facts, to understand the meaning of menstruation for females it is necessary to look at menstrual beliefs within the context of the environment within which they are found (Delaney, Lupton, and Toth 1976; Paige 1973; Snow and Johnson 1977).

Mothers are still the major source of information about menstruation for girls (Research and Forecasts 1981) and there is some evidence that mothers and daughters have similar experiences with the menstrual cycle. Brooks-Gunn and Matthews (1979) found that menstrual distress was related to maternal reports of menstrual distress. It appears that if daughters believed their mothers experienced symptoms of menstrual distress, they too anticipated or reported being negatively affected by menstruation. Dalton (1964) has also reported that even though there are a wide range of premenstrual symptoms, there is a tendency for daughters to have the same ones as their mothers.

Menstrual-cycle beliefs and the experiences of mother-daughter dyads may be similar because of the socialization process. Both mothers and daughters are influenced by such factors as age, age at onset of menarche, knowledge about menstruation, religious and ethnic background, socioeconomic status, and health history. Moreover, because the mother-daughter dyad involves a reciprocal relationship, each influences the others' beliefs and both are affected by their individual experiences.

Brooks-Gunn and Matthews (1979) examined menstrual distress of mothers and daughters, but collected data only from the adolescents. Few studies have been done that use data collected from both mothers and daughters. The purpose of the study described in this chapter was to test the hypotheses that (1) mothers and daughters hold similar beliefs about menstruation and (2) mothers and daughters have similar experiences with the menstrual cycle.

Method

Subjects

The subjects of the study were thirty mother-daughter dyads who resided in central Ohio. The mothers ranged in age from thirty-one to fifty years of age and the daughters ranged in age from twelve to sixteen years of age. All of the subjects were Caucasian and were equally divided in terms of socioeconomic status. The mothers were equally divided between those who worked outside the home and those who worked within the home. None of the mothers nor daughters had any major health problems.

Procedure

The investigator recruited subjects by advertising in a women's campus newspaper and contacting some local women's organizations. The criteria used for sample selection were (1) the daughter had to be between the ages of twelve and sixteen, have had menstrual cycles for at least one year, and not currently be pregnant; (2) the mother must have monthly menstrual periods and be the biological mother of the daughter participating in the study; (3) both mother and daughter must be able to tell the investigator when their last menstrual period started; and (4) both mother and daughter must be willing to participate in the study. The data were collected in the subjects' homes. The mothers and daughters completed the questionnaires in separate rooms and were interviewed individually.

Questionnaires and Interview Schedules

The Menstrual Attitude Questionnaire (MAQ) developed by Brooks, Ruble, and Clark (1977) is a forty-six-item scale that has five dimensions regarding menstruation as: (1) a debilitating event; (2) a positive event; (3) an event whose onset can be predicted and anticipated; (4) a bothersome event; and (5) an event that does not and should not affect one's behavior. The subject responds to each item on a seven-point scale ranging from strongly disagree to strongly agree.

The Moos Menstrual Distress Scale (MDQ) (1977) and eight additional items developed by the investigator that were related to positive correlates of the menstrual cycle comprised the second questionnaire. The MDQ consists of forty-seven items that have been factor analyzed into the following subscales: pain, disturbance of concentration, behavioral decrements, autonomic nervous-system imbalance, water retention, negative affect, arousal, and control. The subject responds to each item on a six-point scale ranging from no experience with the symptom to an acute symptom that occurs during menstruation.

The Interview Schedules were developed by the investigator and included personal and social characteristics, menstrual-cycle history, knowledge concerning menstruation, and menstrual beliefs.

Results

Menstrual Beliefs

The Menstrual Attitude Questionnaire mean scores are show in table 11-1. Possible scores for each dimension are: (1) debilitating 12-84; (2) bothersome 6-42; (3) positive 5-35; (4) predictable 5-35; and (5) denial of effect 7-49. The data suggest that menstruation was seen as slightly debilitating, bothersome, predictable, positive, and having an effect on one's behavior. These results are very similar to the findings of Brooks, Ruble, and Clark (1977) who had Princeton University undergraduate women complete the questionnaire. There were no significant differences between mothers' and daughters' scores. This sample of mothers and daughters held similar beliefs about menstruation.

Responses to the interview schedule revealed that mother-daughter dyads held similar beliefs about what was bad about menstruation and activities one should or should not participate in during menstruation. Some of the things mentioned were cramps, inconvenience, and the curtailment of some physical activities. Approximately 50 percent of the subjects thought there was nothing special that females could or could not do during menstrual periods. The other 50 percent stated that it was necessary to get extra rest, to be extra clean, and exercise. Twenty-five percent of the subjects believed that one should avoid swimming, getting a permanent, sexual

Table 11-1
Means and *t*-tests for Mothers' and Daughters' Scores on the Menstrual-Attitude Questionnaire

Dimension	Total Sample Mean (N = 60)	Mothers' Mean (N = 30)	Daughters' Mean (N = 30)	t-test
Debilitating	46.70	47.86	46.13	.49
Bothersome	18.50	19.13	17.87	.65
Positive	15.30	14.73	15.86	.37
Predictable	15.04	13.44	16.62	1.79
Denial of effects	31.50	32.26	34.93	.44

intercourse, and taking a vacation when menstruating. There was not as much congruence between mothers and daughters regarding what was good about menstruation. Some of the mothers thought that menstruation was good because the process cleansed their bodies and they knew they were not pregnant. None of the daughters gave these responses and many of them could not think of anything good about menstruation.

Menstrual Experiences

The Modified Moos Menstrual Distress Questionnaire scores are shown in table 11-2. Possible scores for each scale are as follows: (1) pain 6-36; (2) water retention 4-24; (3) concentration 8-48; (4) negative affect 8-48; (5) behavior change 5-30; (6) arousal 5-30; (7) autonomic reactions 4-24; (8) control 6-36; and (9) positive affect 8-48. In general, the subjects experienced little difficulty with menstruation, rating most of their responses as barely noticeable or mild. However, the sample experienced the symptoms of pain, water retention, and negative affect during menstruation. They did not experience concentration nor behavioral changes, autonomic reactions, arousal, nor positive affects. On only one subscale, water retention, was there a significant difference between mothers and daughters. The mothers experienced more severe water retention than their daughters.

Discussion

The mothers and daughters in this study held similar beliefs and reported similar experiences with the menstrual cycle. The findings suggest that sex-

Table 11-2
Means and *t*-tests for Mothers' and Daughters' Scores on the Modified Moos Menstrual Distress Questionnaire

Scale Symptom	Total Sample Mean (N = 60)	Mothers' Mean (N = 30)	Daughters' Mean (N = 30)	t-test
Pain	15.00	15.47	14.52	.48
Water retention	11.00	12.82	9.27	2.86[a]
Concentration	9.60	10.51	8.90	1.74
Negative affect	17.80	17.20	18.62	.62
Behavior change	8.37	8.81	7.91	.98
Arousal	7.62	7.82	7.45	.41
Autonomic reactions	5.90	6.32	5.72	.78
Control	7.62	8.01	7.20	.90
Positive affect	10.60	9.80	11.51	1.38

[a]$p < 0.01$

role identity and related behaviors are learned through interaction and observation in the mother-daughter relationship. Thus mothers should be well informed about menstruation, comfortable with the subject, and encourage discussions with their daughters. Accurate information about the menstrual cycle should be provided prior to menarche.

Whether other variables than socialization influence similarities between mother-daughter dyads was not a question addressed here. Further research should consider dietary patterns, life styles, cultural background, and genetic heritage.

References

Brooks, J., Ruble, D., and Clark, A. 1977. College women's attitudes and expectations concerning menstrual-related changes. *Psychosomatic Medicine* 39:288-298.

Brooks-Gunn, J., and Matthews, S.W. 1979. *He and she: How children develop their sex-role identity.* Englewood Cliffs, N.J.: Prentice Hall.

Dalton, K. 1964. *The premenstrual syndrome.* Springfield, Ill.: Charles C. Thomas.

Delaney, J., Lupton, M.J., and Toth, E. 1976. *The curse: A cultural history of menstruation.* New York: E.P. Dutton.

Moos, R.H. 1977. *Menstrual distress questionnaire manual.* Palo Alto, Calif.: Stanford University.

Paige, K.E. 1973. Women learn to sing the menstrual blues. *Psychology Today* 4:41-46.

Snow, L.F., and Johnson, S.M. 1977. Modern day menstrual folklore. *Journal of the American Medical Association* 237:2736-2739.

Sommer, B.B. 1978. *Puberty and adolescence.* New York: Oxford University Press.

Research and Forecasts. 1981. *The TAMPAX Report.*

12 Beliefs and Attitudes of Young Girls regarding Menstruation

Lenore R. Williams

Menstruation is a normal physiologic process that heralds the beginning of the female reproductive cycle. Since it is an exclusively female occurrence, menstruation represents the biological female and is closely associated with female sexuality, womanhood, and female social roles (Frieze et al. 1978; Olesen 1975; Weideger 1977).

A complex set of sociocultural norms influence a woman's psychological response to her body and its function (Freize et al. 1978). Attitudes, beliefs, and practices of women toward menstruation are a reflection of these sociocultural norms. In addition, an individual's body of knowledge and personal experience with regard to menstruation contribute to the perception of the phenomenon of menstruation and thus contribute to one's concept of being female. If the norms regarding menstruation in a particular culture are comprised of myths and taboos and attribute a general negative attitude toward menstruation, the female will acquire these norms and consequently have a devalued sense of self and of being female (Bardwick 1971; Breit and Ferrandino 1977; Clark and Ruble 1978).

In the United States today, there is evidence of a negative ideology associated with menstruation (Breit and Ferrandino 1977; Delaney, Lupton, and Toth 1976; Paige 1973; Weideger 1977) which young girls are incorporating into their concept of menstruation (Clark and Ruble 1978; Ernster 1977; Whisnant and Zegans 1975). Menstruation is defined as an hygienic crisis and the affective importance of menarche is ignored (Paige 1973; Whisnant, Brett, and Zegans 1975). Although other cultures officially acknowledge its unique importance by ceremonies, menarche in U.S. culture is given little formal recognition (Brown 1969; Seiden 1976).

The negative ideology surrounding menstruation can also be seen in the type of research conducted concerning this process. Although there is a large body of literature that deals with menstruation, it has concentrated on physical and emotional symptomatology in relation to cyclic hormonal changes. Research has been limited regarding preadolescent and early adolescent girls' response to the experience of menstruation. Therefore, there is not a large enough data base from which to plan, implement, and evaluate health care for girls in this age group.

139

During pre- and early adolescence, girls are beginning to incorporate a new body image to which has been added internal reproductive organs. Despite the availability of information and emphasis on the intellectualization of the menstrual cycle, there is evidence that young girls have difficulty in the conceptualization and integration of the process of menstruation (Ernster 1977; Whisnant and Zegans 1975).

Studies of U.S. girls have revealed certain ideas and beliefs about menstruation as a physiologic process. For example, menstrual blood is seen as an excess substance or is equated with excrement, and there is thought to be an increased vulnerability to sickness or injury. Mood changes and increased emotionality are also associated with menstruation (Clark and Ruble 1978; Ernster 1977; Whisnant and Zegans 1975).

Three areas of practice with regard to menstruation have been identified in the literature. These include the taboos of communication, activity, and concealment. The most prevalent taboo is that of communication. The communication domain is almost exclusively female (Whisnant and Zegans 1975; Ernster 1977). The activity taboo takes the form of decreased or altered activity. It has been reported that girls felt normal activities should be curtailed (Ernster 1977) or that there would be a disruption of activities (Clark and Ruble 1978). Menstruation as something to hide or be ashamed of is frequently stated in the literature (Clark and Ruble 1978; Ernster 1977; Whisnant and Zegans 1975).

With the onset of menstruation, attention is focused on attitudes relating to feminine sexuality that have accumulated to that point (Shainess 1961). The literature has pointed to several types of attitudes young girls have about menstruation. These include negative notions such as menstruation is a nuisance or is to be feared; positive notions such as a reaffirmation of womanhood; as something to prepare for or anticipate (hygienic crisis); or neutral attitudes such as menstruation has no real effect (Clark and Ruble 1978; Ernster 1977; Whisnant and Zegans 1975).

Differences between pre- and postmenarcheal girls in their knowledge, beliefs, practices, and attitudes regarding menstruation have not been well documented. The research that has been reported is inconclusive and in some conflict. Ernster (1977) concluded that menstrual attitudes may be less negative among postmenarcheal than premenarcheal girls because of the experience with menstruation. Clark and Ruble (1978) found that postmenarcheal girls showed greater dislike for menstruation than premenarcheal. Whisnant and Zegans (1975) reported that premenarcheal girls felt they would be open about menstruation and not ashamed to have family and friends know; whereas , postmenarcheal girls showed more secretive behavior once they began to menstruate. Koff, Rierdan, and Silverstone (1978) in a study of body image of pre- and postmenarcheal girls, reported that postmenarcheal girls drew more sexually differentiated human-figure drawings than did their premenarcheal peers.

The purpose of the study discussed in this chapter was to identify the beliefs, practices, and attitudes of preadolescent girls regarding menstruation. In addition, the study explored knowledge of the anatomy and physiology of menstruation, the sources of information these girls had, and the euphemisms they used for menstruation.

The research questions that guided this research were:

1. What do preadolescent and early-adolescent girls know about the anatomy and physiology of the female reproductive tract particularly in regard to menstruation?
2. What are the beliefs of preadolescent and early-adolescent girls regarding menstruation?
3. What are the practices of preadolescent and early-adolescent girls regarding menstruation?
4. What are the attitudes of preadolescent and early-adolescent girls regarding menstruation?
5. Are there any differences between premenarcheal and postmenarcheal girls in their knowledge, beliefs, practices, and attitudes about menstruation?

Method

Subjects

The sample studied here consisted of seventy-four girls who volunteered and obtained parental permission to participate. They were enrolled in the fourth, fifth, and sixth grades at two suburban elementary schools in the Midwest. Of the girls who participated, sixty-five were premenarcheal and nine were postmenarcheal. The postmenarcheal group comprised 12 percent of the sample and had been menstruating for one to eight months. Subjects ranged in age from nine to twelve years, were predominantly white, born of American parents, and represented all major religions and socioeconomic classes.

Instrument

Data were collected by use of a questionnnaire developed by the investigator. Questionnaire items were based on theory and research findings reported in the literature as well as empirical observations made by the investigator about adolescent behavior and concerns about the menstrual phenomenon.

The questionnaire consisted of four sections. Items in Section I elicited demographic data to describe the sample. Section II measured knowledge of female reproductive anatomy. A figure drawing was used that required the participant to correctly draw and label the uterus, fallopian tubes, vagina, ovaries, and vaginal opening. Section III consisted of five true-false statements about menstrual physiology. Section IV consisted of forty-one statements about beliefs, practices, and attitudes with which the participants could either agree or disagree. Belief items included ideas about menstruation such as, *menstrual blood has a bad odor* and *girls are grouchy just before menstruation.* There were also questions about limiting activities, communication taboos and concealment. Included in the activity taboo were items pertaining to what activities should be prohibited during menses for example, *a menstruating girl should not be active in sports.* The communication taboo included items to determine if it was acceptable to talk with males or in public about menstruation. (*It is all right to discuss menstruation with fathers.*) Items to determine the presence of a concealment taboo included those related to keeping menstruation as unnoticeable as possible, for example, *during menstruation it is best to wear clothes like skirts or dresses.*

Responses to attitude statements were placed in the predetermined categories of positive, negative, neutral, and hygienic crisis. A positive-attitude statement was one that indicated menstruation as a normal function or associated with a positive-feeling state. Negative-attitude items included those items that related menstruation to a negative-feeling state such as disgust or embarrassment. A neutral attitude was ascribed to the respondent if she felt that a girl should act natural during menstruation.

The questionnaire was distributed to the students in a group setting. Each item was read aloud by the investigator and the girls were given time to respond. After the questionnaires were turned in, the investigator held a voluntary group discussion with those who had questions about certain items in the questionnaire or about menstruation in general.

Results

Analysis of Data

Responses to the items were reduced and placed in predetermined categories for the total sample and for the pre- and postmenarcheal groups. For the knowledge variable, responses were scored one for each right answer and zero for each wrong answer. Items in the anatomy category were scored correct if the body part was properly labeled and placed in the outlined figure. The means and standard deviations were calculated for the total sample and for the pre- and postmenarcheal groups. For the variables of belief, practice, and attitude, responses were reported via frequency distributions and modal responses for each predetermined category.

Knowledge of Anatomy and Physiology

On the figure drawing, the range of scores was 0 to 5 correct responses. The mean was 2.68 with a standard deviation of 1.70. There were more correct responses for the vagina and vaginal opening than for internal organs.

The greatest number of correct responses to the five true-false items about menstrual physiology was for the item testing knowledge about the pathway of the menstrual flow. The range of scores was 2 to 5 correct responses. The mean was 3.82 with a standard deviation of .95.

Beliefs about Menstruation

As shown in table 12-1, 89 percent of the respondents believed that increased emotionality was associated with menstruation. Sixty-eight percent believed that menstrual blood has a bad odor. Eighty-six percent did not see the menstruating girl as being avoided by others. And most agreed that their mothers treated them differently after menses began.

Taboos regarding Menstruation

As shown in table 12-2, there were taboos associated with menstruation. Swimming was reported as contraindicated during menstruation by almost half of the respondents. However, hair washing and bathing were generally not restricted. Regarding the communication taboo, most respondents believed that menstruation falls within the female domain and is not a subject for discussion with boys, fathers, or in public. Further, concerning the concealment taboo, the majority of respondents believed that menstruation should be kept as unnoticeable as possible.

Attitudes toward Menstruation

Generally, attitudes toward menstruation were found to be positive. The majority of respondents did not indicate fear, shame, or disgust associated with menstruation. The most frequent response was that of menstruation being exciting since it is related to growing up. (See table 12-3.) The majority also felt it was best to act natural (neutral attitude) and that planning for sanitary protection was an important part of menstruation (hygienic crisis).

Differences between Pre- and Postmenarcheal Girls

Due to the small number of postmenarcheal girls in the study, statistical analysis of the data was not possible ($n = 9$). The differences reported

Table 12-1
Responses to Menstrual-Belief Statements

Category	Agree Number (Percent)	Disagree Number (Percent)
Affective changes		
Girls are more likely to get upset and nervous when they menstruate than when they don't menstruate	66 (89)	8 (11)
As a result of the menstrual cycle, a girl feels especially happy two weeks after menstruation[a]	45 (62)	28 (38)
Girls are grouchy just before menstruation	23 (31)	51 (69)
Characteristics of menstrual blood		
Menstrual blood is old blood that the body doesn't need anymore	40 (54)	34 (46)
If a girl doesn't menstruate every month, she will get sick	25 (34)	49 (66)
Menstrual blood has mysterious powers[b]	21 (15)	79 (58)
Characteristics of a menstruating girl		
There is something dirty or unclean about a menstruating girl[c]	10 (14)	63 (86)
Menstruating girls should be avoided by others	7 (9)	67 (91)
Differential treatment after menses began		
A mother treats her daughter more like an adult once she begins to menstruate[d]	57 (79)	15 (21)
A father treats his daughter more like an adult once she begins to menstruate[e]	36 (49)	37 (51)
Other		
Only older girls and women can use tampons[f]	23 (32)	50 (68)

Note: $n = 74$
[a]$n = 73$
[b]$n = 73$
[c]$n = 73$
[d]$n = 72$
[e]$n = 73$
[f]$n = 73$

must therefore be considered speculative in nature. Knowledge of menstrual anatomy and physiology and menstrual beliefs and practices of the postmenarcheal girls were very similar to those of the premenarcheal girls. The most striking difference between the pre- and postmenarcheal girls in this study was the finding that postmenarcheal girls held a more negative set of attitudes. Postmenarcheal girls indicated more fear, shame, disgust, and less pride and excitement about menstruation.

Table 12-2
Responses to Taboos Associated with Menstruation

Category	Agree Number (Percent)	Disagree Number (Percent)
Activity		
When a girl is menstruating, she should not go swimming	36 (49)	38 (51)
A menstruating girl should not be active in sports	16 (22)	58 (78)
A menstruating girl should not take a bath	13 (18)	61 (82)
A menstruating girl should not wash her hair	4 (5)	70 (95)
Communication		
A girl should not talk about menstruation to boys	63 (85)	11 (15)
One does not talk about menstruation in public	49 (66)	25 (34)
It is alright to discuss menstruation with fathers	44 (59)	30 (41)
Concealment		
Sanitary pads should be disposed of so that blood doesn't show	67 (91)	7 (9)
Deodorant sanitary protection should be worn to hide the odor of menstruation	60 (81)	14 (19)
During menstruation, it is best to wear clothes like skirts or dresses	21 (28)	53 (72)

Note: $n = 74$

Discussion

The results of this study corroborate some findings of other studies concerning the knowledge, beliefs, practices, and attitudes of pre- and early-adolescent girls regarding menstruation. The respondents displayed less knowledge about internal reproductive anatomy than external anatomy, perhaps because the vagina and vaginal opening are external and therefore accessible to the girls. These findings are similar to those of Whisnant and Zegans (1975) but do not corroborate Ernster's (1977) study in which there was confusion about the number and location of body orifices.

The knowledge of the respondents in this study about menstrual physiology was similar on some items and dissimilar on others reported in previous studies. The respondents in two studies (Whisnant and Zegans 1975; Ernster 1977) showed confusion about the amount of blood loss, frequency of flow, and where the flow builds up. The majority of respondents in this study were familiar with the frequency of flow, the pathway of flow,

Table 12-3
Responses to Attitude Statements about Menstruation

Category	Agree Number (Percent)	Disagree Number (Percent)
Positive		
Menstruation is exciting because it means a girl is growing up	64 (86)	10 (14)
Menstruation is a sign that a girl is normal	56 (76)	18 (24)
An important part of being a girl is menstruating[a]	53 (75)	18 (25)
Menstruation is an event to be proud of[b]	43 (59)	30 (41)
Menstruation brings girls closer together	38 (51)	36 (49)
Negative		
Menstruation is embarrassing	27 (36)	47 (64)
Menstruation is a terrible nuisance	21 (28)	53 (72)
Menstruation is disgusting	20 (27)	54 (73)
Menstruation is to be disliked because it is not controllable	17 (23)	57 (77)
Menstruation is something to be afraid of	8 (11)	66 (89)
Menstruation is something to be ashamed of	7 (10)	67 (90)

Note: $n = 74$
       [a]$n = 71$
       [b]$n = 73$

and the uterus as location of the flow build up. However, the findings indicate there was confusion as to the amount of blood loss during menstruation.

The respondents displayed more knowledge about the physiology of menstruation than about female reproductive anatomy. This finding could indicate a lack of specific knowledge about female reproductive anatomy. However, it could also indicate that the girls may be having difficulty incorporating a new body image that now includes internal reproductive organs.

Beliefs about menstruation showed wide variation among respondents. The idea that menstrual blood has a bad odor is evidence of a sociocultural norm that is perpetuated by the feminine-products companies and the reinforced perceived social need to hide any natural body odor. The fact that something has a bad odor makes it undesirable or annoying, which could contribute to a negative ideology about menstruation.

There were several affective changes believed by the respondents to be associated with menstruation. The majority of respondents believed that girls are more nervous and upset during menstruation than at other times in their lives. If a person believes that there is increased emotionality during menses, and there is an associated decreased capacity to function, then the belief could act as a self-fulfilling expectation about menstruation. This finding of increased emotionality agrees with evidence found by Koeske and Koeske (1975) in adults who attributed negative emotions to the menstrual cycle but not positive ones.

Respondents of this study concurred with the findings reported by Whisnant and Zegans (1975) in which mothers were believed to treat daughters differently after menstruation begins. This finding is important in that the girl expects to be treated more like an adult but is given little guidance during childhood as to how to cope with being ushered into approaching adulthood by a single event, menarche.

It is noteworthy that only a small number of postmenarcheal girls participated in the study. This fact could be supportive of the findings in the literature that suggest that postmenarcheal girls become more secretive about menstruation than their premenarcheal peers (Ernster 1977; Whisnant and Zegans 1975). It is possible therefore that if the adolescent denies aspects of menstruation, then she could easily deny the physiology relating to pregnancy and birth control. The current rise in adolescent pregnancies could be in part attributed to this secretive aspect.

There are several major implications of this study. Primarily, there is a need to assess menstrual education and its effectiveness. It seems that the focus of education should be on coping with menarche as a maturational crisis instead of a hygienic crisis. Concrete presentations using anatomical models would aid in the conceptualization of the relationship between internal and external anatomy. Since mothers were named as the major source of menstrual information, a program of formal guidance for parents should also be included.

Considering the respondents adherence to the taboos of concealment and communication, it does not seem logical to include both sexes initially in sex-education programs. It would be more appropriate to have separate male and female programs first and then have a coeducational session.

References

Bardwick, J. 1971. *Psychology of women: A study of biocultural conflicts.* New York: Harper and Row.

Breit, E., and Ferrandino, M. 1977. Demythification of the menstrual taboo. *Nursing Care* 10:30-31.

Brown, J. 1969. Adolescent initiation rites among preliterate peoples. In R. Grinder, ed., *Studies in adolescence.* New York: MacMillan.

Clark, A., and Ruble, D. 1978. Young adolescents beliefs concerning menstruation. *Child Development* 49:231-234.

Delaney, J., Lupton, M., and Toth, E. 1976. *The curse.* New York: E. P. Dutton.

Ernster, V. 1977. Expectations about menstruation among premenarcheal girls. *Medical Anthropology Newsletter* 8:16-24.

Frieze, I.H., Parsons, J.E., Johnson, P.B., Ruble, D.N., and Zellman, G.L., eds. 1978. *Women and sex roles*. New York: W.W. Norton.

Hurlock, E. 1973. *Adolescent development*. New York: McGraw-Hill.

Koeske, R., and Koeske, G. 1975. An attributional approach to moods and the menstrual cycle. *Journal of Personality and Social Psychology* 31:473-478.

Koff, E., Rierdan, J., and Silverstone, E. 1978. Changes in representation of body image as a function of menarcheal status. *Developmental Psychology* 14:635-642.

Olesen, V., ed. 1975. *Women and their health: Research implications for a new era*. Washington: U.S. Department HEW, (Publication No. HRA-77-3138).

Paige, K. 1973. Women learn to sing the menstrual blues. *Psychology Today* 11:41-46.

Shainess, N. 1961. A re-evaluation of some aspects of femininity through a study of menstruation: A preliminary report. *Comprehensive Psychiatry* 2:20-26.

Seiden, A. 1976. Overview: Research on psychology of women: Gender differences and sexual and reproductive life. *American Journal of Psychiatry* 133:995-1007.

Weideger, P. 1977. *Menstruation and menopause*. New York: Dell.

Whisnant, L., and Zegans, L. 1975. A study of attitudes toward menarche in white middle-class American adolescent girls. *American Journal of Psychiatry* 132:809-814.

Whisnant, L., Brett, E., and Zegans, L. 1975. Implicit messages concerning menstruation in commercial educational materials prepared for young adolescent girls. *American Journal of Psychiatry* 132:815-820.

**Part IV
Menarche and Adolescent
Sexuality**

Introduction to Part IV

In addition to its effects on the individual and her family, menarche, because of its link to reproduction, is important to the community-at-large. The age at which a girl becomes sexually mature affects social and sexual behavior, population growth, and economic conditions. In the first chapter in this part, Karen Paige notes the social significance of puberty across different cultures and focuses specifically on the relationship between menarche and the ability to reproduce. She draws an analogy between the different tribal rituals celebrating menarche and the customs guarding daughters' reproductive potential such as purdah, veiling, female-genital mutilation, and virginity tests. These customs, although considered archaic and barbaric, still exist in many parts of the world (Morgan and Steinem 1980). Paige proposes that social-exchange theory can be used to predict the use of chastity-control mechanisms and she would expect to find attention to chastity control in societies where marriage bargains are important and chastity is crucial to the daughter's marriagability. The theory is supported by Paige's presentation of the results of her cross-cultural research, which focused on the relationship between various chastity-control models and the economic resources, fraternal structure, and status distinctions of a particular culture.

John Gagnon addresses the issue of menarche and sexual behavior in the United States. He looks at the relationship between age at first menstruation and the incidence of masturbation, dating, petting, and premarital coitus. Gagnon's research indicates that puberty does not automatically trigger an early sex life. There was no significant relationship between time of menarche and masturbatory experience. However, menarche is an indicator of sexual maturation and as such probably influences the timing of socio-sexual behavior. Gagnon did find that those with younger ages at menarche were more likely to date and pet at an earlier age. And there was some evidence of those with earlier menses beginning premarital coitus earlier as well. These findings are consistent with those of other researchers (Presser 1978; Udry 1979) and have implications for the physical and mental well being of the early maturing girl.

Age at menarche is also of interest to historians who study the family or social structure because it introduces the possibility of procreation; and historians have directed their attention to a wide range of interesting questions (Amundsen and Diers 1973; Bullough and Campbell 1980; Herlihy 1978). For example in an article entitled, "The Age of Slaves at Menarche and Their First Birth," Trussell and Steckel (1978) ask whether slave owners tried to increase their stock of slaves by manipulating the reproductive behavior of their female slaves. Using data about age of menarche among samples of populations around the world and, in addition, shipping manifests that specified slaves' names, sex, age, and height, the authors concluded that menarche occurred by age fifteen. Since the observed mean age at first birth was 20.6, the authors also concluded that slave women did not bear children at the earliest possible age.

Vern Bullough was also interested in age at menarche and questioned the generally held belief that the age of menarche for U.S. girls had dropped from seventeen in the 1900s to about twelve and one-half today. In reevaluating the available historical data, Bullough found that this general assumption came from a 1962 report by Tanner and he suggests that Tanner's data has been misinterpreted. Further, in reviewing a variety of historical sources, Bullough found that many historical documents set the time of menarche between age twelve and fourteen. He discusses the implications of this misunderstanding of historical data, particularly with regard to teen pregnancy.

Teenage pregnancy in the United States is a social and public-health problem of enormous magnitude. The proportion of births to teenage mothers has risen steadily since 1960 (Baumrind 1981) and the number of teenage births in the United States is among the highest in the developed countries (Guttmacher Institute 1981). Teen births are costly to mother, child, and society. The teenage mother often must delay her education and without adequate education or career preparation her opportunities for employment are severely limited. Moreover, both mother and child are at greater risk for such serious health problems as toxemia and low birth weight.

Phyllis Leppert has been involved in the development of the Columbia Presbyterian Medical Center's Young Parents Program for pregnant adolescents. Contrary to common medical beliefs, her research indicates that a substantial number of young women can and do become pregnant within three to nine months after menarche. Leppert suggests that these findings dramatize the need for more effective early sex education and contraceptive advice. Further, she describes factors such as peer referrals, which foster adolescents' use of the contraceptive clinic.

References

Amundsen, D.W., and Diers, C.J. 1973. The age of menarche in Medieval Europe. *Human Biology* 45:363-369.

Baumrind, D. 1981. Clarification concerning birthrate among teenagers. *American Psychologist* 36:528-529.

Bullough, V., and Campbell, C. 1980. Female longevity and diet in the Middle Ages. *Speculum* 55:317-325.

Guttmacher Institute. 1981. *Teenage pregnancy: The problem that hasn't gone away*. New York: The Alan Guttmacher Institute.

Herlihy, D. 1978. The natural history of medieval women. *Natural History* 87:56-67.

Morgan, R., and Steinem, G. 1980. The international crime of genital mutilation. *Ms* 8:65-69.

Presser, H.B. 1978. Age at menarche, socio-sexual behavior, and fertility. *Social Biology* 25:94-101.

Trussell, J., and Steckel, R. 1978. The age of slaves at menarche and their first birth. *Journal of Interdisciplinary History* 8:477-505.

Udry, J.R. 1979. Age at menarche, at first intercourse, and at first pregnancy. *Journal of Biosocial Science* 11:433-441.

13 Virginity Rituals and Chastity Control during Puberty: Cross-Cultural Patterns

Karen Ericksen Paige

The advent of female puberty is of immense social significance in all world societies and there are numerous cultural practices that mark this critical stage of social and biological development. The elaborate puberty rites held in many tribal societies throughout the world are widely recognized as expressions of intense interest in a woman's biological maturity, particularly because they coincide with the onset of first menstruation and are interpreted by ethnographers and their informants as celebrations of this event. One of the best described female puberty rites is Morris Opler's (1941) account of the Chirachua Apache ceremonial, which outlines in detail the considerable amount of time and energy a father spends preparing and executing a large community-wide feast and dance to signify his daugher's menarche. Large numbers of friends and relatives are encouraged to prepare months in advance by making costumes and masks for special dancers and growing food for the feasting. Once menstruation occurs the entire community takes part in weeks of eating, singing, and dancing. A nubile Apache daughter is watched carefully once the ritual takes place so that any marriage arrangements her father has negotiated will not be upset by premarital pregnancy, seduction, or a reputation for promiscuity. Among the Bemba of subsaharan Africa the onset of menstruation is marked by an equally elaborate ritual, the sequence of which was reenacted for Audrey Richards (1956). One important difference between the Apache and Bemba is that Apache daughters' contact with eligible males is strictly controlled after menarche; Bemba daughters, on the other hand, have frequently set up housekeeping with their future spouse prior to their puberty rite although sexual contact may be prohibited until after the rite has been completed. Among the Nayar of south India the premenarcheal *tali-tying* rite is just as elaborate as the Apache and Bemba puberty rites and even includes the ritual defloration of the initiate and a symbolic marriage of the young daughter to a male or representation of a male from the appropriate caste (Gough 1955). The Nayar ritual differs from both the Apache and Bemba rituals by marking the time after which a daughter is free to take on sexual

This research is part of a larger study on world patterns of family honor and female shame funded by the National Institute of Mental Health (#31516). The data were collected with the assistance of Linda Fuller, Mary Haggard, Susan Hahn, and Elisabeth Magnus.

155

partners and bear offspring; a Nayar woman never marries an actual husband and therefore her children are counted as members of her own lineage. Despite the widely different implications puberty rites have for a daughter's subsequent sexual behavior and marriage role, these and other tribal menarcheal ceremonies share one important common characteristic. As Paige and Paige (1981) have demonstrated, public ceremonials coinciding with a daughter's sexual maturity are ritual mechanisms by which father attempts to establish his legitimate claim to allocate rights to his daughter's reproductive capacity, whether those rights are customarily transferred to another male, retained by members of the same lineage, or withheld completely. Puberty ceremonials are occasions on which a father may guage the degree of community support he has for his claims and monitor the behavior of potential disputants. Although disputes over rights to a daughter's fertility and future offspring are chronic thoughout her reproductive span, they are most likely to begin at the time that reproductive span begins. A father's success in mobilizing community opinion in favor of his claims is demonstrated by the success of the puberty rite, just as one's career chances in a large U.S. firm can be tested by guaging the satisfaction of colleagues who attend an aspirant's initial cocktail party.

The social implications of the advent of female puberty are no less profound among societies that do not hold elaborate menarcheal ceremonies. Within the anthropological literature numerous practices are described that can be interpreted as the social-psychological equivalents of puberty rites, since they all serve the purpose of protecting legitimate claims to a nubile daughter's reproductive potential. Such customs as *purdah,* crimes of honor, veiling, female-genital mutilations, and virginity tests have become the focus of increased interest outside of anthropology in recent years, although they are frequently dismissed as archaic, exotic, and barbaric customs of backward societies. One or more of these customs continues to be practiced in some form in many world regions, such as Africa, South America, the Middle East, Mediterranean Europe, South Asia, and parts of Indonesia. Among those societies in which *purdah* is common, women begin to be secluded, chaperoned, and veiled at or near the onset of menarche. Similarly, where genital mutilations (that is, clitoral excision and infibulation) are practiced they are usually performed in late childhood and puberty and almost invariably prior to marriage. Crimes of honor still go unpunished in many of these societies and involve the murder or maiming of daughters and sisters who are suspected of nonconformity with these strict standards of sexual and social behavior. At the time of marriage public virginity tests may be conducted in these societies to provide physical proof that no illegitimate claims to a woman's fertility can be made after those rights have been transferred to her husband. All are mechanisms of chastity control.

All these practices directly anticipate the serious implication of the sexual maturity of daughters, specifically the biological potential for bearing offspring in the absence of publically recognized claims to those offspring in an explicit marriage contract. In this Chapter the major theoretical explanations for these chastity-control mechanisms will be reviewed, followed by a social-exchange theory that attempts to provide a more powerful model about their causes. This model is then tested empirically on a sample of world societies and compared to the explanatory power of the other theories.

There are three important theoretical perspectives that recognize the similarity between the various mechanisms of chastity control. All explain these practices in terms of underlying political and economic dynamics of societies. Jane Schneider (1971) has developed a theory that links concern over chastity with family honor and argues that both function to sustain the internal cohesion of families. Codes of honor and concern with protecting the chastity of daughters and sisters, she argues, represent an alternative to overt violence and are in fact critical indicators of the immense potential for intrafamilial and intracommunity violence. It is the motivation to create and maintain family solidarity under inherently unstable conditions that leads to an obsession with female virginity. For Schneider, instability is most likely when severe limits are placed on the availability of land. This *economic fragmentation* affects a family's autonomy over the allocation of land, which creates serious internal family problems; in particular it creates the potential for conflicts concerning the inheritance of the patrimonial estate among offspring. According to Schneider, "women are a convenient focus . . . around which to organize solidary groups, in spite of the powerful tendencies toward fragmentation" (pp. 21-22). Maintaining the chastity of nubile daughters signifies to others that their families are indeed honorable and solidary. Virginity tests at marriage are a particularly crucial test: if a daughter proves to be a virgin, her family retains its honor, but if she fails her family is shamed and its fragmentation becomes a real possibility. This theory suggests that controls over a daughter's chastity should be most elaborate under conditions of heightened economic fragmentation, such as among agriculturalists and pastoralists as Schneider herself claims, in which family solidarity is always unstable because of the potential for conflict among offspring over the inheritance, as among societies in which land and animals are passed down the family line rather than across kin groups.

Jack Goody's (1976) theory makes a more direct connection between the value of family-owned property, form of inheritance, and chastity control. In particular he argues that a daughter's chastity has real political consequences directly connected with the practice of allowing daughters to inherit property. When daughters as well as sons inherit property, attempts are made to exert maximum control over the marriage partner, since there is always the possibility that the husband's family may usurp that property, thereby fragmenting the patrimonial estate. Control over the choice of marriage partner is greatest when a family can convince others that there are no potential competing claims to their daughter by protecting her sexual reputation. Goody's connection between chastity control and *diverging devolution* (that is, the tendency of families to focus their economic and political interests more on their offspring than on related kinsmen) receives some empirical support. On a large cross-cultural sample he demonstrates moderately strong statistical associations between indicators of high chastity control, such as strong sanctions against premarital sex, and measures of diverging devolution. The crucial link between these two factors is the practice of allowing daughters to inherit real property.

A somewhat different approach to explaining chastity control is taken by Sherry Ortner (1978) who focuses on the relationship between the obsession with female chastity and the development of discreet social classes within state societies. For Ortner it is in the within class-based societies that there is the possibility of hypergamous marriage; it is the possibility of marrying above one's family status that provides a motivation for exerting strong pressures to retain a chaste reputation. Although hypergamy is rare in practice, the very existence of a social ideology of the possibility of hypergamy coupled with the practice of providing a daughter with a dowry to increase her marriage value, reinforces the importance of virginity as a symbol of elite femininity: females withheld, untouched, and exclusive. Harriet Whitehead (1976) broadens Ortner's conception by arguing that the obsession with chastity must be considered within the larger context of status competition among all "rank-conscious" societies. The obsession with loss of chastity, she argues, is inseparable from status loss in such societies. This argument suggests that chastity-control practices should not only appear in class-based state societies as Ortner believes, but in all societies in which wealth and social status are unequally distributed among families.

A Social-Exchange Theory of Virginity Rituals and Chastity Control

The theory tested here proposes that the obsession with chastity and its ritual expressions are a form of bargaining and exchange between families in a society. In particular, cultural practices that demonstrate familial concern with protecting their daughter's social and sexual reputation prior to marriage are implicit political tactics when more direct strategies are either dangerous, impractical, or impossible. Paige and Paige (1981) have argued that reproductive rituals generally are mechanisms for assessing and influencing community consensus about claims to a woman's reproductive capacity as well as implicit devices for monitoring high-stakes bargains over women. In the case of virginity rituals, such as genital mutilations during nubility and public virginity tests at the marriage ceremony, parties to explicit contracts over rights to a woman's sexual and reproductive capacity are provided with explicit demonstration of her family's willingness to comply with the terms of the marriage agreement and offer confirmation to the community as a whole that the bargain will not be upset by the claims of some third party not included in the agreement. Genital mutilations also represent an extreme form of virginity surveillance to ensure a daughter's marriagability. Like virginity tests at marriage, such as the public inspection of the nuptial bed sheets, they represent a means by which the loyalty of the daughter as well as the solidarity of her male kin may be reaffirmed. Ritual reaffirmation of a daughter's chastity by kinsmen, potential affines, and other community members is important throughout nubility since the loyalty of all family members, both male and female, may be threatened by new affinal linkages and by the collective need to make good on a negotiated marriage bargain.

Genital mutilations and virginity tests at marriage both reflect cultural codes of chastity. In the extreme these codes are expressed behaviorally by severe punishment for premarital sexual transgressions, strict supervision of a daughter's social interaction in the form of physical seclusion in the household, chaperonage and veiling in public, and prohibitions against social contact with nonrelated men. These cultural practices and their associated genital-mutilation and virginity-test rituals should be more common among societies in which the economic resource base is valuable enough to reinforce the political solidarity of male kinsmen organized in *strong fraternal interest groups.* Strong fraternal interest groups are coalitions of male kinsmen who are strong enough to take political and military action to assert and defend their claim and to monitor terms of marriage contracts with other fraternal interest groups. The economic systems that provide resources of great enough value to reinforce political solidarity are those based on plow, hoe, irrigation agriculture, and pastoralism (that is, tending herds of camels, cows, sheep, goats, and other large animals). The causal linkages in this theoretical model of chastity control and virginity rituals can be summarized as follows:

Valuable ⟶ Strong Fraternal ⟶ Chastity ⟶ Virginity
Resources   Interest Groups   Control   Rituals

This theory asserts that cultural codes of chastity and their ritual expressions reflect a concern with a daughter's public reputation for chastity to a greater extent than the physical status of her hymen. It also argues that all societies including our own are equally concerned with completing successful marriage bargains and protecting against default on these bargains by protecting the value of a daughter's reproductive capacity. Only among societies and communities in which bargains are negotiated and protected by the parties themselves are such extreme mechanisms of chastity control instituted—especially among those societies in which families have the political power to monitor contract compliance through force if necessary, directed toward the daughter herself, their own kinsmen, or competing kin groups who may be parties to a bargain. It is only among such groups that a daughter's premarital behavior can be monitored successfully by members of a strong fraternal interest group. These group members have a joint interest in protecting her chaste reputation. They also have the power to demonstrate her virginal status through potentially hazardous public rituals and to avenge threats against her reputation through violence.

Method

Sample

The hypothesized relationships outlined above were tested on a subset of 151 societies selected from the Standard Cross-Cultural Sample (SCCS) developed by Murdock and White (1969). The SCCS is a stratified sample of world societies designed to minimize the effects of historical diffusion by including only one society from each of 186 distinct sampling provinces (Murdock, 1968). Each province consists of a cluster of societies with similar culture, language, and location. The subsample used in this study eliminated 35 societies from the original 186 in the SCCS after a pretest revealed a large number of sample societies whose primary source materials contained little or no information about any of the central dependent and intervening variables included in the theoretical model. These variables were constructed from data collected from all source materials on each sample society.

Measures

Female-Genital Mutilations and Virginity Tests. Three different forms of physical manipulation and surgical mutilation of women's genitals were coded: (1) tattooing the genitals or the elongation of the clitoris and/or labia majora; (2) ceremonial defloration prior to marriage, such as digital breaking or stretching of the hymen or piercing vaginal tissue and/or hymen with an instrument; (3) genital surgery in the form of infibulation, clitoridectomy (excision), circumcision, and their variations. In the statistical analysis only the presence or absence of genital surgery was considered, so the mutilation measure was dichotomized into its presence or absence. Virginity tests were coded present if any of the following were reported for a society: (1) public inspection or presentation of tokens of virginity such as blood-stained sheets, cloth, undergarments, or symbolically stained equivalents; (2) physical examination of genitals or public inquiry about the physical status of the hymen by relatives, elders, or ceremonial leaders at or before marriage; (3) husband expected to announce publically the condition of his bride on or after the wedding night. Virginity tests were considered absent if all three of the above events were stated as absent or if the ethnographic materials described wedding ceremonies and marriage agreements without mentioning these practices.

Chastity Control. The set of codes developed to measure kin-group concern with the control of a daughter's chastity measures behaviors that reflect variation in the saliency of chastity or purity belief systems. The measure of *control over premarital sexual behavior* orders the extremity of punishment for premarital sexual activity along a seven-point scale, from death, mutilation, banishment, lasting ostracism, or loss of all marriage chances as a moral imperative (1) or discretionary right (2), to severe disapproval in the form of temporary ostracism, shame, ridicule, beating, or impaired marriage chances (3), to mild disapproval (chastity preferred) (4), to toleration (5), and encouragement (6) of premarital sexual activity. The measure of *control over women's social interaction* is a four-point scale: (1) strict seclusion in the household; (2) can leave household only with a chaperone and male contact forbidden; (3) can leave household without chaperone, but male contact still forbidden; and (4) no restriction on social contact with men other than close kinsmen. Kin group *control over mate selection* is also a four-point scale ranging from two indicators of high kin-group control—(1) women have no choice and (2) women may attempt to circumvent marriage arrangements or be consulted—to two indicators of high female control—(3) women choose but family retains veto power and (4) women always or almost always choose mate.

Economic Resource Base and Fraternal Interest-Group Strength. The two critical antecedent conditions for the strictness of chastity control and ritual practices are the value of the economic resource base and the stength of fraternal interest groups of each society. Each of these variables has already been operationalized by Paige and Paige (1981). In brief, *high* resource base is considered present among pastoralists, and hoe and plow agriculturalists, mounted hunters, fishermen, and hunter-gatherers. Unlike the Paige and

Paige study, peasant economies are integral to the analysis of chastity control; therefore as many peasant societies as possible were included in the sample to investigate the extent to which the introduction of the state affects the control of families over daughters and therefore their virginity-related rituals. Peasants are plow and irrigation agriculturalists who live in so-called large states as defined by the SCCS (Murdock and White 1969).

The strength of fraternal interest groups was measured by summing the codes given each society on three variables: (1) size of the largest effective kin-based political subunit; (2) presence or absence of patrilineality; and (3) ability to make explicit contractual agreements, specifically brideprice payments in marriage bargains. (See Paige and Paige 1981 for a detailed description of this measure).

Social Stratification, Fragmentation, and Diverging Devolution. Three of the major alternative hypotheses about the determinants of worldwide patterns of chastity beliefs and practices require measures of the forms of social stratification, the fragmentation of patrimony, and diverging devolution. The last concept refers to the minimizing of fragmentation of property by allowing daughters to inherit male property, such as through a dowry (Goody 1976). A measure of social stratification has already been developed by Murdock (1967, col. 67) that arranges class stratification along a scale from complex (1), elite (2), and dual (3), to wealth distinctions only (4) and the absence of significant class distinctions (5). Several published codes proved indirect measures of property fragmentation and diverging devolution, but in the present analysis the distribution of inheritance of real property was used (Murdock 1967, col. 74) as the most direct measure of both concepts. This code measures the extent of fragmentation when family ownership of land passed on to offspring (vertical inheritance) is distinguished from *communal* or *horizontal* inheritance, which measures either the absence of inheritance rules or the inheritance across a lineage. It measures diverging devolution when inheritance by daughters is distinguished from inheritance rules excluding daughters.

Results

The extent to which ritual practices (genital mutilations and virginity tests) are statistically associated with three measures of chastity control are examined, as well as the relationships between each of these measures with the two critical predictor variables, resource base and fraternal interest-group strength, to ascertain the empirical support for the theoretical model. The power of the most important alternative theories are also tested by examining the relationship between rituals and chastity control and forms of social stratification and inheritance.

Virginity Rituals and Chastity Control

Of the fourteen societies performing genital mutilations in the sample, half also practiced virginity tests. Of the thirty societies practicing virginity tests, 23.3 percent also practiced genital mutilations (hereafter called excision), and 77.7 percent did not. In this analysis the two rituals are combined, so that a society practicing either or both are classified as performing a virginity ritual and all others are classified as not performing either ritual. This collapse is certainly justified given the small number of excision cases and the equivalence of the two rituals in the theoretical model. Table 13-1 presents the relationships between virginity rituals and the three indicators of chastity control. The presence of virginity rituals is strongly associated with high and moderate control over a daughter's sexual behavior and social interaction. These rituals are over ten times more likely to occur under conditions of high or moderate sexual control as compared to low control ($X^2 = 51.58$, $p < .0001$, $\phi = .645$), so that 41.6 percent of the variance in virginity rituals can be accounted for by severe disapproval of premarital sexual activity. Virginity rituals are as least three times more likely to occur among societies practicing high or moderate control over a daughter's social interaction than among those exerting low control ($X^2 = 9.33$, $p < .005$, $\phi = .30$), with 9 percent of the variance in ritual accounted for by degree of social interaction control alone. Inspection of the tabular distribution of virginity rituals across the three categories of mate-selection control shows a much weaker association, although the trend is in the predicted direction. When the proportion of virginity rituals among societies in which families choose a daughter's mate (high control) is compared to the proportion among societies in which a daughter chooses the mate (moderate and low control), the association is statistically significant ($X^2 = 4.68$, $p < .05$, $\phi = .193$) but weak, accounting for only 3.7 percent of the variance in virginity rituals.

These results provide empirical support for the hypothesis that virginity rituals are expressions of cultural codes of female chastity or purity when those codes lead to familial controls over sexual and social behavior, and to some extent mate selection. Although the three indicators of chastity control are strongly correlated with each other, with zero-order correlations ranging from .74 to .81, the substantial range in the size of the correlation of each indicator with the dependent variable, as expressed by the phi coefficient, suggests that they should be treated separately and not collapsed into an overall index of chastity control.

Political and Economic Antecedents
of Virginity Rituals

The theoretical model proposes that virginity rituals should not only be positively associated with familial control over a daughter's chastity but that both rituals and chastity control should be explained by the political strength of fraternal interest groups in a society and by the economic value of the resource base. Paige and Paige (1981) have already demonstrated a strong, positive association between the economic resource base and fraternal interest-group strength of stateless societies ($r = .66$), and in the present sample, which includes peasants, the association is also strong ($r = .52$).

Table 13-1
Relationship between Virginity Test or Genital Excision and Kin-Group Control over Daughter's Premarital Behavior (Chastity Control)

Virginity Test or Excision	*Chastity-Control Indicators*		
	High	*Moderate*	*Low*
	Control of Sexual Behavior[a]		
Present	69.2%	65.6%	6.3%
	(9)	(21)	(5)
Absent	30.8%	34.4%	93.7%
	(4)	(11)	(74)
Total	100.0%	100.0%	100.0%
	(13)	(32)	(79)
	Control of Social Interaction[b]		
Present	38.9%	35.0%	11.8%
	(7)	(7)	(8)
Absent	61.1%	65.0%	88.2%
	(11)	(13)	(60)
Total	100.0%	100.0%	100.0%
	(18)	(20)	(68)
	Control of Mate Selection[c]		
Present	32.4%	11.8%	22.2%
	(24)	(4)	(4)
Absent	67.6%	88.2%	77.8%
	(50)	(30)	(14)
Total	100.0%	100.0%	100.0%
	(74)	(34)	(18)

Note: *High* represents a score of either 1 or 2 on all three indicators; *moderate* represents a score of 3; and *low* represents a score of 4 on Control of Social Interaction and Control of Mate Selection and 4-6 on Control of Sexual Behavior.

[a] $X^2_{\text{high/moderate versus low}} = 51.58$; $p < .0001$; $\phi = r = .645$; $\phi^2 = .416$
[b] $X^2_{\text{high/moderate versus low}} = 9.33$; $p < .005$; $\phi = r = .30$; $\phi^2 = .09$
[c] $X^2_{\text{high versus moderate/low}} = 4.68$; $p < .05$; $\phi = r = .193$; $\phi^2 = .037$

Table 13-2
Relationship between Virginity Rituals, Resource Base, and Fraternal Interest-Group Strength

Virginity Rituals	Resource Base			Trichotomized Index of Fraternal Strength		
	Low/Unstable	High	Peasant	Weak (0,1)	Moderate (2,3)	Strong (4)
Present	7.4% (5)	43.6% (24)	44.4% (8)	7.4% (6)	47.4% (18)	83.3% (10)
Absent	92.6% (63)	56.4% (31)	55.6% (10)	92.6% (75)	52.6% (20)	16.7% (2)
Total	100.0% (68)	100.0% (55)	100.0% (18)	100.0% (81)	100.0% (38)	100.0% (12)

Table 13-2 presents the relationships between virginity rituals, levels of fraternal interest-group strength, and types of resource base in tabular form. Inspection of this table shows clearly that there is a substantial association between rituals and their predictred political and economic antecedents. The index of fraternal interest-group strength is an ordinal scale along which societies are ordered according to their composite score on each of the three components of political strength. Although their scores can range from 0 to 4, they have been trichotomized in this table (weak = 0,1; moderate = 2,3; strong = 3,4) since the distribution of rituals across each level of strength formed these three distinct clusters. Only a very few of the weakest groups (7.4 percent performed virginity rituals, whereas nearly half of the moderately strong groups (47.4 percent), and the vast majority (83.3 percent) of the strongest groups did. The zero-order correlation between the ordinal index of political strength and virginity rituals was .53.

The distribution of virginity rituals across the three types of economic resource bases shows a similar pattern, with only 7.4 percent of societies with resource bases of low or unstable economic value practicing virginity rituals and about 44 percent of both high resource-base societies and peasants performing the rituals. The zero-order correlation between virginity rituals and resource base is .43 when the latter variable is arranged along an ordinal scale.

These results provide strong empirical support for the theoretical proposition that virginity rituals are surveillance tactics used by the powerful to protect their daughter's social reputation throughout the period of nubility. It is these social groups that have the economic and military capacity to engage in high-stakes marriage bargains that require a demonstration of their ability to deliver a daughter with a chaste reputation and therefore unambiguous rights to her offspring after marriage. A definitive test of the causal linkage between economic base, political strength, and virginity rituals is a statistical demonstration of the extent to which the strong correlation between economy and ritual is due to the strong relationship of each of these variables with political strength. The appropriate empirical test is simply the partial correlation between resource base and virginity rituals when fraternal interest-group strength is held constant. The results of this test show that the association between resource base and rituals drops substantially from .43 to .21, and the amount of variance in rituals explained drops from 18.5 percent to only 4.5 percent. This reduction demonstrates that a substantial proportion of the effects of resource base on the presence or absence of virginity rituals is due to the effects of resource base on political strength of social groups (that is, families).

The Intervening Efffect of Chastity Control

The extent to which a strong cultural concern with protecting the chastity of nubile daughters, particularly her sexual and social activities, provides an important linkage between political strength of families and virginity rituals can be tested in a similar fashion. It has already been shown that all three indicators of chastity control are significantly associated with virginity rituals, with control of sexual activity being the most powerful predictor ($r = .65$) followed by control of social interaction ($r = .30$) and mate selection ($r = .19$). It should be noted that the actual behaviors that correlate most strongly with virginity rituals are acts of violence (that is, death and dismemberment) for premarital sex. If genital mutilations and public tests of virginity at marriage can also be interpreted as physical and social abuse, then the pattern of correlations suggests that the form of chastity control during nubility that best predicts abusive virginity rituals are those that condone violence against a daughter for violation of cultural standard. The lower correlation between rituals and control of social interaction, such as the practice of *purdah,* suggests that among a number of societies strict seclusion of nubile daughters may be an alternative to violence: strict seclusion among other women of the family precludes actual or purported sexual malfeasance and therefore minimizes public demonstrations of a family's ability to control their daughter's virtue through violence or the threat of violence.

For the purposes of the argument presented here the tabular relationships between each indicator of chastity control and the economic and political antecedents need not be described. The zero-order correlations between each indicator and each antecedent condition suffice, before demonstrating the significance of chastity control in linking political strength to virginity rituals. Control over sexual activity has a moderately high correlation with both fraternal interest-group strength ($r = .27$) and resource base (.30). The size of relationship between control over mate selection and each variable is about the same ($r_{strength} = .20; r_{resources} = .34$). Control over social interaction is only weakly associated with political strength ($r = .13$) and moderately correlated with resource base ($r = .26$).

For an indicator to play an important intervening role in linking political strength with virginity rituals it must correlate at least moderately high with both variables. The only indicator that could provide an intervening link, then, is control over sexual activity.

To what extent, then, is the strong positive association between political strength of fraternal interest groups and the practice of virginity rituals due to the common association of these two variables with cultural norms allowing family members to resort to violence against a daughter if she breaks social norms about premarital sex? How much of a reduction in the correlation between strength and rituals occurs when the effects of control of sexual activity are held constant? The results show that in fact the correlation is reduced from .53 to .40, and that the amount of variance in rituals explained by political strength drops from 28 percent to 16 percent, nearly a twofold reduction. Therefore, strong fraternal interest groups are significantly more likely than weak ones to perform genital mutilitations and/or public virginity tests because they allow the use of violence against a daughter for sexual malfeasance throughout her nubility.

Chastity, Social Stratification,
and Inheritance Patterns

Although the variety of practices associated with female puberty have been the focus of much theoretical speculation, four propositions are of particular interest in this chapter since they identify possible social processes that could explain worldwide variation in the chastity-control mechanisms and rituals discussed here. Two theorists argue a concern with female chastity and the institution of mechanisms, including genital mutilations and virginity tests, to control premarital chastity developed in response to social processes that coincided with increased status distinctions between families, such as social stratification and the development of social classes (Ortner 1978; Whitehead 1976). Another two theorists focus on the relationship between chastity control and the development of inheritance rules that pass on valuable real property (that is, land and animals) to sons and daughters, called vertical inheritance. Schneider (1971) proposes that once the patrimonial estate is passed down the family line the protection of female chastity becomes a means of maintaining family solidarity in the face of intense fraternal competition over the control of inheritance. Goody (1976) focuses specifically on the social implications of daughter's being able to inherit property under conditions of vertical inheritance. He believes that among societies in which daughters as well as sons can inherit their father's property there develops an intense concern with control over a daughter's premarital sex behavior and mate choice as a means of controlling the distribution of property after she marries.

An analysis of the empirical data used to test these propositions shows that they complement rather than compete with the social-exchange theory of premarital chastity control outlined above. Table 13-3 presents the distribution of chastity-control indicators and virginity rituals across

Table 13-3
Relationship between Virginity Rituals, Chastity-Control Mechanisms, and Forms of Social Stratification

| | Forms of Stratification | | | |
	None	Wealth Stratification	Dual Stratification	Distinct Classes
	Virginity Rituals			
Present	17.0%	20.0%	43.3%	43.8%
	(9)	(7)	(13)	(7)
Absent	83.0%	80.0%	56.7%	56.2%
	(44)	(28)	(17)	(9)
Total	100.0%	100.0%	100.0%	100.0%
	(53)	(35)	(30)	(16)
	Control over Sexual Behavior			
High	19.6%	42.9%	44.0%	55.6%
	(9)	(15)	(11)	(10)
Low	80.4%	57.1%	56.0%	44.4%
	(37)	(20)	(14)	(8)
Total	100.0%	100.0%	100.0%	100.0%
	(46)	(35)	(25)	(18)
	Control over Social Interaction			
High	33.3%	31.0%	31.6%	60.0%
	(14)	(9)	(6)	(9)
Low	66.7%	69.0%	68.4%	40.0%
	(28)	(20)	(13)	(6)
Total	100.0%	100.0%	100.0%	100.0%
	(42)	(29)	(19)	(15)
	Control over Mate Selection			
High	45.2%	54.8%	55.6%	75.0%
	(19)	(17)	(15)	(12)
Moderate	30.9%	22.6%	37.0%	25.0%
	(13)	(7)	(10)	(4)
Low	23.8%	22.6%	7.4%	0.0%
	(10)	(7)	(25)	(0)
Total	100.0%	100.0%	100.0%	100.0%
	(42)	(31)	(27)	(16)

the major categories of social stratification ordered to the degree of complexity. The sociological distinction between *social stratification* and *social class* is critical in examining these data, since the chastity indicators relate differently to each social form. Social classes coincide with the emergence of the state while families and kin groups can become hierarchically organized on the basis of unequal wealth and status; that is, stratification, among stateless societies. Careful inspection of table 13-3 shows that the presence or absence of distinct classes best predicts the extent to which families will exert high control over a daughter's social interaction and mate selection. Regardless of the level of stratification, only about one-third of classless societies exert high control over social interaction as compared to 60 percent of societies with social classes. When the first three columns are collapsed and compared with the last column (that is, classless versus class societies) the difference in degree of social control is statistically significant ($X^2 = 4.56$, $p < .05$). Similarly the degree of control families exert over mate selection is significantly greater among societies with social classes than those societies without classes ($X^2 = 7.30$, $p < .01$). Control over sexual behavior and virginity rituals, however, appears to be more closely associated with the emergence of stratification systems rather than distinct classes. High control over a daughter's sexual activity involving the use of violence is at least twice as likely to occur once societies begin to develop any form of status distinctions than among those societies that are relatively status homogeneous (for example, compare the first column with the last three columns), with this difference being statistically significant ($X^2 = 8.58$, $p < .01$). Virginity rituals do begin to be more frequent prior to the development of distinct social classses but are significantly more common among societies with a hereditary aristocracy (dual stratification) than societies that only contain wealth distinctions. Societies with either a hereditary aristocracy or distinct social classes are significantly more likely to perform virginity rituals than societies with less complex social forms ($X^2 = 9.84$, $p < .01$). These patterns confirm the general arguments of both Ortner (1978) and Whitehead (1976), although they suggest a much more complex relationship between the form chastity control takes and the development of social groups within a society. These data suggest a historical ordering of the kinds of chastity-control measures families use. Control over a daughter's sexual behavior begins to become most extreme once a society develops some basis of distinguishing the social and economic statuses of families; once a hereditary aristocracy develops, virginity rituals—as well as sexual control—become common. The addition of high control over a daughter's social interaction outside the family and mate choice only appear to be a major concern when states are formed containing complex social classes.

Comparing the social-stratification argument with the theoretical model about the strength of fraternal interest groups the results suggest, first, that virginity rituals and the control over a daughter's sexual behavior are better explained by the social-exchange theory that argues that such practices are violent tactics used to preserve a daughter's reputation for chastity under conditions of high-stakes marriage bargaining. The relationships between each of these practices and the political and economic antecedents proposed by the model are much stronger statistically than those observed with levels of stratification. Second, the social-exchange model is an equally good predictor of control over social interaction and mate selection as the stratification model if the size of the relationships (expressed as X^2 values) in tables 13-2 and 13-3 are compared. The trends in this sample suggest the possibility of an interaction effect between the increased political and military power of kin-based groups within a society and the presence of complex social classes. Although it is beyond the scope of this chapter to explore this possibility in detail, future research should examine the extent to which increased social restrictions and seclusion, as well as familial control over mate choice, are alternative strategies to more violent practices by which a daughter's chastity is preserved in complex states. The development of centralized-state apparatus may reduce interfamily and intrafamily violence but it does not eliminate family control over marriage arrangements. Both sets of chastity-control mechanisms can be interpreted as tactics to protect a daughter's marriagability; whether they take the form of violent practices or social control depends on the presence or absence of a centralized adjudicating procedure.

The analysis of the relationship between each chastity-control practice and types of property inheritance was performed to test the theories of Schnneider (1971) and Goody (1976). If Schneider's theory has any validity then concern with chastity control should be much more intense in societies practicing vertical inheritance of real property; that is, passing property down the family line rather than across the entire community of kinsmen (horizontal inheritance)—and more intense than among societies in which property, if its exists, is owned communally by each succeeding generation of kinsmen. According to Goody's theory, chastity control should become most intense when daughters, as well as sons, begin to inherit property vertically. Therefore vertical inheritance by sons should show the same pattern of chastity control as horizontal and communal inheritance, if Goody's theory is supported. If vertical inheritance by sons alone and by both sexes shows the same pattern of more extreme chastity control than either horizontal or communal inheritance, then Schneider's theory is supported.

The distribution of virginity rituals and indicators of chastity control across each of the four types of inheritance patterns shown in Table 13-4 do not show the consistent pattern observed for stratification. All the relation-

Table 13-4
Relationship between Forms of Property Inheritance, Chastity Control, and Virginity Rituals

| | Inheritance of Real Property | | | |
	Communal	Horizontal	Sons Inherit	Both Sexes Inherit
	Control over Sexual Behavior			
High	21.1%	26.7%	58.9%	36.4%
	(8)	(4)	(20)	(8)
Low	78.9%	73.3%	41.2%	63.6%
	(30)	(11)	(14)	(14)
Total	100.0%	100.0%	100.0%	100.0%
	(38)	(15)	(34)	(22)
	Control over Social Interaction			
High	27.8%	25.0%	53.6%	35.3%
	(10)	(3)	(15)	(6)
Low	72.2%	75.0%	46.4%	64.7%
	(26)	(9)	(13)	(11)
Total	100.0%	100.0%	100.0%	100.0%
	(36)	(12)	(28)	(17)
	Control over Mate Selection			
High	45.9%	42.9%	69.4%	55.6%
	(17)	(6)	(25)	(10)
Moderate	18.9%	50.0%	22.2%	27.8%
	(7)	(7)	(8)	(5)
Low	35.1%	7.1%	8.3%	16.7%
	(13)	(1)	(3)	(3)
Total	100.0%	100.0%	100.0%	100.0%
	(37)	(14)	(36)	(18)
	Virginity Rituals			
Present	10.9%	37.5%	30.2%	53.3%
	(5)	(6)	(13)	(8)
Absent	81.1%	62.5%	69.8%	46.7%
	(41)	(10)	(30)	(7)
Total	100.0%	100.0%	100.0%	100.0%
	(46)	(16)	(43)	(15)

ships conform to Schneider's theory: when families pass down valuable property to their sons they also resort to both violent methods of chastity control, specifically death and mutilation for premarital sex, and non-violent mechanisms of social seclusion and mate choice. The only form of chastity control that conforms to Goody's prediction is the practice of virginity rituals that are much more apparent among societies in which daughters as well as sons are allowed to inherit family property. Control over mate selection, however, is most extreme among societies with either form of vertical inheritance as compared to those societies with horizontal or communal inheritance. All these relationships are statistically significant: (1) vertical inheritance by sons alone is associated with high control over sexual behavior ($X^2 = 10.41$, $p<.01$) and high control over social interaction ($X^2 = 5.93$, $p<.05$); (2) vertical inheritance by both sexes is associated with the practice of virginity rituals ($X^2 = 6.23$, $p<.05$); and (3) both forms of vertical inheritance lead to greater familial control over a daughter's mate choice ($X^2 = 4.12$, $p<.05$). Overall, the results lend most support to Schneider's argument about increased concern by male family members about the behavior of unmarried daughters and sisters during puberty among those societies in which vertical inheritance rules link marriage with property.

Discussion

The empirical tests provide strong support for the social-exchange theory of conditions in world societies that explain the practices of genital mutilations and virginity tests. These rituals mark the beginning and end of a daughter's nubility phase of social development among societies in which her reputation for chastity is so crucial to a marriage bargain that she can even be murdered for actual or suspected sexual misbehavior. Societies that practice virginity rituals are also likely to curtail strongly a daughter's social interactions after puberty and allow her little choice in selecting a husband. The weak connections between virginity rituals and these last two indicators of chastity control show that the seclusion of women at purberty and family-controlled mate selection are not always accompanied by virginity rituals. Extreme sanctions for sexual misbehavior and virginity rituals are most characteristic of societies based on advanced agriculture or pastoralism, economies that promote the development of large and powerful fraternal interest groups. These groups have the economic resources to engage in high-stakes marriage bargains with each other and the military power to protect the terms of these bargains through force if necessary. When the stakes in a marriage bargain are high, default on its terms can have serious consequences. In these societies any suspicion about a daughter's virginal status is considered default on a bargain since it creates ambiguity about the future husband's rights to exclusive claims to her sexual and reproductive capacity. Only when such claims can be guaranteed through public consensus will he be willing to transfer large amounts of property (called a bride price) to her family.

The results also suggest that a full explanation of chastity control should consider the role of status distinctions between families in a society, as well as inheritance patterns. It is possible that the same characteristics of valuable economic resource bases that produce strong fraternal interest groups also produce unequal access to these resources among families; social and economic inequality, in turn, motivates families to retain control over resources by means of vertical inheritance of the patrimonial estate and to form marriage alliances only with families of equal or greater socioeconomic status. Although a precise accounting of family social and economic resource control is often difficult to ascertain, its demonstrated success in protecting nubile daughters against a reputation for promiscuity can be used to estimate its success in protecting other valuable resources.

The responses to female sexual maturity examined in this chapter can be interpreted as a familial strategy for protecting claims to their nubile daughters' marriage value that is an alternative to sponsoring large menarcheal ceremonies. The ceremonial strategy has already been shown to be a characteristic of weak fraternal interest groups in societies where economic resources are of little or no value (Paige and Paige 1981). Expansion of this empirically based model of pubertal practices in nonindustrial societies to further understand U.S. responses to puberty will require an examination of the similarities in practices between our society and strong fraternal interest-group societies. Although our society is industrialized, it has distinct social classes and a peasant heritage in which disputes over familial property can be intense and a daughter's premarital conduct and mate selection are a source of considerable parental concern. Theoretical linkages may begin to be made by considering similarities in parental socialization practices. Although we do not practice the apparently elaborate forms of sexual and social control observed in strong fraternal interest-group societies, strong pressure begins to be exerted by parents, especially in the middle class, toward so-called ladylike behavior in daughters once they reach puberty. Although modesty socialization has been a seriously neglected research area in social and developmental psychology (Nelson 1977), there are some empirical studies that show an important shift in parental practices and peer pressure once a daughter reaches puberty (for example, Block 1975; Blyth and Simmons 1981). Inspection of the kinds of female behaviors that become differentially reinforced at puberty shows a pattern of strong emphasis on conformity to normative standards of sexual modesty, monitoring of cross-sex activities, and pressures toward ladylike demeanor that is similar to the socialization practices observed in strong fraternal interest-group societies. Preliminary analysis of the relationships between fraternal interest-group strength and the shift in socialization emphasis in late childhood toward self-restraint, sexual restraint, and obedience shows strong correlations (between .24 and .38) with the variables in our social-exchange model. Future research should attempt to identify what ladylike behavior in the United States implies and examine the broad range of parental socialization practices within the context of social and economic dynamics discussed here.

References

Block, J. 1975. Another look at sex differentiation in the socialization behaviors of mothers and fathers. Draft of paper for Conference on New Directions for Research on Women, Madison, Wisconsin.

Blyth, D., and Simmons, R. 1981. The social and psychological effects of puberty. Paper presented at the Conference on Female Pubertal Development, La Jolla, California, March 1981.

Goody, J. 1976. *Production and reproduction*. Cambridge, Eng.: Cambridge University Press.

Gough, E. 1955. Female initiation rites on the Malabar Coast. *Journal of the Royal Anthropological Institute* 85:45-80.

Murdock, G.P. 1967. Ethnographic atlas: A summary. *Ethnology* 6:109-236.

_____ .1968. World sampling provinces. *Ethnology* 7:305-326.

Murdock, G.P., and White, D. 1969. Standard cross-cultural sample. *Ethnology* 8:239-269.

Nelson, K. 1977. Modesty socialization in sexual identity. Unpublished doctoral dissertation, University of California at Berkeley.

Opler, M. 1941. *An Apache life-way*. Chicago: University of Chicago Press.

Ortner, S. 1978. The virgin and the state. 4:19-35.

Paige, K.E., and Paige, J.M. 1981. *The politics of reproductive ritual*. Berkeley: University of California Press.

Richards, A. 1956. *Chisungu*. New York: Grove Press.

Schneider, J. 1971. Of vigilance and viergins: Honor, shame, and the access to resources in Mediterranean society. *Ethnology* 10:1-24.

Whitehead, H. 1976. The dynamics of chastity and the politics of mutilation. Paper presented at the Symposium on Social Structure Ideology and Women's Choice, American Anthropological Association Meetings.

14

Age at Menarche and Sexual Conduct in Adolescence and Young Adulthood

John H. Gagnon

The relation between the changes that take place in an individual at puberty and his or her subsequent sexual conduct is not well understood (Gagnon 1977). There are those persons who infer from differences between the adolescent sexual conduct of females and males that there are possible gender-related biological or biosocial factors operating in this period that shape sexual conduct (Meyer-Bahlburg 1980). Still other researchers suggest from these gender differences that age at puberty may be implicated as well. Most of these inferences, however, rest upon gross differences in the sexual conduct of males and females in the contemporary United States that are assumed to be either strongly or weakly related to hormonal differences. At the present time there is no study of either females or males that has carefully assessed in a prospective design various levels of sexual conduct near in time to the various physiological and anatomical changes associated with puberty in either males or females. As a consequence the majority of current knowledge is speculative in character.

The research that is being reported does not meet these strong methodological strictures either and its limitations will be apparent as its goals and research design are described. Despite these constraints it offers some new empirical evidence about the relation between age at menarche and youthful sexuality. In the spring of 1967 a sample of twelve nonsectarian, coeducational, accredited four-year colleges and universities was drawn from the National Opinion Research Center's list of such schools. A probability sample of students was interviewed: a total of 100 males and females at each institution, stratified equally by years in school. Within each year in school there was a restriction by age: seventeen to nineteen for first-year students, eighteen to twenty for second-year students, and so forth. The outcome of this interviewing produced a total sample of 1177 students, 593 males and 584 females. The completion rate, calculated to include both those students not able to be contacted (the majority) and refusals (a minority), was just shy of seventy-five percent. The goal of this study was to examine the role

The research program on which this chapter is based was codirected by Professor William Simon of the University of Houston. Support for the research was provided by NICHD grants numbers HD02257 and HD 04157. Support for this chapter also came from PHS/Biomedical Grant #431-H172.

of sexuality in the psychosocial development of young people and represented a pilot study of the possibility of using conventional survey sampling and interviewing techniques to study sexual matters (Simon and Gagnon 1965).

The age at menarche reported by the subjects ranged from nine to twenty and as usual heaped in the years twelve and thirteen. This distribution appears quite comparable to those from other retrospective studies of age at menarche (Kinsey et al. 1953). The median age at menarche for the entire sample was 12.89 and the mean was 12.29. The differences between the year in school groups were small (from the first to the fourth year the medians were 12.75, 13.06, 12.93, and 12.89). However much distortion in recall there is, it is not associated with age at report, thus whatever effects that are found will not be the result of different distributions of reported ages of menarche in each class in school.

There are data on three different types of sexual conduct usually for two points in time, more immediately for the college years and more retrospectively for the high-school period. For this earlier period recall differences can be examined by year in school as with age at menarche. In addition, there are data on masturbation in high school and college, genital petting in high school, and premarital coitus during high school and college. Further there are data on orgasm associated with petting and coitus.

These different types of sexual expression can be used to test a number of different hypotheses about the relation between age at menarche and sexuality. Thus one could suppose that earlier ages of menarche might indicate a greater biological readiness not only for reproduction but also for sexual activity (Diamond 1976). As a result there should be a linear-inverse rela-

Table 14-1
Age at First Menses

Age	Percent	Cumulative Percent
9	2.1	2.1
10	3.8	5.9
11	17.2	23.1
12	29.9	53.0
13	32.7	85.7
14	11.1	96.8
15	2.6	99.4
16	.2	99.6
17	.2	99.8
18	.0	99.8
19	.0	99.8
20	.2	100.0

Note: $N=581$; missing data = 3.

tionship between age at menarche and sexual conduct. An earlier age at menarche should result in higher levels of sexual activity across all types of conduct. Support for such a view would still be possible if there were a linear-inverse relationship solely between age at menarche and masturbation incidences and frequencies since masturbation would be less mediated by social opportunities and constraints than sociosexual conduct such as petting or intercourse.

A social-psychological hypothesis would be that the visible secondary sexual characteristics that usually occur close in time to first menses are indicants to the young girl and others around her of a new sexual status (Gagnon and Simon 1973). The young girl with a more womanly shape is defined as being ready for participation in heterosocial and heterosexual conduct. The earlier such preliminaries as dating and hugging and kissing occur the sooner more extensive sexual experimentation would follow. Support for such a view would exist if sociosexual conduct showed a relation to age at menarche and would be further strengthened if neither age at menarche nor sociosexual conduct were related to masturbation.

An alternative social-psychological hypothesis would predict a U-shaped relationship in which young women who had earlier or later ages at menarche shared some common experience of being different than those who were socially more "normal." Thus girls who had to manage the experience of menarche well in advance of peers as well as those for whom it was delayed could share a sense of alienation from normal development, making them vulnerable to other deviant experience. Rossi (1962)[1] has suggested that women who went to graduate school during the 1950s were more likely to have either an early or late first menses. In addition she argued that such women (who by their pursuit of unconventional goals; that is, those ends other than marriage and children, could be construed as deviant) also tended to extreme responses to other items—they loved their parents very much or very little, and so forth. Their "outlier" status on many dimensions suggested a cumulative experience of difference that made them vulnerable to nonconforming conduct. If the outlier hypothesis were true in this case then we would expect young women with both earlier and later ages at menarche to be similar. While it is somewhat problematic to view sexual experimentation among the young as an expression of nonconformity or deviance, particularly when rates of such experimentation are high, it is possible to consider outliers as having a special potential for alternative or different patterns of development.

Masturbation is one of the ubiquitous forms of sexual conduct, yet except for the Kinsey studies (and a series of studies earlier in time) research is extremely sparse (DeMartino 1979). The general findings for this study are consonant with earlier research that reports that male rates of masturbation, both incidence and frequencies, are substantially higher than those of women. There is evidence that there is an environment among young males that is productive of sexual fantasy and sexual experimentation that does not exist among young women (Quartararo, Gagnon and Simon, submitted for publication). As a result, as one can see in table 14-2, only about half of the female sample report ever masturbating, about four in ten in high school and three in ten in college. There are minimal differences by age at first menarche except for the rather odd finding that the early menstruators also have the lowest incidence of masturbation in high school.

When the frequency of masturbation is examined, the rates for high school and college do not differ for the two periods. While there are differences among the various age at menarche groups they are neither strong nor consistent. The problem may be that the frequencies are very low and unstable, which may indicate that masturbation does not represent a salient form of conduct for most women. It is clear that these data do not offer support for a view that early ages of menarche are associated, by whatever mechanism, social or biological, with higher rates of masturbatory conduct.

A number of authors have suggested that there could be an association between discomfort from menses and the use of masturbation to relieve such discomfort (Kinsey 1953). The question about discomfort was not retrospective and must be assumed to refer to the time of the interview. Further there is no measure of intensity of discomfort, only its presence or absence and its source. As a consequence it is only possible to examine the relation between type of discomfort and the incidence and frequency of masturbation in college. It should be noted that 27 percent of the total sample reported no discomfort, 39 percent physical discomfort only, 29 percent physical and mental discomfort, and 6 percent mental discomfort only. Over the four years of college there is a slight decrease in the proportion reporting no discomfort and solely physical discomfort with a concomitant increase in proportion reporting both mental and physical discomfort. About 10 percent more of those women who reported only mental discom-

Table 14-2
Incidence of Masturbation by Age at First Menses

Age at First Menses	Incidence of Masturbation			
	Ever	High School	College	N
9-11	46.3	33.6	30.6	134
12	54.0	44.2	35.6	174
13	47.4	44.2	29.5	190
14-20	49.4	44.4	33.3	81

Note: Missing data = 5.

fort masturbated during college. However, among those who did masturbate, higher rates are reported by those who reported both mental and physical or solely mental discomfort. While the findings cannot be considered
conclusive there is some indication that some women who experience menstrual discomfort that they define as having a psychological component
masturbate more frequently than those who report no discomfort or only
physical discomfort. Though this connection was not made explicitly in the
interview, masturbation may well be specifically used by some women as a
source of relief from menstrual discomfort.

In contrast to masturbation, any sexual conduct that requires a partner
or partners neccessitates the possession and management of a wide variety
of social skills that need to be brought to bear on a number of persons in
several social contexts. As a result any effects that age of menses has on
such forms of sexual conduct as petting or coitus are surely mediated by a
number of other important variables, particularly the age-appropriateness
of the conduct (which includes the values and expectations of the individual
as well as the opportunities afforded). In this society such factors as dating,
falling in love, relations with parents, religious constraints, and educational
aspirations all play a role in determining the speed and extent with which
young people move into sexual experimentation.

Age at menses is unassociated with most of these social variables,
whether they are reviewed as facilitating or constraining of the sexual activity of young women. Thus strong attachment to parents and frequent
church attendance, which are predictive of minimal sexual activity in high
school and college, were not associated with age at menarche. Similarly
such a facilitator as falling in love was also unrelated to age at menarche.
There was, however, a weak negative association between frequency of dating and age at menarche with those with an earlier age at menarche more
likely to date frequently. For the most part whatever effects age of menarche has on various aspects of socio-sexual conduct in this study, except
for the effects of dating, they are not a result of an association with these
important mediating social factors.

About one-quarter of the young women in the sample reported involvement in genital petting during high school, either as a recipient or a pro-
vider. Few of them reported that it occurred with any great frequency, even
though among those young women who experienced genital petting about
one-half experienced orgasm as least once. A slightly larger proportion of
the young women with the earliest ages at menarche reported genital petting
than did those with later ages. (see table 14-3). There were, however, no differences among the older age groups. The differences are not very large and
could be due to the slightly higher rates of dating found for this group. The
weakness of this finding may result from the instability of patterns of sexual
conduct among young people interviewed during this historical period. As a

Table 14-3
Age at Menarche and Incidence of Genital Petting in High School

Age at First Menses	Done to Respondent	Done by Respondent	N
9-11	35.3	27.1	133
12	26.0	18.5	173
13	20.9	15.5	183
14-20	24.7	18.5	81

Note: Missing data = 8.

consequence it might be that some effects might not be present that would be found in a more recent sample, which would have a larger proportion with extensive sexual experience (Chilman 1979).

In addition to these findings for petting during high school the data for premarital coitus also show some modest effects that seem to be related to age at menarche, though the results are not easily explainable. From table 14-4 it can be observed that a somewhat smaller proportion of women with oldest ages of menarche had intercourse in high school. Recalling that women with earlier ages at menarche also had higher rates of dating in high school these rates were controlled.

What is apparent in table 14-5 is that young women with high rates of dating are equally likely to have intercourse regardless of age at menarche. However for those with lower rates of dating there is a small, but observable, increase in the proportion with coital experience among those with earlier puberty. In this case there might be an independent effect of early puberty in increasing these rates.

However from table 14-4 it also can be observed that a somewhat larger proportion of women with later menarche have *ever* had premarital coitus,

Table 14-4
Incidence of Premarital Coitus and Coital Frequency in College by Age at First Menses

Age at First Menses	Incidence				Frequency			
	In High School	In College	In High School or College	N	Rare	Sometimes	Frequent	N
9-11	9.7	34.3	36.3	134	30.4	41.3	28.3	46
12	8.6	30.1	32.8	173	23.1	51.9	25.0	52
13	8.6	22.4	25.3	188	33.3	47.6	19.0	42
14-20	4.8	43.4	44.6	83	47.2	33.3	19.4	36
Total	8.6	30.7	32.6	578				

Note: Missing data = 6.

Table 14-5
Proportion of Respondents with Intercourse during High School by Frequency of Dating and Age at First Menses

| | Age at First Menses | | | | | | | |
| | 9-11 | | 12 | | 13 | | 14-20 | |
Frequency of Dating	Percent	(Number)	Percent	(Number)	Percent	(Number)	Percent	(Number)
High	14.0	(50)	25.5	(47)	16.4	(55)	13.0	(23)
Medium	11.9	(42)	1.7	(60)	6.3	(63)	0.0	(28)
Low	7.3	(41)	3.0	(67)	4.2	(72)	3.1	(32)

even though fewer of them had had intercourse while in high school. Thus the incidence in high school for the oldest age at menarche group was about half that of the other three younger age categories (about five percent in contrast to ten). However, about ten percent more of this oldest group had had intercourse by the end of college. Data on age of onset of coitus show that intercourse begins earliest in the youngest age at menarche groups, with a division between the two next younger groups and the oldest group.

When the relation between the year in school in which intercourse first took place and the age at menarche is examined, controlling for the year in school of the respondent, these differences between the three groups aged thirteen and under and the group aged fourteen and over become more apparent.

The small number of cases make the cell entries unstable, however there is a clear-cut tendency for sophomores through seniors with menarche at fourteen and over to be more likely to have had intercourse in college *and* especially in the latter years of college. There does not seem to be any particularly satisfying reason for this finding nor for the finding that the groups with a larger proportion beginning coitus early do not continue this pattern in college.

The larger proportion having had intercourse among those who have the oldest age at menarche does not result in higher frequencies of coitus during college (see table 14-4). Those young women with earlier ages at menarche report higher rates of coitus during college, perhaps as a consequence of their earlier ages of onset. That is, if intercourse begins earlier the likelihood is that it will continue with reasonable regularity during the college years, though perhaps in a number of relationships. Those women who begin coitus late in college share a pattern of sporadic sexual activity that young people who began earlier, experienced earlier. This sporadic pattern of intercourse is likely the cause of the other finding related to intercourse and menarche; that is, women with earlier ages at menarche are more likely to have orgasm more frequently in intercourse in college. (see table 14-7). It is not that early menarche produces higher rates of orgasm but that those women who have more coital experience are more likely to report higher

Table 14-6
Incidence of Premarital Intercourse by Age at
First Menses and Year in School

Year in School	Age at First Menses	Never	High School	First Year	Second Year	Third Year	Fourth Year	Number
First	9-11	81.8	12.1	6.0	—	—	—	33
year	12	78.3	13.0	8.7	—	—	—	46
	13	83.3	11.9	4.8	—	—	—	42
	14-20	78.8	7.1	14.2	—	—	—	14
Total		81.2	11.5	7.2	—	—	—	135
Second	9-11	62.1	13.8	6.9	17.2	—	—	29
year	12	69.8	9.3	11.6	9.3	—	—	43
	13	79.7	6.8	11.9	1.7	—	—	59
	14-20	55.0	10.0	10.0	25.0	—	—	20
Total		70.2	9.5	10.6	10.0	—	—	151
Third	9-11	58.6	10.3	13.8	13.8	3.4	—	29
year	12	68.8	6.3	6.3	10.4	8.3	—	48
	13	62.8	11.6	4.7	11.6	9.3	—	43
	14-20	59.3	3.7	3.7	14.8	18.5	—	27
Total		63.3	8.2	6.8	12.2	9.5	—	147
Fourth	9-11	55.8	9.3	9.3	7.0	9.3	9.3	43
Year	12	48.6	5.4	10.8	13.5	18.9	2.7	37
	13	71.7	4.4	6.5	8.7	8.7	0.0	46
	14-20	36.4	0.0	4.5	18.2	31.8	9.1	22
Total		56.1	5.5	8.1	10.8	14.9	4.7	148

rates of orgasm. The fact that those women with early ages of menses start coitus earlier and that those women with late ages begin late in college both contribute to this effect.

From this examination of these data it appears that there is no relation between age at menarche and the incidence and frequency of masturbation in high school and college. There is a slight elevation in the proportion experiencing genital petting in high school among those women with earliest menarche, but this increase is not reflected in the frequency and orgasm rate of genital petting during high school. There is some evidence that young women with early ages of menarche (eleven and under) begin coitus somewhat earlier than their peers and young women who have much older ages at menarche (fourteen and older) have much later starts in coitus. As a result, women with earlier ages at menarche have histories of more frequent coitus and in consequence report higher rates of orgasm. In all cases when differences are found they tend to be small.

From these data it would be difficult to support any of the hypotheses about the relation between menarche and sexual conduct except for the rela-

Table 14-7
Orgasm in Premarital Intercourse in College by Age at First Menses

Age at First Menses	Orgasm			
	None	Rarely/ Sometimes	Often/ Always	Number
9-11	9.1	38.6	52.3	44
12	5.7	50.9	43.4	53
13	16.3	51.2	32.6	43
14-20	25.0	36.1	38.4	36
Total	13.1	44.9	42.0	176

tively weak assertion that early menses may contribute in some minor ways to early start-up of heterosocial and heterosexual conduct. The delay in onset for those women older at menarche could be accounted for in the same way. But, the most unexpected finding, the large increase of the proportion experienced in coitus in the same group during the later years of college, seems less immediately understandable. The outlier hypothesis receives no support from these data and a strong case cannot be made for a biological argument either (particularly since the masturbation data show no differences). What is most likely is an interaction between social and biological factors with the former accounting for most of the effects found.

That these data do not support a strong connection between age at first menses and sexual behavior does not mean that such a connection could not be found either in a more sensitive design aimed specifically at this question or if similar research were conducted in a different social context for sexual learning. The data reported here suffer from being gathered for quite different purposes and because the questions asked did not target either the measures of puberty or the sexual items in such a way that the questions could be framed precisely. It is also possible that historical changes in the timing of sexual experimentation during adolescence might make the changes associated with puberty more closely related to youthful sexuality.

In recent years, age at first intercourse has declined (more dramatically for those not attending college, but somewhat for those attending college) (Chilman 1979). The closer to the age at first menses that first coitus (or other forms of sexual experimentation) comes the more influential the former will be, particularly in sociological and psychological terms. In recent data from Sweden Klackenberg-Larsen and Bjorkman (1978) report that age at first coitus for young girls in the first year of high school is now lower than that for young men. This finding is, of course, a reversal of the usual findings from the past. The reasons for this reversal appear to be threefold: intercourse has become relatively widespread among all youthful females in Sweden, eliminating the old good-girl/bad-girl distinctions (where the many stay virtuous while the minority absorb male sexual attentions); intercourse is now experienced under conditions of greater expressions of love and affection, more often expressive of young women's expectations; and young women continue to expect to have intercourse with males who are slightly older. The first two factors eliminate the phenomenon of a minority of young girls having intercourse with many males while other girls have intercourse at later ages in association with mate selection. However as the general pool of sexually active females grows both larger and younger the preference of a young woman for a slightly older partner has not changed. This latter factor will result in an absence of eligible females for young males; for example, if girls fourteen prefer boys sixteen, those thirteen, boys fifteen, with whom will the fourteen-year-old boy have intercourse? The lack of intercourse for this group could be tolerated when no one this age is having coitus but is likely to be experienced as unbearable if a majority of age-mate females are having coitus. Then the pressure for young boys to seek out girls who are in the midst of pubertal changes is very likely to ensue. In this situation the timing of the changes associated with puberty, changes that indicate sexual availability to the self and others, will begin to influence more directly the ages at early sexual participation.

These findings, then, of a limited relationship between menarche and youthful sexuality should be read noting both the limitations of the research design and the historical context in which the data were gathered. Both may serve to attenuate whatever social or biological factors might come into view when the timing of menarche and sexual experimentation are more closely linked in the research design or in historical time.

Note

1. Rossi, A. Personal communication, 1962.

References

Chilman, C. 1979. *Adolescent sexuality in a changing American society.* Washington, D.C.: DHEW Publication NIH 79-1426.
DeMartino. S.F. 1979 *Human autoerotic practices.* New York: Human Sciences Press.
Diamond, M. 1976. Human sexual development: Biological foundations for social development. In F.A. Beach, ed., *Human sexuality in four perspectives.* Baltimore: Johns Hopkins.

Gagnon, J.H. 1977. *Human sexualities.* Glenview, Ill.: Scott, Foresman.

Gagnon, J.H., and Simon, W. 1973. Sexual conduct. New York: Aldine.

Kinsey, A.C., Pomeroy, W.P., Martin, C.M., and Gebhard, P.H. 1953. *Sexual behavior in the human female.* Philadelphia: Saunders.

Klackenberg-Larsen, I. and Bjorkman, K. 1978. Tonaringars sexdebu, *Socialmedicinsk tidskrift* 5-6:333-340.

Meyer-Bahlburg, H. 1980 Sex hormone changes during puberty and sexual behavior. In J.M. Samson, ed., *Enfance et sexualite.* Montreal: Editions Etudes Vivants.

Quartararo, J.D., Gagnon, J.H., and Simon, W. Masturbation in adolescence and young adulthood. (Submitted for publication.)

Simon, W., and Gagnon, J.H. 1965. On the study of psychosexual development. Bloomington: Institute for Sex Research, 40 pp., (mimeo).

15 Menarche and Teenage Pregnancy: A Misuse of Historical Data

Vern L. Bullough

Until recently historical data on the age of menarche were probably only of interest to a few specialists. In recent years, however, it has had political and social repercussions, and this, in part, has been due to misinformation. The focus of much of the current publicity about the historical age of menarche has to do with the belief that modern U.S. girls are entering menarche at increasingly younger ages and this lowered age is a major factor in their increasing sexuality and the "growing national problem of teenage pregnancy." Stories to this effect have appeared in almost every kind of popular journal from *Newsweek* to the *Nation*, in books dealing with child development, and in both popular and semischolarly literature. A recent article in *Newsweek* (1 September 1981) is a good summary of the political implications. The article, which deals with the rising tide of sexual precocity, lays part of the explanation on the fact that the age of menarche has dropped from 17 years to 12.5 years—spawning a breed of young people whose sexual awareness outruns their emotional development. The outcome, according to *Newsweek*, is the demise of the adolescent virgin. The inevitable result is a belief that teenage pregnancy is a runaway national problem.

Quite frankly, *Newsweek* and the popular literature are wrong on every account. Teenage pregnancy is not a greater problem now than it ever has been, and menarche has dropped much less radically over the past hundred years than is supposed. In short, the publicity about teenage pregnancy is based upon poor scholarship and inaccurate statistics.

Menarche

In the United States the mean age at normal menarche is 12.3 years (some would say 12.5 or 12.6) with a range between 9 to 17 years. Age differences for menarche are attributed to general health and nutrition, heredity, psychosocial development, and a number of other factors. Pediatricians would normally do a diagnostic work up for girls who have not begun menstruating by 16 (Vaughan and McKay 1969; Kaplan 1964; Hughes 1967; Smith 1977). The broad range of menarche is important to emphasize because in the past each clinician reporting did so, with a few exceptions, on the basis of a very small sample—and any historical data can be skewed because of this factor. The informed guesses and best estimates of the past can be tested against the age of mothers at first pregnancy, marriage date, and other factors that traditionally have been dependent upon menarche.

Roman law, for example, assumed that females were mature at the age of twelve, and the classical writers who examined menarche put it as taking place somewhere between twelve and fourteen (Hopkins, 1964-1965), not too different from modern authorities. Medieval authorities tended to agree, although much of our information comes from the later Middle Ages. One of the best indicators of medieval assumptions is in the gynecological text, *De passionibus mulierum*, attributed to Dame Trotula, extant copies of which date from the thirteenth century. There are numerous copies of the English provenance, eighteen at Oxford alone. Twelve of the English manuscripts include tables on menarche, and the ages appear to vary according to the scribe's personal knowledge. Most of the Oxford copies put the beginning of menstruation at age fourteen, although a minority put it at thirteen (Post 1971). Other medieval writers set the age of menarche with the same range, thirteen or fourteen (Bullough and Campbell 1980). In Islamic countries, it was a criminal act to have sex with a woman before she had menstruated. Marriage also could not be consummated. In fact the Arabic term *nikah* used for marriage literally means sexual intercourse. Before marriage and intercourse could happen, women were to examine the girl to see that she was physically prepared. Arabic law set a range of ages between twelve and thirteen for this. (Koran II; abu-Bakr 1957; Levy 1957.)

Some of the nineteenth- and early twentieth-century data puts menarche slightly later than classical or medieval authorities. J. Whitehead writing in the 1840s put the age of menarche for Manchester working women at 15 years and 7 months while the age for "educated ladies" was 14 years and 6 months (Whitehead 1847). E.W. Murphy reported that obstetric patients in University College Hospital, London, had begun menstruating at 14 years and 4 months in 1830 while Rigden in 1855 estimated their age as 15 years and 5 months (Murphy 1844; Rigden 1869). Menarche for London middle-class women was set at 15 years in 1880 by another observer (Giles 1901). Scottish women in 1980 ranged between 15.5 and 16.5 with upper class having a lower age than lower class (Duncan 1871). In Germany menarche in 1869 was estimated to begin at 15 years and 7 months (Ploss, Bartels, and Bartels 1936). U.S. women, however, seemed consistently to begin menstruation earlier than European, perhaps because of better nutrition. Edward B. Foote, the author of the best-selling home medical manual in the last part of the nineteenth century, set the age of menarche as between 12 and 14 and most U.S. authorities followed suit (Foote 1871). Statistical data gathered in 1905 led one authority to set menarche at 14 as the average age,

(Mills 1937; Mills 1950) while another set it at 15 years and 7 months (Fluhmann 1956). Those girls who menstruated before 12.5 were considered precocious (Harris 1871).

Where then does the age of seventeen become established as the age of menarche in the nineteenth century. The source of this statement turns out to be one of the major authorities on physical development, J.M. Tanner, who in this instance was not particularly careful in checking his data or in qualifying his statements. In 1962, Tanner wrote that the "age at menarche has been getting earlier by some 4 months per decade in Western Europe over the period 1830-1960." (Tanner 1962, p. 152.) Tanner uses a figure to

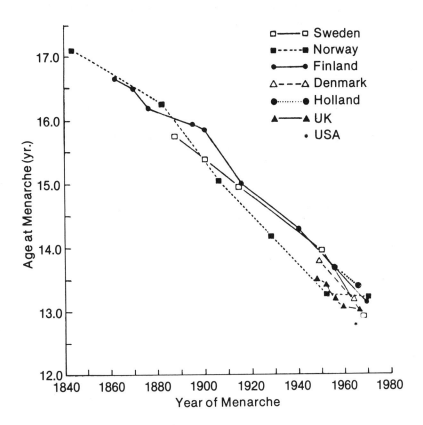

Source: Diagram in P.B. Eveleth and J.M. Tanner, *Worldwide variation in human growth* (Cambridge University Press, Cambridge, England, 1976), figure 168(a), page 218. Reproduced by permission of the publisher. Many slight variations of this diagram have been published.

Figure 15-1. Trend toward Earlier Median Age of Menarche in Europe from 1840 to 1970

illustrate this statement but a close reading both of the graph and of his data indicates that this reasoning is not the case. Instead, Tanner's data demonstrate that the average of menarche in Europe in the nineteenth century as reported in his sources, some of whom are mentioned above, was between 14 and 15. Only one of his sources reports menarche at 17, and this source is for Norway in 1844 (Backman 1948). Elsewhere he reports that Norwegian girls in 1950 began menstruating at 13.5 years (Tanner 1973). Apparently he uses the Norwegian data and ties it in with the U.S. data where menarche begins, as indicated above, at an average of 12.3 years. The Norwegian data, however, cannot be so utilized since there is still a disparity between U.S. women and Norwegian women. Some of Tanner's figures from Finland also put the age of menarche at 16 but there is only the one isolated piece of data setting menarche anywhere at 17. Tanner apparently recognizes his own difficulty but then relies upon G. Backman and other Scandinavian data to argue for the rather radical drop in the age of menarche when neither his English nor any U.S. data support this kind of statement. In plotting his graph, Tanner entirely ignores the non-Scandinavian data for the nineteenth century (see figure 15-1). It might well be that Tanner emphasized 17 in his menarche table because earlier he discusses changes in height and weight and used the age of 17 for this particular graph. It is also possible that he carried the same mindset over into his graph on menarche. Whatever the reason, Tanner has solidified into the literature the age of 17 for menarche in the nineteenth century with only one isolated report to support such an age. One case that goes against the other recorded data falls within the normal range but rather than regarding it as part of a range Tanner compounded the difficulty by using it as an average. Undoubtedly there has been a drop in menarche in the United States from about 14 or 15 in the nineteenth century to under 13 in the 1980s but how much of a drop is debatable since so many variables are present (Frisch 1978). Moreover, recent research has found that Tanner's data for Norway is also wrong (Brudevoll, Liestøl, and Walløe 1979).

Unfortunately the erroneous conceptions about menarche fitted well into assumptions about teenage pregnancy, since lowering the age of menarche would likely increase teenage pregnancy. This hypothesis is also erroneous. It is true that teenage pregnancy has increased in the last thirty years but the increase is entirely due to the increase in the number of teenagers. For example, there were 6.6 million women between fifteen and nineteen in 1960 and 10.4 million in 1976. Pregnancy rates per teenager, however, have fallen from a peak reached in 1960. The rate in 1960 was 89.1 births per thousand women between fifteen and nineteen years of age; in 1976 the rate had dropped to 53.5, a 40-percent reduction. Since, however, birth rates of children to women over twenty have dropped even more precipitously, the total percentage of teenage births has increased from

14 percent of all births in 1960 to 18 percent in 1976.[1] There is also one major difference between teenage births in 1960 and those today and that difference is the decline in the marriage rate among teenagers. In 1960 teenage brides accounted for 48 percent of all first marriages compared to 38 percent in 1976 (Millman & Mosher 1980). By implication more babies born to teenagers today are born out of wedlock than in the past. More positively there are simply fewer forced marriages.

Conclusion

What seems obvious is that the popular media and some semischolarly analysts have jumped on teenage pregnancy as a major problem in our society. I do not deny that it is a problem. It is, however, no more or less a problem now than in the past, and though there is some age drop in menarche it is debatable how much this drop has caused teenagers to be more sexually precocious now than in the past. Though there seems to be no change in sexual activity of adolescent boys, there has been some in adolescent girls—in part because they no longer marry so young and in part because there has been a lessening of the double standard. Overall, however, it seems that teenagers of today are acting no less responsibly in the field of sex than their parents were when they were in their teens. To imply otherwise is to distort the data, which unfortunately is what has happened.

Note

1. I realize that pregnancy and births are not always the same thing. The difficulty is that the birth figures are reliable and the pregnancy ones are not. We are not certain of the number of abortions in 1960 and estimates vary. I would also argue that the data about pregnancy until at least the middle of the 1970s is also debatable.

References

Backman, G. 1948. Die beshleunigte Entwocklung der Jugend. Verfrühte Menarche, verspätete Menopause, verlängerte Lebensdauer. *Acta Anatomica* 4:421-480.

abu-Bakr, A. 1957. *The hedaya or guide: A commentary on Mussulman laws,* Charles Hamilton, ed. West Pakistan: Premier Books House.

Brudevoll, J.E., Liestøl, K., and Walløe, L. 1979. Menarcheal age in Oslo during the last 140 years. *Annals of Human Biology* 6:407-416.

Bullough, V.L. 1981. Age of menarche: A misunderstanding. *Science* 213:365-366.

Bullough, V.L., and Campbell, C. 1980. Female longevity and diet in the Middle Ages. *Speculum* 55:317-325.

Duncan, J.M. 1871. *Fecundity, fertility, sterility and allied topics.* Edinburgh: Adam and Charles Black.

Fluchmann, C.F. 1956. *The management of menstrual disorders.* Philadelphia: Saunders.

Foote, E.B. 1871. Plain home talk . . . *embracing medical common sense.* New York: Wells and Company.

Frisch, R.E. 1978. Population, food intake, and fertility. *Science* 199:22-30.

Giles, A.E. 1901. The factors which lead to variations in the age of puberty and the clinical characteristics of menstruation. *Medical Chronicle* 34:161-179; 254-264.

Harris, R.P. 1871. *American Journal of Obstetrics* 3:611.

Hopkins, M.K. 1964. The age of Roman girls at marriage. *Population Studies* 1964-1965, 18:309-327.

Hughes, J.G. 1967. *Synopsis of pediatrics.* St. Louis: C.V. Mosby.

Kaplan, S. 1964. *Growth disorders in children and adolescents.* Springfield, Ill.: Charles C. Thomas.

Koran. Many editions. The book is broken down into surahs. The references come from the second surah, known as the Cow.

Levy, R. 1957. *The social structure of Islam.* Cambridge, Eng.: Cambridge University Press.

Millman, S. and Mosher, W.D. 1980. *Advance data from vital and health statistics.* HHS Publication No. 1 (PHS), 80-1250.

Mills, C.A. 1937. Geographic and time variations in body growth and age at menarche. *Human Biology* 9:43-56.

———. 1950. Temperature influence over human growth and development. *Human Biology* 22:71-74.

Murphy, E.W. 1844. *A report on the obstetric practice of University College Hospital.* London: *Dublin J. Medical Science* 26:177-229.

Newsweek. 1 September 1980, p. 51.

Ploss, H., Bartels, M., and Bartels, P. 1936. *Woman: An historical gynecological and anthropological compendium,* E.J. Dingwall, ed. St. Louis: C.V. Mosby.

Post, J.B. 1971. Ages at menarche and menopause: Some medieval authorities. *Population Studies* 25:83-87.

Rigden, W. 1869. On the age at which menstruation commences. *Transactions of the Obstetrical Society of London* 11:243.

Smith, D.W. 1977. *Growth and its disorders.* Philadelphia: W.B. Saunders.

Tanner, J.M. 1962. *Growth at adolescence.* 2d ed. Oxford: Blackwell.

_____ . 1973. Growing up. *Scientific American* 229:43.

Trotula. 1940. *The diseases of women.* Elizabeth Mason-Hohl, ed. Los Angeles: Ward Ritchey Press.

Vaughan, V.C., and McKay, R.J. 1969. *Nelson textbook of pediatrics.* 10th ed. Philadelphia: W.B. Saunders.

Whitehead, J. 1847. *On the causes and treatment of abortion and sterility.* London: Church.

16 Menarche and Adolescent Pregnancy

Phyllis C. Leppert

More than one in ten teenagers become pregnant each year and that ratio is predicted to rise to one in four, primarily because of an increase in the number of teenagers in the population and the increase in the number of sexually active teenagers. In 1978, 1,100,000 adolescents became pregnant (Guttmacher Institute 1981). Of these, 434,000 ended in abortion, 362,000 resulted in births conceived out of wedlock, and 192,000 of the pregnancies ended in births conceived after marriage (Guttmacher Institute 1981). The remaining pregnancies ended in miscarriage. These pregnancies occurred in all regions of the United States and among all socioeconomic groups.

Focusing on girls under the age of fifteen, between 1973 and 1978, there were thirty thousand pregnancies in the United States. These are the teenagers who are most at risk for pregnancy complications such as low-birth-weight infants, pregnancy-induced hypertension, and iron-deficiency anemia. These young girls, most apt to be the closest in year interval from menarche, are truly children having children. Infants born to these mothers are much more likely to die in the first year of life (American College of Obstetricians and Gynecologists 1979).

Obviously, in addition to the health hazards, the most distressing consequence of adolescent pregnancy is the interruption of education that results in a vicious cycle of limited opportunity to learn marketable skills, to compete in society, inability to get good jobs, low family income, poverty, and more pregnancies. All these side effects hurt the children of teenage parents. These children are more apt to have lower IQ and achievement scores than children of parents in their twenties and thirties, and when they become adults they are more likely than others to become teenage parents themselves (Elster and McAnarney 1980).

While the overall adolescent pregnancy rate has been rising at a slower rate than the adolescent sexual-activity rate because of greater and more successful use of contraception among teenagers, more than one-fifth of first pregnancies in adolescents occurred in the first month after initial sexual intercourse. Fifty percent of pregnancies occur in the first six months of sexual activity. National figures are not available as to the percentage of boys and girls under thirteen who are sexually active. However, 18 percent of boys and 6 percent of girls aged thirteen to fourteen have had intercourse (Guttmacher Institute 1981). A survey conducted of 408 females in a tempo-

rary detention home in New York City cited the mean age of initial intercourse to be twelve years (Hein 1978). It is this group of younger teenagers
who are more likely to become pregnant during the first months of sexual
exposure. They are the least likely of all teenagers to use adequate contraception. Therefore, decreased fertility following menarche due to
anovulatory cycles is eliminated by the fact that these young girls have not
sought contraceptive information or used contraception.

The Washington Heights community that surrounds Columbia-Presbyterian Medical Center is a community that has changed radically over the
past fifteen years. A stable, middle-income community has become a
younger, poorer, highly mobile, multiethnic community. Adolescents in the
community are experiencing pregnancy rates 50 percent higher than the national averages (Jones, Rothenberg and Philliber 1981). Columbia-
Presbyterian Medical Center and The Department of Obstetrics and
Gynecology provide a Young Parents Program for pregnant adolescents
planning to give birth to their infants and a Young Adult Clinic for family
planning and ambulatory gynecology. These programs have been in existence for several years and now cooperate with a newly formed Division of
Adolescent Medicine in the Department of Pediatrics. During the first nine
months of 1980 a total of 4,251 visits were made by teenagers to the Young
Adult Clinic for contraception, and from September 1980 to April 1981,
305 pregnant teenagers were enrolled in the Young Parents Program.

A survey was conducted during April 1981 to ascertain the gynecological age at first pregnancy of young women enrolled in the Adolescent
Pregnancy Program. This number reflects the interval between onset of
menses and the first pregnancy. The smaller the gynecological age the
higher the risk of poor pregnancy outcome. Forty adolescents aged 15 to 21,
median age 16 years, who attend the Adolescent Pregnancy Program were
surveyed (see table 16-1). Ten percent of the group were delivered or were
expected to deliver within 1 year of menarche. Fifteen percent of the group
were or were expected to be 1.5 years beyond menarche at the time of their
first delivery. This 15 percent represents young women who conceived three
to nine months after their menarche, or had gynecological ages less than 1
year at the time of conception. The median age of menarche in the survey
was 12.2 years (range 9 to 16 years). Of those who conceived three to nine
months after menarche the median age of first menses was slightly older or
13 years (range 12 to 15 years). None of the young teenagers who had
menarche at age 9 or 10 had a pregnancy within one year. The median interval for first pregnancy in this group of seven was 6 years (range 3 to 8
years). While this group had used some contraception the survey did not
provide detailed information as to effectiveness of use. Although this sample is small the survey supports the nationwide statistics revealing that a
considerable number of younger adolescents become pregnant.

Table 16-1

Gynecological Age (Menarche to First Pregnancy) in Forty Patients Seen in April 1981 in the Young Parents Program at Columbia Presbyterian Medical Center

(aged thirteen to twenty-one)

Age of Menarche	Age of First Pregnancy				
	13 or Younger	*13-14*	*15-16*	*17-18*	*19 or Older*
9-10		2	5	1	1
11-12		3	8	1	2
12-13	1	3	2	3	3
14 or older			3	2	

Data obtained in 1980 from the Young Adult Family Planning Program at Columbia-Presbyterian Medical Center demonstrate that the 442 new patients who had never used contraception prior to their first visit had a median interval of nine months from first intercourse to first visit to the clinic. Twenty-five percent of this group had waited two years or longer after initial intercourse to seek contraception. Of the 4,251 visits by teenagers in the first nine months of 1980, 361 were by girls fifteen years old or younger (see table 16-2). Forty-eight or 13 percent of these young girls were found to be pregnant on their second visit to the clinic. The majority of these were unintended pregnancies, although a few were using contraceptives.

Teenagers, especially the very young teenagers, tend to repeat pregnancies during adolescence. From 1977 to 1980, 54 percent or 2,123 of new patients to the Young Adult Clinic had been pregnant at least once prior to coming to the clinic; 10 percent of those who had been pregnant had had two or more live births and 5 percent had had two or more abortions, while 13 percent had had both live births and abortions. (See table 16-3.)

Table 16-2

Age of New Patients at First Visit to Young Adult Family Planning Clinic, October 1977-September 1980

Age	*Total Number*	*Percent*
15 or younger	591	14%
16-17	1182	28%
18-19	1320	32%
20 or older	1087	26%

Source: Adapted from the Adolescent Reproductive Health Care Program, A Three-Year Report, Center for Population and Family Health, Columbia University.

Table 16-3
Pregnancy Histories of the New Female Patients

Ever Pregnant	Number	Percent
Yes	2123	54%
No	1804	46%
Of those who had been pregnant		
One live birth only	725	34%
One abortion only	534	25%
One live birth and one abortion	279	13%
Two or more live births only	201	10%
Two or more abortions only	97	5%
Live birth and abortion	277	13%

With teenagers, especially the younger teenagers, it becomes apparent that teaching contraceptive information alone is not adequate education in sexuality. Many young girls either subconsciously wish to become pregnant or, as may often be the case, they are not yet intellectually developed enough to reason abstractly and plan for contingencies, or they take risks and do not use contraceptives because they believe nothing will happen to them as individuals. Some believe a baby will provide them with love.

At Columbia-Presbyterian Medical Center a study of clinic visits revealed that the younger teenager was more apt to come to the evening clinics and to be referred by friends. Referrals from health professionals and teachers were less common in the teenager under fifteen years of age.

Recently, a community teenage-education and outreach program has been initiated using same age peers as the educators in an effort to reach more young people. The Young Parents Program has successfully demonstrated since 1969, as have other similar programs across the nation, that when comprehensive obstetric services are offered to pregnant adolescents their reproductive outcome is similar to that of women in their twenties. The low-birth-weight babies and toxemia rates are reduced to a minimum. The unfinished business, however, is that the social consequences to the teenager and the detrimental consequences to the offspring of teenage parents have not been reduced to the lowest level possible. Thus, it becomes necessary to examine the age at which teenagers are educated about reproduction, family life, and contraception, including the teaching of responsible sexuality. Apparently the teenager is being reached too late; education should start at menarche or before and facts are not enough. The idea of teenagers working with younger teenagers has potential. However, adults, especially adults who are not the teenager's parents, but rather other relatives or friends, also can help adolescents to understand and accept their sexuality and to deal with it responsibly. Teenagers do take risks, challenge parents, tend not to think of the consequences. They are also very idealistic people who tend to have stable relationships with their sexual partners. Perhaps sex-education programs need to appeal to that idealism.

References

American College of Obstetricians and Gynecologists. 1979. *Adolescent prenatal health: A guidebook for services*. Chicago: American College of Obstetricians and Gynecologists.

Elster, A., and McAnarney, E.R. 1980. Medical and psychosocial risks of pregnancy and childbearing during adolescence. *Pediatric Annals* 9:11.

Guttmacher Institute. 1981. *Teenage pregnancy: The problem that hasn't gone away*. New York: Alan Guttmacher Institute.

Hein, K. 1978. Age at first intercourse among homeless adolescent females. *Journal of Pediatrics* 93:147.

Jones, J., Rothenberg, P.R., and Philliber, S.G. 1981. *The adolescent reproductive health program: A three-year report*. New York: Center for Population and Family Health, Columbia University.

Part V
Menarche as Portrayed
in Literature

Introduction to Part V

Menarche has been said to be almost absent in literature (Delaney, Lupton, and Tooth 1976). However, there have been a few scattered descriptions: first, by such French nineteenth-century authors as Emile Zola and Edmond de Goncourt, and, more recently, in the work of U.S. writers. Elizabeth Kincaid-Ehlers is quick to point out that heretofore women's lives in general have not been well described. Perhaps this omission is because of the under-representation of women writers; perhaps it is because of menstrual taboos. Certainly there is a notable lack of reference to menstruation in most books. And, if menarche is an important part of a woman's life, one cannot help but reflect on its omission in the books we read.

In this chapter Kincaid-Ehlers discusses the taboos and silence that have kept menarche out of literature until relatively recently. She describes the negative, sometimes mystical, presentation of menstruation by men. She speculates about some of the codes or literary euphemisms for menstruation, such as *the blush*, and *headaches*. And she concludes that in the recent, women-created literature, we have moved from taboo and secrecy to openness and even the possibility of celebration.

References

Delaney, J., Lupton, M.J., and Toth, E. 1976. *The curse: A cultural history of menstruation*. New York: Dutton.

17

"Oh dear me! Why weren't we all boys, then there wouldn't be any bother": Menarche and Popular American Fiction

Elizabeth Kincaid-Ehlers

In 1977, in *The Women's Room*, Marilyn French unmasked the disguised lives of numberless U.S. women. Working through the process of the life of one woman in a transitional generation, detailing other female lives that touched upon the central one, French broke the silence, speaking the unspeakables. One of these unspeakables has always been the female cycle of menarche, menstruation, and menopause. The surrounds of silence, embarrassment, and shame indicate the presence of an incredibly strong taboo. Currently women are engaged in a communal effort to break free from stunting restraints, including taboos. Anthropologists, psychologists, biologists, literary specialists—we try to locate causes and publish them to produce change. Literature reflects as well as illuminates life. Creative writers, who are more sensitive and more perceptive about our shared human experience, offer imaginative re-creations of that experience that can serve as models, as representatives of what we have been and what we are becoming.

Mira, Marilyn French's central character, knows that her parents (and thus society, culture, history) lie to her. "She asked her mother about an ad in magazines, and her mother said she did not know what sanitary napkins were. She asked her mother what *fuck* meant; she had heard it at the schoolyard. Her mother said she did not know, but later, Mira heard her whisper to Mrs. Marsh, 'How can you tell a child a thing like that?' "[1]

> At the end of her fourteenth year, Mira began to menstruate and was finally let in on the secret of sanitary napkins. Soon afterward, she began to experience strange fluidities in her body, and her mind, she was convinced, had begun to rot. She could feel the increasing corruption, but couldn't seem to do anything to counter it. . . . images rampaged through her head. These images were always, horrifyingly, of the same things. She had a code word for the decaying condition: she called it *boys* (French 1977, pp. 25, 26).

Mira looks around and sees that everybody despises boys: at home and at school they are "troublesome," always "fighting and showing off and mak-

205

ing noise." But boys turn into men, and everyone admires men. Men stride "purposefully to the center of the stage" and take up "the whole surface of every scene" (French 1977, p. 27). Mira realizes that her desire to be like "Bach and Mozart and Beethoven and Shakespeare and Thomas E. Dewey" is "somehow inappropriate" (French 1977, p. 28). Thus begins for Mira the painful, heretofore inevitable split of personality that is built into the process of growing up female in the United States.

A new kind of consciousness comes to girls at menarche, one that contains a heightened awareness both of the realities of the world out there and of the discrepancy between female internal drives and the possibilities of their external realization. This new consciousness is linked with a self-conscious sexuality. The self and the world become terrifying at once. Nothing is what we had thought it to be. Tragically, and typically, a girl has no place to look for help. She doesn't know where her terrible confusion originates and cannot begin to ask the questions that would earn her the grail of understanding. Even if she could, by some witch-given fairy-godmother power, form language into a perfect instrument for grace, her heroics would be futile: the world would respond, as it always has done, with silence, lies, evasions, and punishment.

Literature begins as a part of the world out there, becoming a part of our internal world only through the creative process of imaginative and responsive reading. Caught in the confusions commencing with menarche, one could, ideally, look to literature to function as an agent for clarity—and even sanity. Mira, as French writes,

> turned to literature. She looked for books about adolescents, books she could find herself and her problems in. There were none. She read every thin, saccharine "girl's book" she could find, and gave up. She began to read trashy novels, anything she could find in the library that looked as if it were about women. She swallowed them whole. She read, without making distinctions among them, Jane Austen and Fanny Burney and George Eliot and Gothic novels of all sorts, Daphne de Maurier and Somerset Maugham and Frank Yerby and John O'Hara, along with hundreds of nameless mystery tales, love stories, and adventures. But nothing helped. Like the person who gets fat because they eat unnourishing foods and so is always hungry and so is always eating, she drowned in words that could not teach her to swim (French 1977, p. 29).

American literature simply does not reflect female experience. Not surprisingly, what we know about initiation into maturity we know from male writing about male experience. Being a child in American literature is largely a matter of being a boy: growing up in American literature is growing up male. In life, we are indoctrinated in complex ways to believe that our transformation from girl to woman occurs at the moment the first drop of menstrual blood incarnadines our once pure and innocent white pants. Even if we were to grant that being a woman is merely, or even mostly, a matter of being a body in a state of potential fertility—an identity we emphatically reject—we would find that our literature has reflected that moment in silence. Its rare incarnations occur either in codes and torturous symbolic disguises, or in situations reflecting associations with sickness, disease, sin, guilt, dirt, evil, odor, avoidance, denial, negation, humiliation, and shame.

In life, the state of being a man is defined in terms of certain kinds and qualities of action. American literature copiously narrates the process by which boys operate on their own experience to arrive at manhood. Male terminologies associate the process with the heroic—the true, the good, the brave. William Faulkner, one of our acknowledged great writers, concerned himself in major work after major work with the process of growing-up male. In *Go Down, Moses*, 1940, young Isaac McCaslin, descendant and heir of the great men who crossed the barrier mountains and subdued the land, goes hunting with his mentor, the mixed-breed Sam Fathers. They wait in the stand, patiently. At last, the buck appears.

> "Now," Sam Fathers said, "shoot quick, and slow." The boy did not remember that shot at all. . . . He didn't even remember what he did with the gun afterward. He was running. Then he was standing over the buck. . . . with Sam Fathers beside him again, extending the knife. "Don't walk up to him in front," Sam said. "If he ain't dead, he will cut you all to pieces with his feet. Walk up to him from behind and take him by the horn first, so you hold his head down until you can jump away. Then slip your other hand down and hook your fingers in his nostrils."
>
> The boy did that—drew the head back and the throat taut and drew Sam Fathers' knife across the throat and Sam stooped and dipped his hands in the hot smoking blood and wiped them back and forth across the boy's face. . . . then the men, the true hunters—Walter Ewell whose rifle never missed, and Major de Spain and old General Compson and the boy's cousin, McCaslin Edmonds,. . . . sitting their horses and looking down at them: at the old man of seventy. . . . and the white boy of twelve with the prints of the bloody hands on his face, who had nothing to do now but stand straight and not let the trembling show.
>
> "Did he do all right, Sam?" his cousin McCaslin said.
>
> "He done all right," Sam Fathers said.[2]

Notice how marking the boy's face with blood is central to this ceremony of initiation into manhood. What are the ceremonies for initiation into womanhood? Anthropologists and historians can tell of other cultures that did and do incorporate ceremony into a process of initiation into womanhood; for instance, enforced seclusion, the isolated menstrual hut, the special dance, however they may have become perverted or degraded, did give public recognition to a significant event in a girl's transformation process. One remnant of what might possibly have been an ancient ceremony survives in certain eastern European traditions and is also reported in some contemporary Jewish mores. In this tradition, when a girl reports that she has entered menarche, her mother slaps her face. This phenomenon fascinates, on a number of counts. Metaphorically, it enacts perfectly the traditional psychological experience associated with menarche, which functions as the consciousness-raiser, the great slap-in-the-face that ends the girl child's innocent dreams. Physically, this slap quite literally brings blood to the face, calling attention to the blood's presence and insisting upon it. This physical, literal level of experience is so striking that it almost demands a symbolic accounting. Surely there is a link between the blood-bringing slap to the girl's face and the ritual face-blooding of Faulkner's boy's initiation.

Possibly this concordance of blood's coming to the face, or showing in the face, reveals a code for menarche in earlier American literature. On the explicit level, menarche, or menstruation, has no existence there. Even in works by women about women these body functions remain part of the pervasive silence about women's lives and stories. However, another seemingly unrelated phenomenon about women recurs insistently and in increasingly fascinating relationship to other behaviors and perceptions. This other phenomenon, itself a sudden rush of blood to the face, is *the blush*. Menarche, initiation into adulthood, and blushing are associated. Literary blushing became epidemic during the nineteenth century: to investigate its contexts there, we can begin with what has been our longest-lasting favorite book about growing-up female in the United States—*Little Women*.

The phrase that begins the title of this chapter is uttered in exasperation by the adolescent female more loved by more of us than any other ever—Jo March. "Oh, dear me! Why weren't we all boys, then there wouldn't be any bother" (Alcott 1962, p. 228). Jo's exasperation arises from her sister Meg's increasing preoccupation with John Brooke, the male intruder threatening the bonds of sisterhood. Meg has become sexually conscious: Jo has not. When Jo goes to New York, partly to make her own way, but also partly to escape complication, "'Are these your only reasons for this sudden fancy?'" asks her mother. "'No, Mother.' 'May I know the others?' Jo looked down, then said slowly, with sudden color in her cheeks, 'It may be vain and wrong to say it, but—I'm afraid—Laurie is getting too fond of me.'" Jo's sexual consciousness is rising. When Jo is going back home and invites Professor Friedrich Bhaer to visit to attend Laurie's commencement, we get the following passage:

> Jo looked up then, quite unconscious of anything but her own pleasure in the prospect of showing them to one another. Something in Mr. Bhaer's face suddenly recalled the fact that she might find Laurie more than "a best friend," and simply because she particularly wished not to look as if

anything was the matter, she involuntarily began to blush, and the more she tried not to, the redder she grew (Alcott 1962, p. 396).

Jo's blushing relates to menarcheal self-conscious sexuality. When Professor Bhaer comes, these two meet, ostensibly accidentally, in town, in the rain. Mr. Bhaer says, "politely, 'You haf no umbrella. May I go also, and take for you the bundles?' 'Yes, thank you.' Jo's cheeks were as red as her ribbon. . . . Her bonnet wasn't big enough to hide her face, and she feared he might think the joy it betrayed unmaidenly" (Alcott 1962, p. 519). She shops in confusion, while he stands by, equally confused, "watching her blush and blunder" (Alcott 1962, p. 521). As Alcott says, "Mr. Bhaer could read several languages, but he had not learned to read women yet" (Alcott 1962, p. 520). Only when Jo cries does Friedrich read the signal correctly and propose.

This kind of blush signals sexual awakening and functions as a simulacrum of menarche and/or menstruation. The silence surrounding our body cycle in literature and in life has deeper, more complex causes than can be explained by literary, or even genteel, conventions. Writers felt they couldn't discuss this crux in a woman's life—it was simply not to be talked about, mentioned, alluded to. But women know how crucial menarche in fact is; inevitably, they have developed a code to mark the event in their literature.

Other codes suggest themselves as well. For instance, consider all the women in novels who lie down with headaches. The damp cloth goes on the head to draw the heat off the blood; headache may be a literary marker for menstruation, with the locus of the show of blood again displaced to the head. The camphor or vinegar-soaked cloths compressing the blood-filled foreheads of my childhood come back, and I wonder if they weren't bleaching the blood in some way we have not yet explained. Or consider the literary (and literal) preference for fair skin and blondness: all those fair good women and dark bad ones. The conflict between the supposed sexiness of blondes and their opposing, perhaps even bleached, symbolic bloodlessness typifies the confusion of the whole subject.

Such male writers as mention menstruation at all, tend to use the tropes of sickness, or absence and negation, and to view the menses solely as they thwart the gratification of their own immediate sexual desires. Probably knowing nothing about menarche, they do not deal with it at all. How could they learn about what cannnot be mentioned? Nothing in literature has enriched boys' experience of girls and women in the way that it has expanded our experience of them. For instance, we know about deflowering virgins from the male perspective and first visits to whorehouses from the john's point of view—all these are part of the male process of sexual self-awareness and initiation. What could boys learn about us from our point of view? As Miller Williams admits, in a cocky poem called "Getting Experience," he lacked even rudimentary information. In his first real job as delivery boy for Jarman's drugstore

> *a cloudy woman with pentecostal hair*
>
> *softly asked for sanitary napkins.*
> *She brought the Kleenex back unwrapped in twenty minutes.*
>
> *Shame said Mr. Jarman, we shouldn't make a joke*
> *of that and made me say I'm sorry and fired me.*
>
> *When I found out what the woman wanted*
> *I had to say I did what everyone said I did.*
>
> *That or let them know I hadn't heard of Kotex.*
> *Better be thought bad than known for stupid.*[3]

In her 1943 novel about growing up Irish, female, and poor in the city in the early twentieth century—*A Tree Grows in Brooklyn*—Betty Smith made real progress, dealing directly with Francie Nolan's first period and with the accompanying sexual awareness as well. In her thirteenth year, Francie writes in her diary: "Sept. 24. Tonight when I took a bath, I discovered that I was changing into a woman. It's about time" (Smith 1943, p. 222). Immediately following this passage, Smith describes the ways in which kids in the Williamsburg section of Brooklyn learn about sex. That chapter is followed by the famous scene in which the perverted child murderer attacks Francie in the hall, managing to touch her leg with what she describes as his "wormy white exposed part," before her mother, Katie, shoots him in that very place. When he falls, blood is "all over that part of him that had been worm white" (Smith 1943, p. 230).

Francie's menarche actually commences directly after a scene in which neighborhood women stone Joanna, a young girl who is pushing her illegitimate baby in its carriage. Katie had told Francie earlier: "Let Joanna be a lesson to you" (Smith 1943, p. 208). So Francie does not smile at Joanna and doesn't try to stop the women from throwing stones at her, in what I begin to recognize is a counterceremony, or anticeremony. When one stone hits the tiny baby girl's forehead and draws blood—now what shall we do with this image of a sudden rush of blood to the infant face?—Francie suffers a terrible guilt and waves of hurt. She curls up in the cellar, "in the darkest corner," and tries to figure out the lesson of Joanna.

> The waves had almost stopped passing over Francie when she discovered to her fright that something was wrong with her. She pressed her hand over her heart trying to feel a jagged edge under the flesh. She had heard papa

sing so many songs about the heart; the heart that was breaking—was aching—was dancing—was heavy laden—that leaped for joy—that was heavy in sorrow—that turned over—that stood still. She really believed that the heart actually did those things. She was terrified thinking her heart had broken inside her over Joanna's baby and that the blood was now leaving her heart and flowing from her body.

She went upstairs to the flat and looked into the mirror. Her eyes had dark shadows beneath them and her head was aching. She lay on the old leather couch in the kitchen and waited for Mama to come home.

She told Mama what had happened to her in the cellar. She said nothing about Joanna. Katie sighed and said, "so soon? You're just thirteen. I didn't think it would come for another year yet. I was fifteen."

"Then . . . then . . . this is all right what's happening?"

"It's a natural thing that comes to all women."

"I'm not a woman."

"It means you're changing from a girl into a woman."

"Do you think it will go away?"

"In a few days. But it will come back again in a month."

"For how long."

"For a long time. Until you are forty or even fifty." She mused awhile. "My mother was fifty when I was born."

"Oh, it has something to do with having babies."

"Yes. Remember always to be a good girl because you can have a baby now." Joanna and her baby flashed through Francie's mind. "You mustn't let the boys kiss you," said Mama.

"Is that how you get a baby?"

"No. But what makes you get a baby often starts with a kiss." She added, "Remember Joanna."

Now Katie didn't know about the street scene. Joanna happened to pop into her mind. But Francie thought she had wonderful powers of insight. She looked at Mama with new respect.[4]

Francie remembers most clearly the terrible lesson of the counterceremony, the celebration of destruction rather than creation: menarche, sexual awareness, and the gender-specific psychic split again have occurred simultaneously.

Remember Joanna. Remember Joanna. Francie could never forget her. From that time on, remembering the stoning women, she hated women. She feared them for their devious ways, she mistrusted their instincts. She began to hate them for this disloyalty and their cruelty to each other. Of all the stone-throwers, not one had dared to speak a word for the girl for fear that she would be tarred with Joanna's brush . . . Most women had one thing in common: they had great pain when they gave birth to their children. This should make a bond that held them all together; it should make them love and protect each other against the man-world. But it was not so. It seemed like their great birth pains shrank their hearts and their souls. They stuck together for only one thing: to trample on some other woman . . . Men were different. They might hate each other but they stuck together against the world and against any woman who would ensnare one of them.

Francie opened the copybook she used for a diary. She skipped a line under the paragraph that she had written about intolerance and wrote:

"As long as I live, I will never have a woman for a friend. I will never trust any woman again, except maybe mama and sometimes Aunt Evy and Aunt Sissy" (Smith 1943, pp. 213-214).

Toni Morrison, writing almost thirty years later, in *The Bluest Eye*, about growing up black and female and poor in a small midwestern city, deals with Pecola's first period early in the book. Pecola, temporarily a ward of the county, is staying with Claudia, aged nine, and Frieda, aged ten. She is about Frieda's age, or a little older. Claudia is the point-of-view character, the "I" of the first person part of the narrative. Their mother has been haranguing about the amount of milk that is disappearing—Pecola is a totally deprived child—and the three girls are making themselves scarce on the porch steps.

Suddenly Pecola bolted straight up, her eyes wide with terror. A whinnying sound came from her mouth.

"What's the matter with *you*?" Frieda stood up too. Then we both looked where Pecola was staring. Blood was running down her legs. Some drops were on the steps. I leaped up. "Hey. You cut yourself? Look. It's all over your dress."

A brownish-red stain discolored the back of her dress. She kept whinnying, standing with her legs far apart.

Frieda said, "O Lordy! I know. I know what that is!" "What?" Pecola's fingers went to her mouth.

"That's ministratin.'"

"What's that?"

"You know."

"Am I going to die?"

"Noooo. You won't die. It just means you can have a baby!"

Pecola was crying. "What you crying for? Does it hurt?"

She shook her head.

"Then stop slinging snot."

Frieda opened the back door. She had something tucked in her blouse. She looked at me in amazement and pointed to the jar. "What's that supposed to do?"

"You told me. You *said* get some water."

"Not a little old jar full. Lots of water. To scrub the steps with, dumbbell!"

Here was something important, and I had to stay behind and not see any of it. I poured the water on the steps, sloshed it with my shoe, and ran to join them.

Frieda was on her knees; a white rectangle of cotton was near her on the ground. She was pulling Pecola's pants off. "Come on. Step out of them." She managed to get the soiled pants down and flung them at me. "Here."

"What am I supposed to do with these?"

"Bury them, moron."

Frieda told Pecola to hold the cotton thing between her legs.

"How she gonna walk like that?" I asked.

Frieda didn't answer. Instead she took two safety pins from the hem of her skirt and began to pin the ends of the napkin to Pecola's dress.

I picked up the pants with two fingers and looked about for something to dig a hole with. A rustling noise in the bushes startled me, and turning toward it, I saw a pair of fascinated eyes in a dough-white face. Rosemary was watching us. I grabbed for her face and succeeded in scratching her nose. She screamed and jumped back.

Mrs. MacTeer! Mrs. MacTeer!" Rosemary hollered. "Frieda and Claudia are out here playing nasty! Mrs. MacTeer!"

Mama opened the window and looked down at us.

"What?"

"They're playing nasty, Mrs. MacTeer. Look. And Claudia hit me 'cause I seen them!"

Mama slammed the window shut and came running out the back door.

"What you all doing? Oh. Uh-huh. Uh-huh. Playing nasty, huh?" She reached into the bushes and pulled off a switch. "I'd rather raise pigs than some nasty girls. Least I can *slaughter* them!"

We began to shriek. "No, Mama. No, ma'am. We wasn't! She's a liar! No, ma'am, Mama! No, ma'am, Mama! No, ma'am, Mama!"

Mama grabbed Frieda by the shoulder, turned her around, and gave her three or four stinging cuts on her legs. "Gonna be nasty, huh? Naw you ain't!"

Frieda was destroyed. Whippings wounded and insulted her.

Mama looked at Pecola. "You too!" she said. "Child of mine or not!" She grabbed Pecola and spun her around. The safety pin snapped open on one end of the napkin, and Mama saw it fall from under her dress. The switch hovered in the air while Mama blinked. "What the devil is going on here?"

Frieda was sobbing. I, next in line, began to explain. "She was bleeding. We was just trying to stop the blood!"

Mama looked at Frieda for verification. Frieda nodded. "She's ministratin'. We was just helping."

Mama released Pecola and stood looking at her. Then she pulled both of them toward her, their heads against her stomach. Her eyes were sorry. "All right, all right. Now, stop crying. I didn't know. Come on, now. Get on in the house. Go on home, Rosemary. The show is over."

That night, in bed, the three of us lay still. We were full of awe and respect for Pecola. Lying next to a real person who was really ministratin' was somehow sacred. She was different from us now—grown-up-like. She, herself, felt the distance, but refused to lord it over us.

After a long while she spoke very softly. "Is it true that I can have a baby now?"

"Sure," said Frieda drowsily. "Sure you can."

"But . . . how!" Her voice was hollow with wonder.

"Oh," said Frieda, "somebody has to love you."

"Oh."

Then Pecola asked a question that had never entered my mind. "How do you do that? I mean, how do you get somebody to love you?" But Frieda was asleep. And I didn't know.[5]

The anticeremony of the whipping is redeemed by the loving-mother figure and the supportive admiration of the younger girls. However, the menarcheal sexual awareness is located in the world out there and Pecola is subsequently raped by her father, Cholly Breedlove; the resulting baby dies. Pecola goes quite mad, becoming the perfect scapegoat, "searching the garbage" on the edge of town (Morrison 1972, p. 160).

The psychic split inherent in American females characteristically leads to physical self-disgust. Jane, in Gail Godwin's 1974 novel *The Odd Woman*—in the United States, astonishing numbers of women consider themselves to be odd—observes the loss of the blond hair of infancy, the "Engelshaar" of the "pure soul," with horror. "And there was worse to come. Soon, on other parts of her body, dark hair began to grow as well. She was alarmed and shaved herself with a razor and got down on her knees at night and prayed it would not come back. It came back. Darker and thicker than before. Her guilt pressed upon her'' (Godwin 1974, p. 237). Her grandmother, discovering the pudendal shaving, tells her about menarche and menstruation. As Edith speaks, her face curls "down into an expression of disgust Jane had seen before, the same expression she got when smelling milk or meat that was 'off' . . . At that moment, Jane was disgusted with her budding womanhood. She wished more than anything to have it over with, to be respectable and old, with no taint of men and the blood that seemed to go with them" (Godwin 1972, p. 238).

This female predicament finally begins to be overtly expressed in books like Alix Kates Shulman's *Memoirs of an Ex-Prom Queen*.

> They say it's worse to be ugly. I think it must only be different. If you're pretty, you are subject to one set of assaults; if you're plain you are subject to another.

> Pretty or plain, by the time you survive puberty, your job in life is pretty much cut out for you. In either case, you must somehow wheedle back into that humanity from which you have been systematically excluded since you learned to walk. Among the ruling fraternity whose members can often barely hide their contempt for you, you must find one sponsor willing to brave ridicule for love of you. You must make him desire you more than manliness. For boys are taught that it is weak to need a woman, as girls are taught it is their strength to win a man.

> The Blue Fairy had blessed my face all right, but suddenly there was my body. I loathed it . . . People were always ready to make fun of it. They made fun of it for not having breasts, and then they made fun of it for having them . . . I hated walking on the street inside it. On the slightest provocation I blushed crimson, and then they made fun of it for that. My very blood betrayed me. What had my body to do with me inside?

> One day I got out of the bath bleeding *down there*, and from the nervous way my mother said it was "natural" after I screamed for her from the bathroom, I knew for sure I was a freak.

> I was way past being upset. I was so horrified by my sudden wound that I was detached, as though I were watching a mildly interesting home movie of myself . . .

> Seated on the toilet, I looked down at myself. It was hard to see, not like my brother's. The mysteries were inside—to keep us, I guessed, from seeing them. To use a mirror, even in this crisis, would have been suspect (suppose she walked in and saw me?), though indeed it might have helped, as my father had taught me it helped to watch the dentist in a mirror drilling out tooth decay.

> My mother's textbook words droned on and curdled like sour milk. *Every month*? If it happened once a month for a lifetime, why had I never seen these bandages before?

> " . . . and passes through the vagina."

> In our family we had never called it anything, and now she was calling it a "vagina." Unutterable word. It was better than "cunt" or "pussy"—boys'

words—but for me they were all unutterable. Twelve years old and I had never called it anything but "down there."

Finished and self-satisfied, my mother put her arm around me and kissed the tip of my nose. "My sweet Sasha, one night you go to sleep a little girl, and the next day you wake up a young woman. You'll be a lovely woman, Sasha." But I knew I was not a woman. I was a child, frightened, unable to comprehend what was happening. Nothing had been explained; everything had at least two meanings. I tried to pass as normal, but inside I knew I was a freak.[6]

As women generally, and women writers in particular, have become more outspoken about female experience, insisting on its validity and on the value of symbolic re-creations of it, men have reacted. In *Carrie*, Stephen King, a very popular male writer, reacts atavistically, throwing us back to an earlier age we had thought mercifully gone, accessible only to anthropologists, in which the power-to-create implicit in our mysterious bleeding cycle is misperceived as a power-to-destroy and treated accordingly (consider the witches and how they burned). In this 1974 novel, King has embodied a male projection of feared power: Menarche is the generating event and near total destruction the consequence. King's menarcheal counterceremony is a holocaust.

Carrie White, the butt of all jokes—the scapegoat—is standing dazed in the shower in the girls' locker room when the book opens. She grunts a "strangely froggy sound," and turns off the water. "It wasn't until she stepped out that they all saw the blood running down her leg" (King 1974, p. 5).

Carrie has "telekinesis, the ability to move objects by effort of the will alone." This power "comes to the fore only in moments of extreme personal stress."

"*Per*-iod!"

The catcall came first from Chris Hargensen. It struck the tiled walls, rebounded, and struck again.

"*PER*-iod!"

It was becoming a chant, an incantation. Someone in the background . . . was yelling, '*Plug it up!*' with hoarse, uninhibited abandon.

"*PER*-iod, *PER*-iod, *PER*-iod!"

Carrie stood dumbly in the center of a forming circle, . . . like a patient ox, aware that the joke was on her (as always), dumbly embarrassed but unsurprised.

Sue felt welling disgust as the first dark drops of menstrual blood struck the tile in dime-sized drops. "For God's sake, Carrie, you got your period!" she cried. "Clean yourself up!"

Carrie looked down at herself.

She shrieked.

The sound was very loud in the humid locker room.

A tampon suddenly struck her in the chest and fell with a plop at her feet. A red flower stained the absorbent cotton and spread.

Then the laughter, disgusted, contemptuous, horrified, seemed to rise and bloom into something jagged and ugly, and the girls were bombarding her with tampons and sanitary napkins, some from purses, some from the broken dispenser on the wall. . . . the chant became: "Plug it *up*, plug it *up*, plug it *up*, plug it . . . "

The gym teacher . . . slapped Carrie smartly across the face. She hardly would have admitted the pleasure the act gave her, and she certainly would have denied that she regarded Carrie as a fat, whiny bag of lard.

Carrie flinched away. At the same instant, a rack of softball bats in the corner fell over with a large, echoing bang. They rolled every which way, making Desjardin jump.

The blood was dark and flowing with terrible heaviness. Both of Carrie's legs were smeared and splattered with it, as though she had waded through a river of blood.

"It hurts," Carrie groaned. "My stomach . . . "

'That passes,' Miss Desjardin said. Pity and self-shame met in her and mixed uneasily. "You have to . . . uh, stop the flow of blood. You . . . "

There was a bright flash overhead, followed by a flashgun-like pop as a lightbulb sizzled and went out. Miss Desjardin cried out with surprise, and it occurred to her (the whole damn place is falling in).[7]

As the climactic joke, Carrie is asked to the prom by one of the most popular boys. They are voted an outstanding couple; when they go on stage, buckets of pig's blood are dumped on Carrie from high in the stage rigging. In bloody rage, Carrie destroys the school, almost all of the students, and much of the town. In the process, she also kills her mother, by simply stopping her heart, after her mother has stabbed her. Eventually, Carrie bleeds to death on the highway.

King explicitly connects Carrie's power to the female line and to witchery. As her mother remembers, on the night of the prom:

First had come the flow of blood and the filthy fantasies the Devil sent with it. [for example, Carrie's menarcheal sexual awareness] Then this hellish Power the Devil had given to her. It came at the time of the blood and the time of hair on the body, of course . . . Her own grandmother had it. She had been able to light the fireplace without even stirring from her rocker by the window. It made her eyes glow with (thou shalt not suffer a witch to live) a kind of witch's light. And sometimes, at the supper table the sugar

bowl would whirl madly like a dervish. Whenever it happened, Gram
would crackle crazily and drool and make the sign of the Evil Eye all
around her. . . .First the blood, then the power, (you sign your name you
sign it in blood) [King 1974, pp. 120-121].

King ends this book with a letter written 3 May 1988, describing a little girl
who is able to play with her brother's marbles without touching them. She is
only two and "awful pretty and her eyes are as brite as buttons. I bet she'll
be a world beeter someday." (King 1974, p. 198). We are meant to feel the
threat of that potentially destructive blood; sometime around the year 2000
we can expect to endure, if we survive them, the effects of that child's
menarche. King may genuinely fear that women are going to destroy men's
marbles. Certainly he has conjured a destructive counterceremony of his
own, complete with appalling distortions of mother/daughter and woman/
woman relationships. As the so-called feminist wave gains strength and
community of purpose can we expect more and more of this kind of sensa-
tional backlash?

Where shall we look for hope? In a new kind of fiction specifically
directed toward girls at the age of menarche. In *The Long Secret*, a sequel to
the very popular *Harriet the Spy*, Louise Fitzhugh devotes an entire chapter
to Beth Ellen's menarche. In so doing, however, Fitzhugh forges a disturbing link between Beth Ellen's impending and then actual menarche and the
child's compulsion to send anonymous poison-pen letters throughout the
community. This crazy/witch connotation distresses in a book directed
toward girls who are themselves on the brink of everything.

A better book, Judy Blume's *Are You There God? It's Me, Margaret*,
arrived in 1970. Margaret Simon has moved from New York City to Morn-
ingbird Lane in Farbrook, New Jersey. Befriended immediately, Margaret
helps form a group of four girls who call themselves Pre-Teen Sensations.
One club rule states that "the first one to get her period has to tell the others
all about it. Especially how it feels" (Blume 1970, p. 33).

Getting ready for a fancy class party to be held at a boy's house,
Margaret moves her desk chair over to the dresser and stands "naked in
front of the mirror." She is "starting to get some hairs." Turning
sideways, she looks and looks—and still looks the same. "Are you there
God?" she says. "It's me, Margaret. I hate to remind you, God . . . I
mean, I know you're busy. But . . . Isn't it time, God?" Margaret wants a
figure.

In school, girls are shown a film prepared by the Private Lady Company, a manufacturer of sanitary supplies. The film is affected ("say men
stroo-ate"; "remember, it's menstrooation"), somewhat evasive, and, as
Margaret comments, "like one big commercial" (Blume 1970, p. 97). The
girls vow never to buy that brand, ever. Boys are not shown the film.

Gretchen "gets it" first. Margaret records a special meeting of the PTS Club:

"I got it last night. Can you tell?" she asked us.

"Oh, Gretchen! You lucky!" Nancy shrieked. "I was sure I'd be first. I've got more than you!"

"Well, that doesn't mean much," Gretchen said, knowingly.

"How did it happen?" I asked.

"Well, I was sitting there eating my supper when I felt like something was dripping from me."

"Go on—go on," Nancy said.

"Well, I ran to the bathroom, and when I saw what it was I called my mother."

"And?" I asked.

"She yelled that she was eating."

"And?" Janie said.

"Well, I yelled back that it was important."

"So . . . so . . . " Nancy prompted.

"So . . .uh . . . she came and I showed her," Gretchen said.

"Then what?" Janie asked.

"Well, she didn't have any stuff in the house. She uses Tampax herself—so she had to call the drugstore and order some pads."

"What'd you do in the meantime?" Janie asked.

"Kept a wash cloth in my pants," Gretchen said.

"Oh—you didn't!" Nancy said, laughing.

"Well, I had to," Gretchen said.

"Okay—so then what?" I asked.

"Well . . . in about an hour the stuff came from the drugstore."

"Then what?" Nancy asked.

"My mother showed me how to attach the pad to the belt. Oh . . . you know . . . "

Nancy was mad. "Look Gretchen, did we or did we not make a deal to tell each other absolutely everything about getting it?"

"I'm telling you, aren't I?" Gretchen asked.

"Not enough," Nancy said. "What's it *feel* like?"

"Mostly I don't feel anything. Sometimes it feels like it's dripping. It doesn't hurt coming out—but I had some cramps last night."

"Bad ones?" Janie asked.

"Not bad. Just different," Gretchen said. "Lower down, and across my back."

"Does it make you feel older?" I asked.

"Naturally," Gretchen answered. "My mother said now I've gained too much weight this year. And she said to wash my face well from now on—with soap."

"And that's it?" Nancy said. "The whole story?"

"I'm sorry if I've disappointed you, Nancy. But really, that's all there is to tell. Oh, one thing I forgot. My mother said I may not get it every month yet. Sometimes it takes a while to get regular."

When I went home I told my mother. "Gretchen Potter got her period."

"Did she really?" my mother asked.

"Yes," I said.

"I guess you'll begin soon too."

"How old were you Mom—when you got it?"

"Uh . . . I think I was fourteen."

"*Fourteen*! That's crazy. I'm not waiting until I'm fourteen."

"I'm afraid there's not much you can do about it, Margaret. Some girls menstruate earlier than others. I had a cousin who was sixteen before she started."[8]

Margaret maintains a private colloquy with God throughout most of the book:

> *Are you there God? It's me, Margaret. Gretchen, my friend, got her period. I'm so jealous God. I hate myself for being so jealous, but I am. I wish you'd help me just a little. Nancy's sure she's going to get it soon, too. And if I'm last I don't know what I'll do. Oh please God. I just want to be normal* (Blume 1970, p. 100).

Nancy reports that she "got it" too, causing Margaret to despair. However, it turns out that Nancy has lied. "I want my period, too," Margaret thinks, "but not enough to lie about it."

When a severe battle between grandparents over Margaret's religion causes her to decide never to talk to God again, a lonely period of time ensues. Feeling reckless, Margaret goes to a drugstore with Janie and, facing the boy clerk at the check-out counter with desperate courage, buys some

"Teenage Softies" and a pink belt. Sneaking the supplies into her closet, Margaret practices putting on belt and pad in the dark. She likes the feeling.

Toward the end of the school year, after turning in a simple letter telling about her religious investigations for her year's project, instead of a big, thick folder like everybody else, Margaret flees to the girl's room, crying, wondering what's wrong with her. She never used to cry.

Just after the last day of school, Margaret deliberately encounters Moose, a "special" boy. Going inside to the bathroom, she thinks of how she likes "to stand close to him." Then she looks down at her underpants—there it is. She's got it. Laughing and crying, she calls her mother.

"Are you sure, Margaret?" my mother asked.

"Look—look at this," I said, showing her my underpants.

"My God!" You've really got it. My little girl! Then her eyes filled up and she started sniffling too. "Wait a minute—I've got the equipment in the other room. I was going to put it in your camp trunk, just in case."

"You were?"

"Yes. Just in case." She left the bathroom.

When she came back I asked her, "Is it that Private Lady stuff?"

"No, I got you *Teenage Softies*."

"Good," I said.

"Now look, Margaret—here's how you do it. The belt goes around your waist and the pad . . . "

"Mom," I said. "I've been practicing in my room for two months!"

Then my mother and I laughed together and she said, "In that case, I guess I'll wait in the other room."

Are you still there God? It's me, Margaret. I know you're there God. I know you wouldn't have missed this for anything! Thank you God. Thanks an awful lot (Blume 1970, pp. 147-149).

Margaret feels that what she has received is not a curse, but a blessing. The story contrives to make narrative force and moral tension out of subject matter that until a very, very short time ago was altogether unmentionable.

Regarding menarche, then, in literature, we have moved from silence, total taboo, shame and secrecy, through indirection and coded allusion, to openness, matter-of-factness, and a hint of celebration. At least in women-created literature we have so moved. Menarcheal sexual consciousness and sexual self-awareness can be openly recognized and even enjoyed. As the gap between female desires and real female possibilities lessens, growing up female in the United States becomes less painful and produces more healthily integrated female psyches. As American literature finally begins to reflect a more representative American experience, however, the split heretofore processed into the female psyche now develops more blatantly between the genders. Creative female ceremonies meet with increasingly destructive male counterceremonies. We, male and female, are only now writing the literature of this phase of our progress.

Notes

1. Marilyn French, *The Women's Room* (New York: Summit Books, 1977), p. 21. All quoted material reprinted by permission.
2. William Faulkner, *Go Down, Moses* (New York: Random House, 1940), pp. 163-165. Reprinted by permission.
3. M. Williams, *Why God Permits Evil* (Baton Rouge: Louisiana State University Press, 1977), p. 48. Reprinted with permission.
4. From pp. 212-213 in *A Tree Grows in Brooklyn* by Betty Smith. Copyright 1943 by Betty Smith. All quoted material by permission of Harper & Row Publishers, Inc.
5. Toni Morrison, *The Bluest Eye* (New York: Pocket Books, 1972), pp. 25-29. All quoted material printed by permission.
6. Alix Kates Shulman, *Memoirs of an Ex-Prom Queen* (New York: Bantam Books, 1972), pp. 40-45. Reprinted by permission of Random House, Inc.
7. Excerpts from *Carrie* by Stephen King, pp. 120-121. Copyright © 1974 by Stephen King. Reprinted by permission of Doubleday & Company, Inc.
8. Copyright © 1970 from *Are You There, God? It's Me, Margaret* by Judy Blume, pp. 97-100. Reprinted with permission of Bradbury Press, Inc. Scarsdale, N.Y.

References

Alcott, L.M. 1962. *Little women, or Meg, Jo, Beth and Amy, Parts I and II.* New York: Macmillan. (Little Women, Part I, 1868: *Goodwives, Part II, 1869).*
Blume, J. 1970. *Are you there, God? It's me, Margaret.* New York: Dell.
Faulkner, W. 1940. *Go down, Moses.* New York: Random House.
Fitzhugh, L. 1965. *The long secret.* New York: Dell.
French, M. 1977. *The women's room.* New York: Jove.
Godwin, G. 1974. *The odd woman.* New York: Knopf.

King, S. 1974. *Carrie* New York: Doubleday & Company, Inc.

Morrison, T. 1972. *The bluest eye.* New York: Pocket Books.

Shulman, A.K. 1972. *Memoirs of an ex-prom queen.* New York: Bantam Books.

Smith, B. 1943. *A tree grows in Brooklyn.* New York: Harper & Row Publishers, Inc.

Williams M. 1977. *Why God permits evil.* Baton Rouge: Louisiana State University Press.

**Part VI
Clinical Aspects of Menarche**

Introduction to Part VI

The average age of menarche in the United States today is about 12.8 years. When a girl deviates a great deal from this norm, both she and her parents become concerned and often seek medical counsel. In the next chapter, Michelle Warren reviews normal pubertal development, explaining the hypothalamic-pituitary-gonadal axis. She notes some of the disorders that advance or retard menarche, such as obesity, blindness, acute or chronic illness, ulcerative colitis, uremia, congenital heart disease, and cystic fibrosis. And she discusses the effects of athletic training, weight loss, and anorexia nervosa on the menstrual cycle. In addition to early or delayed menarche, the cessation of menstrual periods or alterations of menstrual function are common clinical problems among adolescents.

Another significant problem is dysmenorrhea. Dysmenorrhea affects about 50 percent of women and is especially common in young women (Moos 1968; Research and Forecasts 1981). For most, the discomfort is mild to moderate. However, of those women who experience pain about 10 percent are incapacitated for one to two days because of it (Budoff 1981). Until recently, dysmenorrhea was thought to be a psychosomatic problem. However, the research of W.Y. Chan and others has clearly demonstrated a relationship between high levels of menstrual prostaglandins and dysmenorrhea. Moreover, Chan has shown that dysmenorrhea can be effectively treated with prostaglandin-inhibiting drugs such as ibuprofen (Motrin), naproxen sodium (Anaprox), and mefenamic acid (Ponstel).

There is evidence that psychological factors also play a role in dysmenorrhea. In a study of a large group of adolescents and college students, Jeanne Brooks-Gunn and Diane Ruble found a reliable though low correlation between poor preparation and/or negative menarcheal experiences and reports of dysmenorrhea. They also found that premenarcheal girls expect to have more severe pain than their postmenarcheal peers actually experience. Thus cultural beliefs and expectations may influence reports of dysmenorrhea or responses to it and a multicausal model in which both physiological and sociocultural variables are taken into account is proposed.

In the last chapter in this section, Shawky Badawy and his colleagues sound a cautionary note with regard to the use of oral contraceptives by young women. Badawy found a relationship between the use of oral contraceptives and hyperprolactinemia in women under the age of twenty-five. He emphasizes the need to monitor young women who are on the pill for pituitary dysfunction and hyperprolactinemia in addition to the customary screening for cardiovascular, genital, and liver effects.

References

Budoff, P.W. 1981. *No more menstrual cramps and other good news*. New York: Penguin.
Moos, R.H. 1968. The development of the Menstrual Distress Questionnaire. *Psychosomatic Medicine* 30:853-867.
Research and Forecasts. 1981. *The TAMPAX Report*.

18 Clinical Aspects of Menarche: Normal Variations and Common Disorders

Michelle P. Warren

Menarche marks a complex series of biologic events that occur fairly late in the maturational process known as puberty. At present the initiating events that trigger pubertal development are still unknown. A number of processes will advance or retard menarche in normal girls. For example, the progressive decline in the age of menarche noted in Western Europe and the United States is thought to be due to improvement in socio-economic conditions, nutrition, and general health (Frisch, Revelle, and Cook 1973; Tanner 1973). The average age of menarche in the United States is stated to be 12.8 years according to a recent study (National Center for Health Statistics 1973).

The premenarchial years in girls are marked by extraordinary physical changes that include a rapid gain in fat (an average of 11 kilograms) a growth-spurt, and the development of secondary sexual characteristics (Frisch, Revelle, and Cook 1973; Friis-Hanson 1965; Pierson and Lin 1972). (See figure 18-1.) Proportional changes in body composition also occur: lean body mass, skeletal mass, and body fat are equal in prepubertal boys and girls, but adult women have twice as much body fat as men, while men have almost 1.5 times the lean body mass and the skeletal mass of women (Cheek 1974; Forbes 1975). In fact the increase in body mass starts at six years in females and is the earliest change in body composition at puberty. Fat accumulation can be preceded or accompanied by the development of a body odor thought to be related to adrenal androgen secretion. A progressive increase in plasma dehydroepiandosterone and dehydroepiandosterone sulfate occurs in both boys and girls by eight years of age, which continues through ages thirteen to fifteen. Dehydroepiandosterone and its sulfate are thought to originate from the adrenal gland and are the earliest hormonal changes to be secreted in puberty. These precede the increase in secretion of gonadotropins from the pituitary gland and sex steroids from the gonads (Hopper and Yen 1975; Reiter, Fuldauer, and Roat 1977).

A growth spurt also occurs prior to menarche. If it is significantly delayed, pubertal obesity may result. Females grow a mean of 25 centimeters, with the time of most rapid growth being prior to the first menstrual periods—growth slows rapidly after menarche and growth potential in a

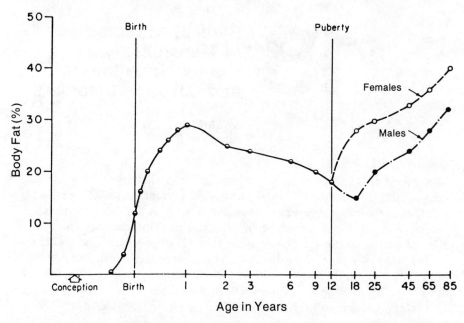

Source: J. Brozek (Ed.) *Human body composition*. Oxford: Pergamon Press, 1965, pp.
191-209. Reprinted with permission.
Figure 18-1. Changing Body Composition from Gestation through Adult
             Life

postmenarcheal girl is definitely limited (Tanner et al. 1976). Body proportions are also altered. The upper-to-lower (U/L) ratio in particular is changed.
This ratio is defined as length from top of pubic ramus to top of head divided
by the distance from the top of pubic ramus to floor. Early puberty is marked
by elongation of the extremities. Later the growth spurt equalizes growth of
both the torso and lower extremities so that the mean U/L ratio decreases.
The triggering factors for all of these changes are still unknown although
growth-hormone secretion from the anterior pituitary and gonadal sex hormones appears to be important, as well as adrenal androgens, which may play
a less important role (Tanner et al. 1976; Styne and Grumbach 1978).

   The important bony changes that occur prior to menarche include epi-
pheseal fusion of different bone centers and osseous maturation as is evidenced by X-ray. Bone age is a very accurate index of physiologic maturation
and correlates closely with menarche. It is a valuable tool in the evaluation of
children with delayed puberty, and bone age can also be used to predict
final height (Styne and Grumbach 1978).

   Menarche is preceded physically by adrenarche, or the development of
body hair, and thelarche, or breast development. Some debate still remains

as to which is the first event seen in adolescents, but either the appearance of downy labial hair or a breast bud are the first visible signs of puberty (Marshall and Tanner 1969; Zacharias, Wurtman, and Schatzoff 1970). A large individual variation for these two pubertal events has been noted among normal girls, suggesting that there may be independent central mechanisms. Pubarche may be related to androgen secretion—and in particular androgen secretion from the adrenal gland. An unidentified pituitary adrenal androgen-stimulating hormone may be responsible for adrenarche (Grumbach et al. 1977). Recent work on the hormones that stimulate the adrenal gland, adrenocorticotropin (ACTH), indicates that they are secreted in association with brain peptides, which contain opioid-like properties. These brain peptides include B-endorphin, B-lipotropin, or fragments of these that may in fact modulate adrenal secretion of androgens, in particular dihydorepiandosterone (DHEA), one of the first hormones to increase in puberty (Givens et al. 1980).

Breast development, or thelarche, is influenced by the secretion of estrogen, in particular estradiol from the ovary, but other factors may also be important. The secretion of hormones from the anterior pituitary gland such as prolactin most likely play a role in maturation of the breast. Common indices of estrogen secretion include:

1. Body fat distribution
2. Breast development
3. Bone maturation
4. Vaginal cell cornification
5. Cervical mucous
6. Proliferative endometrium present on biopsy
7. Withdrawal bleeding after the administration of progesterone
8. Plasma estradiol measurement

These indices are the clinical measures used in evaluating girls to determine if estrogen secretion is present. Particularly valuable in the adolescent girl is the presence of a cornified vaginal smear and a bone age.

The ovary is filled with primary follicles at birth, which contain oogonia in an arrested phase of development. A girl is born with approximately 400,000 follicles—all the follicles she will ever have. Only a limited number will ever develop; during the entire reproductive years, 400 oogonia will be used in the ovulatory process while the majority undergo atresia after a period of aborted growth (Baker 1972; Odell 1979).

Ovarian follicular development is stimulated by the pituitary gonadotropins LH and FSH. The gonadotropins are present in high concentration in early life. Levels decrease in the fetus as term is reached. At birth and in the neonatal period LH and FSH are present at significant levels but subsequently drop to barely measurable levels. Later, perhaps beginning as early as age eight or nine serum gonadotropins rise with maturation, with FSH increasing earlier than LH (Faiman and Winter 1971; Winter and Faiman 1972). As puberty progresses in the female there is a change from the constant low-grade secretion of gonadotropins in the prepubertal patterns to a striking sleep-associated rise, particularly of LH. This sleep-associated increase in gonadotropins is not present in either the prepubertal child or the adult (Boyar et al. 1972; Swerdloff 1978).

The prepubertal gonad appears to have a restraining influence on the secretion of gonadotropins. The gonad has a dampening effect on the hypothalamic pituitary axis and, with maturation, a decreased sensitivity to these effects develops and frees the gonad to secrete increasing amounts of sex steroids. A large body of evidence indicates that the central nervous system, and not the pituitary gland or gonads, prevents the pubertal activation of the hypothalamic-pituitary-gonadal system (Critchlow and Bar-Sela 1967). The inhibitory effect appears to be mediated by the hypothalamus and its neurosecretory neurons. These neurons synthesize and secrete luteinizing hormone-releasing hormone (LRH)—the hormone essential for the release of both FSH and also LH. The cell bodies of these neurons are located mainly in the medial basal hypothalamus in a region called the *arcuate nucleus*.

The axons of these specialized neurons end in the central portion of the hypothalamus called the *median eminence*. Most probably it is at this site that a chemical transmitter is released into the pituitary vascular portal system and travels to the anterior pituitary. Other evidence indicates that extrahypothalamic central-nervous-system structures may influence gonadotropin secretion. Biogenic amines such as norepinephrine, dopamine, and serotonin may have significant effects on LRH release. Thus the systems that stimulate or inhibit the hypothalamic-pituitary-gonadal axis are influenced by complex neural pathways that integrate a complicated system of extrinsic and intrinsic stimuli. The initial events that release the hypothalamic-pituitary-gonadal unit from its inhibitors by sex steroids are still unknown. Research has shown that in addition to nocturnal spurting of gonadotropins, the pubertal years are marked by an enhanced release of FSH, and later LH, in response to intravenous LRH. The pattern of LRH stimulation also appears to be important as intermittant LRH injections can initiate puberty in humans (Styne and Grumbach 1978; Swerdloff 1978; Valk et al. 1980). Full maturity of the CNS hypothalamic-pituitary-gonadal unit in the female is marked by the development of an adult pattern of episodic release of gonadotropins and eventually in normal menstrual cyclicity (Grumbach et al. 1974; Styne and Grumbach 1978).

One of the most common disorders of young adolescent girls is anovulatory bleeding. This disorder usually manifests itself as the absence of regular menses and ovulation and may last as much as two years after menarche. The irregular bleeding may occasionally be heavy and, rarely, a hemorrhage will occur. This age group is also prone to prolonged follicular or preovulatory phases of the menstrual cycle. Presumably, the immature ovary takes longer than fourteen days to produce a mature follicle that will initiate an estrogen peak necessary to induce ovulation (Swerdloff 1978).

A variety of factors can delay or advance menarche.

Conditions shown to *advance* menarche include:

1. Blindness
2. Obesity
3. Urban residence
4. Hypothyroidism
5. Bedridden retarded children.

Those shown to *retard* the age of menarche include:

1. Food shortage, poor nutrition
2. Altitude
3. Number of children in family
4. Thyrotoxicosis
5. Muscular development
6. Ballet dancing.

A common cause of delay is the so-called constitutional delay of puberty. Examination of the history and a growth chart will help to make this diagnosis. Typically, bone age will be retarded over chronological age. Treatment is often not necessary and reassurance and continued observation will confirm the diagnosis as onset of puberty, and menarche will eventually occur.

Another common abnormality includes an early puberty and menarche, particularly in obese children. Menarche is generally not considered premature in North American girls unless its onset is below age eight (Styne and Grumbach, 1978). Occasionally premature puberty is due to premature maturation of the hypothalamic-pituitary-gonadal axis and is called true precocious puberty (Styne and Grumbach 1978). A variety of pathologic conditions may also cause premature puberty and menarche. These conditions include central-nervous-system tumors, encephalitis, head trauma, and virilizing conditions.

Acute and chronic illness such as uremia, regional enteritis, ulcerative colitis, congenital heart disease, cystic fibrosis, and diabetes mellitus, can cause delay in menarche. This delay is generally due to the effects of malnutrition. Some of these conditions may be unsuspected as the cause of the problem. The timing of the onset of the illness appears to be important. For example, recent studies indicate that girls who develop diabetes mellitus prepubertally have a fairly normal menarche. If the disease manifests itself in the initial pubertal period, however, menarche is significantly delayed. Similar observations have been made in girls with leukemia. Leukemia, in most cases, is associated with pubertal development at a normal age. Girls with onset of leukemia in late childhood may have a delay in pubertal development. This delay may be associated with suppressed serum gonadotropins (Siris, Leventhal, and Vaitukaitis 1976). This pattern is different from gonadal failure with elevated circulating gonotropin levels sometimes found in leukemic patients treated with chemotherapy. In these cases ovarian, rather than hypothalamic-pituitary, failure appears to be at fault (Belhorsky et al 1960; Uldall, Kerr, and Tacchi 1972; Warne et al. 1973). The mechanism for drug-induced ovarian failure is not understood, although in one study a leukemic patient had many primordial follicles with maturation arrest beyond the primary follicular stage. In this case, follicular resistance to gonadotropin stimulation may occur (Siris, Leventhal, and Vaitkaitis 1976).

Recent studies indicate that adolescent girls are particularly prone to developing behavioral changes during puberty, in particular aberrant nutritional behavior leading to obesity and/or undernutrition due to dieting (Garell 1965; Coates and Thorensen 1980). In extreme cases the syndrome of anorexia nervosa may ensue. This condition may, of course, delay puberty and menarche, or cause amenorrhea if menarche has already occurred. Anorexia nervosa is a syndrome that combines bizarre behavioral manifestations with self-induced weight loss and amenorrhea (Warren and Vande Wiele 1973). This illness is occurring with increasing frequency. One in one hundred girls age sixteen to eighteen were diagnosed to have this illness in Great Britain, while partially recovered anorexia was the most common cause of amenorrhea in another report (Crisp, Palmer, and Kalucy, 1976; Kendell et al. 1973). Diet-related amenorrhea may be more common in girls who pursue activities where there is emphasis on body image (ballet, gymnastics, modeling, athletics), and some work shows that ballet dancers appear to be a unique at-risk group for the development of anorexia nervosa. A recent survey of professional dance companies has put the incidence at 5 percent (Garner and Garfinkel 1978). The frequency of weight-loss, diet-related amenorrhea among young women suggests that amenorrhea in this setting may represent a very mild form of the severe hypothalamic disorder seen in anorexia nervosa (Jacobs et al. 1975; Knuth, Hull, and Jacobs 1977). On the other end of the scale, a *thin-fat syndrome* has been used to describe individuals whose psychological orientation is similar to patients with anorexia nervosa, but who have little if any weight loss (Crisp 1977).

Girls with anorexia nervosa have a variety of behavioral abnormalities, which include an abnormal attitude toward food and abnormal handling of food. In addition, perceptual abnormalities develop and there is a distortion of body image (Bruch 1973; Feighner et al. 1972; Halmi 1974). These changes are accompanied by a multitude of endocrine changes that are thought to be hypothalamic in origin (Warren and Vande Wiele 1973). The hallmark of the endocrine abnormalities is amenorrhea, which may occur prior to or during the development of psycho-physiological abnormalities (Fries 1977). The high incidence of anorexia nervosa at puberty would suggest that the young adolescent is particularly prone to this illness for reasons that remain unexplained (Warren and Vande Wiele 1973).

Athletic training and exercise in combination with low body weight can delay breast development, menarche, and perturb menstrual cyclicity (Warren 1980). Girls who engage in intensive physical activity in early adolescence have a significant delay in puberty and menarche and a high incidence of amenorrhea that cannot be explained by weight change alone (Malina et al. 1973; Warren 1980). This phenomenon has been observed in young ballet dancers (see figure 18-2) and Olympic athletes. Women engaging in long-distance running have a high incidence of secondary amenorrhea that is directly related to the energy drain in the form of weekly mileage (Feicht et al. 1978).

This energy drain is suggested by the endocrine profiles, which show low gonadotropin secretion and a delay in bone age. The prepubertal state in dancers appears to be prolonged (Warren 1980). The gonadotropin pattern in those dancers who develop amenorrhea shows a reversion to the premenarchial pattern except that when gonadotropin suppression occurs, the suppression of LH is more marked than that of FSH. This pattern is also typical of girls who become amenorrheic in the setting of weight loss and in severe nutritional deprivation such as anorexia nervosa (Warren et al. 1975; McArthur et al. 1976; Vigersky et al. 1977). The dancers have a low body weight that is 10 percent to 15 percent below the norm for their age. The delay in pubertal development and menarche and the occurrence of secondary amenorrhea is more prominent in the dancers with lower weights and body fat. This fact suggests that an energy drain such as exercise has a modulatory effect on body weight and these two variables work together in affecting hypothalamic-pituitary function (Warren 1980). The occurrence of lower weights and body fats in runners with amenorrhea has also been noted recently (Dale, Gerlach, Wilhite 1979).

Dancers in this study also had a dichotomy in breast and pubic-hair development. A fairly normal pubarche occurs but there is a remarkable delay in thelarche. This finding suggests that the mechanism for pubic-hair development is not affected, or possibly enhanced, by exercise while the mechanism affecting both breast development and menarche is definitely

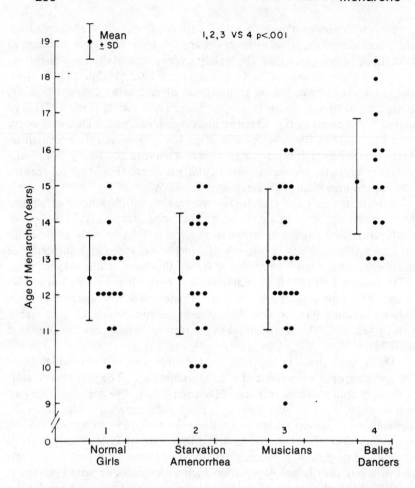

Source: Warren, M.P. The effects of exercise on pubertal progression and reproductive function in girls. *Journal of Clinical Endocrinology and Metabolism*, 1980, 51:1150-1157. © 1980, The Endocrine Society. Reprinted with permission.

Figure 18-2. Ages of Menarche in Ballet Dancers Compared to Those in Three Other Age Groups

suppressed (Warren 1980). Pubarche may be related to androgen secretion and higher testosterone levels have been reported in runners; its source is unclear but may be adrenal, ovarian, or due to a decrease in aromatization of androstenedione to estrone as a result of a decrease in adipose tissue, where this conversion takes place (Schindler, Ebert, and Friedrich 1972).

Another interesting observation is that the delay in menarche may influence long-bone growth. Dancers have a decreased upper-to-lower body ratio and a significantly increased arm span when compared to the female members of their family, although their final heights do not differ (Warren 1980). Nutritional deprivation may delay bone age and epiphyseal closure (Dreizen, Spirakis and Stone 1967) but on the other hand, the ballet may be attracting girls with these physical characteristics. Other authors have suggested that the physical characteristics associated with later maturation in females are more suitable for successful athletic performance and in another study the group of women with later menarche were more successful runners (Espenschade 1940; Malina et al. 1978; Feicht et al. 1978).

Physical exercise and varying metabolic requirements may affect the reproductive system, but there is little data on the mechanism involved. Dancers have a delay in menarche and achieve reproductive maturity at a weight and a body fat that is higher than for most normal children, suggesting that the triggering mechanism responsible for the onset of puberty and menarche and normal cyclical reproductive function may be modified by the large energy drain (Warren 1980). Recent studies do suggest that a curbing of physical activity may advance menarche. Inactive, retarded, bedridden children reach menarche at an earlier age and at a lower body fat than their active retarded counterparts (Osler and Crawford 1973).

Children who do not participate in interscholastic sports have an earlier menarche than their athletic classmates or that of the general population (Malina et al. 1973). The younger age of menarche in blind children (Zacharias & Wurtman 1964) may in fact be due in part to their confined activity. Further investigations will be needed before these mechanisms are understood.

Altered nutritional states, whether caused by starvation, either self-induced or accidental, appear to cause suppression of the hypothalamic-pituitary- ovarian axis and abnormalities of its central regulating mechanism. As shown in particular in studies on anorexia nervosa, this condition is manifested by suppression of gonadotropin secretion, absence of episodic secretion, and reversion in severe cases to prepubertal twenty-four-hour patterns (Boyar et al. 1974).

A unique feature of the effects of altered nutritional states and illness on the reproductive system is that reversibility occurs with recovery from illness or weight gain. Studies done on patients with anorexia nervosa reveal that gonadotropin levels return to normal and the blunted response to LHRH reverts to a normal pattern (Warren et al. 1975). The recovery of the response can be directly correlated to the weight gain. If the weight loss has been very severe, twenty-four studies reveal that patients progress from completely suppressed gonadotropin secretion to a normal pubertal nocturnal episodic pattern and finally to normal fluctuating levels) Boyar, et al. 1974). Unfortunately, completely normal cyclicity with estrogen secretion and a menstrual pattern may not return even with weight gain. The central regulation of gonadotropic function, which undoubtedly alters in these conditions, may not recover completely although the pattern of secretion may approach normal.

Mild forms of the starvation syndrome include self-induced weight loss of a mild degree, strenuous exercise, or a combination of food restriction and strenuous exercise. These forms appear to be more easily reversible, but the neuro-endocrine mechanisms for these changes have yet to be elucidated.

The events that precede and initiate menarche are presently the subject of active research. Further study into the basic mechanisms that govern these changes will provide therapeutic modalities in the treatment of menstrual disorders. Cessation or alteration of menstrual function remains a common clinical problem.

References

Baker, T.C. 1972. Oogenesis and ovulation. In C.R. Austin and R.V. Short, eds., *Germ cells and fertilization: Reproduction in mammals I*. Cambridge, Eng.: Cambridge University Press, pp 14-45.

Belhorsky, B., Siracky, J., Sandor, L., and Klauber, E. 1960. Comments on the development of amenorrhea caused by meleran in cases of chronic myelosis. *Neoplasma* 7:397-403.

Boyar, R.M., Finkelstein, J., Roffwarg, H., Kapen, S., Weitzman, E., and Hellman, L. 1972. Synchronization of augmented luteinizing hormone secretion with sleep during puberty. *New England Journal of Medicine* 287:582-586.

Boyar, R.M., Katz, J., Finkelstein, J.W., Kapen, S., Weiner, H., Weitzman, E., and Hellman, L. 1974. Anorexia nervosa: Immaturity of the 24-hour luteinizing hormone secretory pattern. *New England Journal of Medicine* 291:861-865.

Bruch, H. 1973. *Eating disorders, obesity, anorexia nervosa, and the person within*. New York: Basic Books.

Cheek, D.B. 1974. Body composition hormones, nutrition, and adolescent growth. In M.M. Grumbach, G.D. Grave, and F.E. Mayer, eds., *Control of the onset of puberty*. New York: John Wiley and Sons, pp. 424-447.

Coates, T.J., and Thorensen, C.E. 1980. Obesity among children and adolescents. In B. Takey and A.E. Kazden, eds., *Advances in clinical child psychology*, vol. 3. New York: Plenum, pp. 109.

Crisp, A.H. 1977. Some psychological aspects of adolescent growth and their relevance for the fat/thin syndrome (anorexia nervosa). *International Journal of Obesity* 1:231-238.

Crisp, A.H., Palmer, R.L., and Kalucy, R.S. 1976. How common is anorexia nervosa? A prevalence study. *British Journal of Psychiatry* 128:549-554.

Critchlow, V., and Bar-Sela, M.E. 1967. Control of the onset of puberty. In L. Martini, and W.F. Ganong eds., *Neuroendocrinology*, vol. II. New York: Academic Press, pp. 101-162.

Dale, E., Gerlach, D.H., and Wilhite, A.L. 1979. Mentrual dysfunction in distance runners. *Obstetrics and Gynecology* 54:47-53.

Dreizen, S., Spirakis, C.N., and Stone, R.F. 1967. A comparison of skeletal growth and maturation in undernourished and well-nourished girls before and after menarche. *Journal of Pediatrics* 70:256-263.

Espenschade, A. 1940. Motor performance in adolescence. *Monographs of the Society for Research and Child-Development* 5:1-126.

Faiman, C., and Winter, J.S.D. 1971. Sex differences in gonadotropin concentrations in infancy. *Nature* 232:130-131.

Feicht, C.B., Jonson, T.S., Martin, B.J., Sparkes, K.E., and Wagner, W. W. 1978. Secondary amenorrhea in athletes. *Lancet* 2:1145-1146.

Feighner, J.P., Robins, E., Guze, S.B., Woodruff, R.A., Winokur, G., and Munoz, R. 1972. Diagnostic criteria for use in psychiatric research. *Achives General Psychiatry* 26:57-63.

Forbes, G.B. 1975. Puberty: Body composition. In S.R. Berenberg, ed., *Puberty, biological and psycho-social components*. Leiden: Stenfert Koese, pp. 132-145.

Fries, H. 1977. Studies on secondary amenorrhea, anorectic behavior, and body image perception: Importance for the early recognition of anorexia nervosa. In R. Vigersky, ed., *Anorexia nervosa*. New York: Raven Press, pp. 163-176.

Friis-Hanson, B. 1965. In J. Brozek, ed., *Human body composition: Approaches and applications*. (Symposia of the Society for the Study of Human Biology, 7), Oxford, Eng.: Pergamon Press, pp. 191-209.

Frisch, R.E., Revelle, R., and Cook, S. 1973. Components of weight at menarche and the imitation of the adolescent growth spurt in girls: Estimated total water, lean body weight, and fat. *Human Biology* 45:469-483.

Garell, D.C. 1965. Adolescent medicine: A survey in the United States and Canada. *American Journal of Diseases in Children* 109:314-317.

Garner, D.M., and Garfinkel, P.E. 1978. Sociocultural factors in anorexia nervosa. *Lancet* 2:674.

Givens, J.R., Wiedeman, E., Anderson, R.N., and Kitabchi, A.E. 1980. B-endorphin and B-lipotropin plasma levels in hirsute women: Correlation with body weight. *Journal of Clinical Endocrinology and Metabolism* 50:975-976.

Grumbach, M.M., Richards, H.E., Conte, F.A., and Kaplan, S.A. 1977. Clinical disorders of adrenal function and puberty: An assessment of the role of the adrenal cortex in normal and abnormal puberty in man and evidence for an ACTH-like pituitary adrenal androgen stimulating hormone. In M. Serio, ed., *The endocrine function of the human adrenal cortex, Serono Symposium*. New York: Academic Press, pp. 583-612.

Grumbach, M.M., Roth, J.C., Kaplan, S.L., and Kelch, R.P. 1974. Hypothalamic pituitary regulation of puberty in man: Evidence and concepts derived from clinical research. In M.M. Grumbach, D. Grave, and F.F. Mayer, eds., *Control of the onset of puberty*. New York: John Wiley and Sons, pp. 115-166.

Halmi, K.A. 1974. Anorexia nervosa: Demographic and clinical features in 94 cases. *Psychosomatic Medicine* 36:18-26.

Hopper, B.R., and Yen, S.S.C. 1975. Circulating concentrations of dehydroepiandosterone and dehydroepiandosterone sulfate during puberty. *Journal of Clinical Endocrinology and Metabolism* 40:458-461.

Jacobs, H.S., Hall, M.G.R., Murray, M.A.F., and Franks, S. 1975. Therapy-oriented diagnosis of secondary amenorrhea. *Hormone Research* 6:268-287.

Kendell, R.E., Hall, D.J., Harley, A., and Babigan, H.M. 1973. The epidemiology of anorexia nervosa. *Psychological Medicine* 3:200-203.

Knuth, U.A., Hull, M.G.R., and Jacobs, H.S. 1977. Amenorrhea and loss of weight. *British Journal of Obstetrics and Gynecology* 84:801-807.

Malina, R.M., Harper, A.B., Avent, H.H., and Campbell, D.E. 1973. Age at menarche in athletes and nonathletes. *Medicine and Science in Sports* 5:11-13.

Malina, R.M., Spirduso, W.W., Tate, C., and Baylor, A.M. 1978. Age at menarche and selected menstrual characteristics in athletes at different competitive levels and in different sports. *Medicine and Science in Sports* 10:218-222.

Marshall, W.A., and Tanner, J.M. 1969. Variations in pattern of pubertal changes in girls. *Archives of Disease in Childhood* 44:291-303.

McArthur, J.W., O'Laughlin, K.M., Bertus, I.Z., Johnson, L., Hourihan, J., and Alonso, C. 1976. Endocrine studies during the refeeding of young women with nutritional amenorrhea and infertility. *Mayo Clinic Proceedings* 51:607-616.

National Center for Health Statistics. 1973. Age at menarche. U.S. *Vital and Health Statistics*, series II., no. 133.

Odell, W.D. 1979. The physiology of puberty: Disorders of the pubertal process. In L.J. DeGroot, ed., *Endocrinology*, vol. 3. New York: Grune and Stratton.

Osler, D.C., and Crawford, J.D. 1973. Examination of the hypothesis of a critical weight at menarche in ambulatory and bedridden mentally retarded girls. *Pediatrics* 51:675-679.

Pierson, R.N., Jr., and Lin, D.H. 1972. Measurements of body compartments in children: Whole-body counting and other methods. *Seminars in Nuclear Medicine* 2:373-382.

Reiter, E.O., Fuldauer, V.G. & Roat, A.W. 1977. Secretion of the adrenal androgen, dehydroepiandrosterone sulfate during normal infancy, children with endocrinologic abnormalities. *Journal of Pediatrics* 90:766-770.

Schindler, A.E., Ebert, A., and Friedrich, E. 1972. Conversion of androstenedione to estrone by human fat tissue. *Journal of Clinical Endocrinology and Metabolism* 35:627-630.

Siris, E.S., Leventhal, B.C., & Vaitukaitis, J.L. 1976. Effects of childhood leukemia and chemotherapy on puberty and reproductive function in girls. *New England Journal of Medicine* 294:1143-1146.

Styne, D.M., & Grumbach, M.M. 1978. Puberty in the male and female: Its physiology and disorders. In S.S.C. Yen, and R.B. Jaffe, eds., *Reproductive endocrinology, physiology, pathophysiology and clinical management*. Philadelphia: B. Saunders, p. 193.

Swerdloff, R.S. 1978. Physiological control of puberty. *Medical Clinics of North America* 62:351-366.

Tanner, J.M. 1973. Trend towards earlier menarche in London, Oslo, Copenhagen, the Netherlands, and Hungary. *Nature* 243:95-96.

Tanner, J.M., Whitehouse, R.H., Hughes, P.C.R., & Carter, B.S. 1976. Relative importance of growth hormone and sex steroids for the growth at puberty of trunk length, limb length, and muscle width in growth hormone deficient children. *Journal of Pediatrics* 98:1000-1008.

Tanner, J.M. Whitehouse, R.H., Marubini, E., and Resele, L.F. 1976. The adolescent growth spurt of boys and girls of the Harpenden Growth Study. *Annals of Human Biology* 3:109-126.

Uldall, P.R., Kerr, D.N.S., & Tacchi, D. 1972. Sterility and cyclophosphamide. *Lancet* 1:693-694.

Valk, T.W., Corley, K.P., Kelch, R.P., and Marshall, J.C. 1980. Hypogonadotropic hypogonadism: Hormonal response to low dose pulsatele administration of gonadotropin-releasing hormone. *Journal of Clinical Endocrinology and Metabolism* 51:730-738.

Vigersky, R.A., Anderson, A.E., Thompson, R.H., and Loriaux, D.L. 1977. Hypothalamic dysfunction in secondary amenorrhea associated with simple weight loss. *New England Journal of Medicine* 297:1141-1145.

Warne, G.L., Fairley, K.F., Hobbs, J.B., and Martin, F.I.R. 1973. Cycle phosphamide-induced ovarian failure. *New England Journal of Medicine* 289:1159-1162.

Warren, M.P. 1980. The effects of exercise on pubertal progression and reproductive function in girls. *Journal of Clinical Endocrinology and Metabolism* 51:1150-1157.

Warren, M.P., Jewelwicz, R. Dyrenfurth, I., Ans, R., Khalaf, S., and Vande Wiele, R.L. 1975. The significance of weight loss in the evaluation of pituitary response to LHRH in women with secondary amenorrhea. *Journal of Clinical Endocrinology and Metabolism* 40:601-611.

Warren, M.P., and Vande Wiele, R.L. 1973. Clinical and metabolic features of anorexia nervosa. *American Journal of Obstetrics and Gynecology*, 117:435-449.

Winter, J.S.D. and Faiman, C. 1972. Pituitary-gonadal relations in male children and adolescents. *Pediatric Research* 6:126-135.

Zacharias, L., and Wurtman, R.J. 1964. Blindness: Its relation to age of menarche. *Science* 29:1154-1155.

Zacharias, L., Wurtman, R.J., and Schatzoff, M. 1970. Sexual maturation in contemporary American girls. *American Journal of Obstetrics and Gynecology* 108:833-846.

19 Prostaglandins in Primary Dysmenorrhea: Basis for the New Therapy

W.Y. Chan

Primary dysmenorrhea, which once was thought to be principally a psychosomatic disorder, has now been found to have a physiologic cause. The recognition that prostaglandin (PG) released from the endometrium is a major cause of dysmenorrhea has led to the introduction of PG synthetase inhibitors for its treatment. The identification of the PG etiologic factor in dysmenorrhea has revolutionized the treatment of this common gynecologic disorder.

Although PG was discovered in the early 1930s (Goldblatt 1935; von Euler 1936), its presence in the menstrual blood was not identified until 1965 (Pickles et al. 1965). Because the PGs, $PGF_{2\alpha}$ and $PGE_{2\alpha}$, have powerful uterine-stimulating action and their systemic side effects resemble the somatic symptoms commonly seen in dysmenorrhea, it was postulated that dysmenorrhea may be caused by an elevated level of PG production from the endometrium.

In 1971, aspirin and related nonsteroidal anti-inflammatory drugs used in the treatment of rheumatoid arthritis were found to inhibit PG synthesis (Smith and Willis 1971; Vane 1971). It was discovered that these nonsteroidal anti-inflammatory drugs are inhibitors of PG synthetase (cyclo-oxygenase), the enzyme involved in the biosynthesis of PG. With this new information, trials of PG synthetase inhibitors in dysmenorrhea were soon to follow. The first specific use of PG synthetase inhibitor for the treatment of dysmenorrhea appeared to be that of flufenamic acid reported in 1974 (Schwartz et al. 1974). Since that time, a number of nonsteroidal anti-inflammatory drugs have been investigated. These drugs include ibuprofen, indomethacin, mefenamic acid, and naproxen. All were found highly effective in alleviating dysmenorrheic symptoms. The results of clinical trials of these drugs have recently been reviewed (Jacobson et al. 1979; Ylikorkala and Dawood 1978).

We studied ibuprofen (Motrin) in a double-blind, ibuprofen-placebo crossover clinical trial. Ibuprofen 400 mg or placebo were given at the first sign of menses; two tablets for the first dose and then one tablet four times a day for three days. Clinical evaluations of dysmenorrhea were made between the second and third day of menstruation. Severity and relief of dysmenorrhea were rated by a categoric scoring method that awarded points to specific symptoms, including extrauterine symptoms. Based on this scoring system, the severity of dysmenorrhea ranged from none with 0 points to very severe with a maximum of 40 composite points. Figure 19-1 shows the remarkable efficacy of ibuprofen. In this trial, eight patients were studied in forty menstrual cycles. There was good to excellent relief of dysmenorrheic symptoms in sixteen of the twenty ibuprofen-treated ccyles. There was poor or no relief of dysmenorrhea in all but four of the twenty placebo-treated cycles. Ibuprofen was clearly far superior to the placebo in alleviating dysmenorrhea (Chan, Dawood and Fuchs 1981).

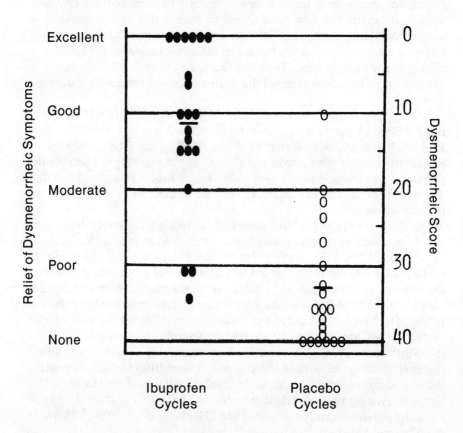

Source: Chan, W.Y., Dawood, M.Y., and Fuchs, F. Prostaglandins in primary dysmenorrhea. Comparison of prophylactic and nonprophylactic treatment with ibuprofen and use of oral contraceptives. *American Journal of Medicine*, 1981, 70:535-541. Reprinted with permission.

Note: Each circle represents one monitored menstrual cycle. Eight subjects were studied in this double-blind, ibuprofen-placebo crossover trial. The bar in each group indicates the mean dysmenorrheic score.

Figure 19-1. Relief of Dysmenorrheic Symptoms by Ibuprofen or Placebo Therapy

We also studied naproxen sodium (Anaprox) 275 mg and obtained similar good results. No significant side effects were observed in either trials.

The effectiveness of PG synthetase inhibitors in alleviating dysmennorrhea strongly supports the hypothesis that primary dysmenorrhea is caused by high levels of menstrual PGs. However, it should be recognized that these clinical trials though highly successful, provide no direct evidence for a PG etiology of dysmenorrhea. To prove the PG theory of dysmennorhea, it is necessary to demonstrate a correlation between menstrual PG levels and the severity of dysmenorrheic symptoms. No such correlative data were obtained in these clinical trials. There was no evidence that the salutary effects of nonsteroidal anti-inflammatory drugs in dysmenorrhea was indeed related to their PG synthesis inhibitory activity since the effect of these drugs on menstrual PG levels was not determined in these clinical drug trials. Menstrual PGs were not measured in most of the early clinical trials because of the difficultly in collecting menstrual specimens. Such procedures as taking endometrial biopsies or collecting menstrual blood by the jet-wash technique or by cervical cup are not acceptable to most patients due to their invasive nature.

We developed a new sampling-extraction method that can measure menstrual PG in a single tampon specimen (Chan and Hill 1978). This procedure not only is totally noninvasive but also makes it possible to monitor menstrual PG release continuously as well as to determine the total amount of menstrual PG released during menstruation in a subject. With this new method, it becomes possible for the first time to monitor and relate menstrual PG levels to symptoms of dysmenorrhea.

Figure 19-2 shows the menstrual PG release patterns of a nondysmennorheic subject, a subject on oral contraceptives and a dysmenorrheic subject. It is apparent that the dysmenorrheic subject had a significantly higher level of menstrual PG release. It should be noted, however, that not all the dysmenorrhea subjects whom we have monitored have high levels of menstrual PG. But, the majority do.

Figure 19-3 shows the effect of ibuprofen and oral-contraceptive therapy on menstrual PG release. Ibuprofen therapy markedly suppressed menstrual PG release compared to the control level. This reduction in menstrual PG release was associated with good to complete relief of dysmenorrheic symptoms.

Placebo treatment had little effect on menstrual PG release. It also produced little or no relief of dysmenorrhea.

In two dysmenorrheic subjects, menstrual PG release was measured while they were on oral-contraceptive therapy. During these cycles, they were free of dysmenorrheic symptoms and their menstrual PG release was low. The two subjects then stopped their oral-contraceptive therapy. Two cycles later, their menstrual PG levels were again measured. Very high levels were found. Significantly, dysmenorrhea recurred in these cycles.

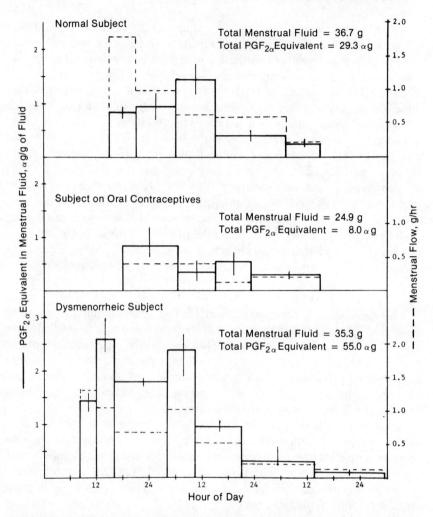

Source: Chan, W.Y., and Hill, J.C. Determination of menstrual prostalandin levels in non-dysmenorrheic and dysmenorrheic subjects. *Prostaglandins*, 1978, 15:365-375. Reprinted with permission.

Figure 19-2. Menstrual PG Release Patterns in a Normal Nondysmenor-rheic Subject, a Subject on Oral Contraceptives, and a Dysmenorrheic Subject

These studies demonstrate clearly that dysmenorrhea is associated with a high level of menstrual PG release. When menstrual PG release is reduced by either PG synthetase inhibitors such as ibuprofen, or by oral contraceptives, dysmenorrhea is alleviated.

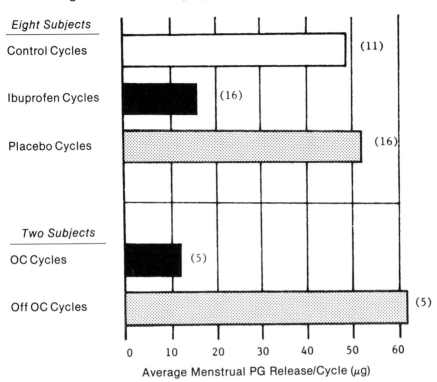

Figure 19-3. Effects of Ibuprofen and Oral-Contraceptive (OC) Therapy on Menstrual PG Release

Note: Eight dysmenorrheic subjects were studied in the ibuprofen treatment trial. The number in the parenthesis indicates the number of monitored menstrual cycles. Double-blind, ibuprofen-placebo crossover protocol. Bottom half of the figure shows the levels of menstrual PG release of two dysmenorrheic subjects when they were on and off OC therapy.

Although these two classes of drug produce similar beneficial effects in the treatment of dysmenorrhea, they have very different mechanisms of action. PG synthetase inhibitors specifically inhibit the enzyme involved in PG synthesis and thus suppress PG production. Oral contraceptives inhibit ovulation and produce hypoplasia of the endometrium and thus reduce the capacity of the endometrium to produce PG during menstruation. Oral contraceptives have many endocrine and metabolic effects, they should not be used for the treatment of dysmenorrhea unless contraception is also desired. It is also irrational to give a patient long-term endocrine therapy for the relief of pain that occurs only for one or two days a month.

Figure 19-4 illustrates the relationship between menstrual PG levels and dysmenorrheic symptoms. In this series of study, menstrual PGs were mea-

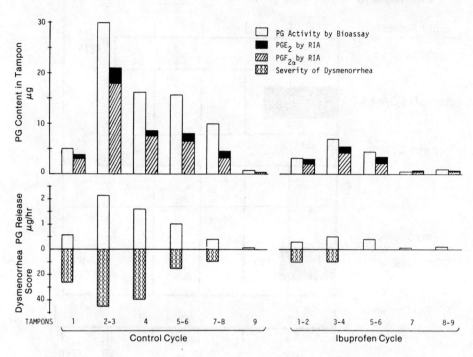

Source: Chan, W.Y., Dawood, M.Y., and Fuchs, F. Prostaglandins in primary dysmenorrhea. Comparison of prophylactic and nonprophylactic treatment with ibuprofen and use of oral contraceptives. *American Journal of Medicine*, 1981, 70:535-541. Reprinted with permission.

Note: Consecutive tampons from a patient were measured for PG content and rate of release in a control cycle and in an ibuprofen-treated cycle. The upper panel shows PG content in the tampon measured by bioassay and by radioimmunoassay. The lower panel shows the correlation between the severity of dysmenorrhea and the rate of PG release for the corresponding period.

Figure 19-4. Menstrual PG Activity Measured by Bioassay and by Radioimmunoassay, and Its Relationship to Dysmenorrhea

sured by parallel bioassays and radioimmunoassays. Radioimmunoassays showed that $PGE_{2\alpha}$ is the principal PG in the menstrual blood.

In individual patients, there was a positive correlation between the severity of dysmenorrhea and the level of menstrual PG released during the corresponding period.

Our studies have thus provided the scientific evidence showing that primary dysmenorrhea has a physiologic basis. In the majority of the patients, dysmenorrhea is associated with a high level of menstrual PG release. PG synthetase inhibitors such as ibuprofen, mefanamic acid, and naproxen suppress endometrial PG synthesis and, therefore, are effective and specific agents for the treatment of dysmenorrhea.

All currently available PG synthetase inhibitors suffer one common shortcoming. Although they are relatively specific inhibitors of the enzyme PG synthetase, they lack selectivity. There is no evidence that these agents are uterine selective. Their pharmacologic action is not confined to the uterus. Indeed, therapy with these agents suppresses total-body PG synthesis. Although no serious side effects have been reported in their use in dysmenorrheic therapy, these agents are potentially toxic and should be used judiciously.

References

Chan, W.Y., Dawood, M.Y., and Fuchs, F. 1981. Prostaglandins in primary dysmenorrhea. Comparison of prophylactic and non-prophylactic treatment with ibuprofen and use of oral contraceptives. *American Journal of Medicine*, 70:535-541.

Chan, W.Y., and Hill, J.C. 1978. Determination of menstrual prostaglandin levels in non-dysmenorrheic and dysmenorrheic subjects. *Prostaglandins* 15:365-375.

Goldblatt, M.W. 1935. Properties of human seminal fluid. *Journal of Physiology* 84:208-218.

Jacobson, J., Davalli-Bjorkman, K., Lundstrom, V. Nilsson, B., and Norbeck, M. 1979. Prostaglandin synthetase inhibitors and dysmenorrhea. A survey and personal clinical experience. *Acta Obstetricia et Gynecologica Scandinavica*, supplement 87:73-79.

Pickles, V.R., Hall, W.J., Best, F.A., and Smith, G.N. 1965. Prostaglandins in endometrium and menstrual fluid from normal and dysmenorrheic subjects. *British Journal of Obstetrics and Gynecology* 72:185-192.

Schwartz, A., Zor, U., Lindner, H.R., and Naor, S. 1974. Primary dysmenorrhea. Alleviation by an inhibition of prostaglandin synthesis and action. *Obstetrics and Gynecology* 44:709-712.

Smith, J.B., and Willis, A.L. 1971. Aspirin selectively inhibits prostaglan- production in human platelets. *Nature* (New Biology) 231:235-237.

Vane, J.R. 1971. Inhibition of prostaglandin biosynthesis as a mechanism of aspirin-like drugs. *Nature* (New Biology) 231:232-235.

von Euler, U.S. 1936. On the specific vasodilating and plain muscle stimulating substance from accessory genital glands in man and certain animals (prostaglandin and vesiglandin). *Journal of Physiology* 88:213-234.

Ylikorkala, O., and Dawood, M.Y. 1978. New concept in dysmenorrhea. *American Journal of Obstetrics and Gynecology* 130:833-847.

20 Dysmenorrhea in Adolescence

Jeanne Brooks-Gunn and
Diane N. Ruble

Menstrual distress is believed to affect most women at least sometime during their cyclic life (Novak, Jones, and Jones 1965). Cultural beliefs have been shown to play an important role in the development and maintenance of menstrual symptomatalogy (Parlee 1978, Ruble and Brooks-Gunn 1979; Sherif 1980). For example, cross-cultural research indicates menstrual distress varies as a function of culture, religion, and sex roles as well as whether or not a women knows that menstruation is the focus of study (WHO Task Force 1975; Paige 1973; Englander-Golden, Whitmore, and Dienstbier 1978). Menstrual distress has been characterized as not only affecting the vast majority of women but as being debilitating in nature, being directly linked to and/or totally accounted for by hormonal fluctuations, and affecting women's ability to function effectively in the workplace. These beliefs are not necessarily supported by the available research. For example, most college women do not perceive menstruation as very debilitating (although they do see it as bothersome, Brooks-Gunn and Ruble 1980a), prospective studies find much less evidence of menstrual distress than do retrospective studies (Ruble and Brooks-Gunn 1979), and performance decrements associated with menstruation in general have not been documented (Sommer 1973).

Gradually, the view of menstrual distress as either a biologic or sociocultural event has been replaced by a multicausal model in which distress is best understood by a complex interplay of cultural expectations, socialization factors, and actual experience (Brooks-Gunn and Ruble 1982a; Peterson and Taylor 1980). The study of the emergence and maintenance of menstrual distress has been undertaken to explore the contribution of various factors (Golub and Harrington 1981; Brooks-Gunn and Ruble 1980b).

Dysmenorrhea, or menstrual pain, is the most frequently reported menstrual symptom, the one that is rated as most severe and is the most robust, in that it is the only symptom that is seen in all prospective studies

Preparation of this chapter and the research reported were supported by the National Science Foundation (SOC-76 02137 and SOC-76 02129) and by Educational Testing Service. We wish to thank Linda Worcel and Al Rogers for their assistance in data collection and analysis. Requests for further information about this research should be addressed to Dr. Jeanne Brooks-Gunn, Educational Testing Service, Princeton, New Jersey 08541.

251

(Ruble and Brooks-Gunn 1979). Interestingly, it is also the one symptom in which a link with a hormone has been found, specifically prostaglandin, a locally acting hormone (Chan, Dawood, and Fuchs 1979; Halbert, Demers, and Jones 1976). In addition, dysmenorrhea is the symptom that has been implicated in school and work absences. For example, the 1969 National Health Examination Survey indicates that 14 percent of all adolescents missed school due to dysmenorrhea (Klein and Litt in press, b) and a Finnish survey suggests that 23 percent of all adolescents have been absent from school for this reason (Widholm 1979). At the same time, more sociopsychological factors play a role in the expression of dysmenorrhea, as we shall see in the present chapter.

Taken together, these findings suggest that dysmenorrhea is influenced by both biologic and psychologic factors. To better understand the contribution of these factors, the development of dysmenorrhea during adolescence may be explored by examining the interplay of expectations, experience, and socialization. In addition, if menstrual pain is implicated in school absence, it is important to explore the sociocultural determinants to better help teenagers cope with this problem (on the biologic side, Klein and Litt [in press, a] have shown that prostaglandin inhibitors are as effective in reducing dysmenorrhea in adolescent girls as they are in adult women).

A Definition of Dysmenorrhea

Given that so much is known about dysmenorrhea, it is surprising that disagreement exists as to its definition, incidence, and severity. For example, primary dysmenorrhea, which unlike secondary dysmenorrhea occurs in the absence of organic disorders in the pelvic region, usually includes abdominal, back, and upper leg pain, and cramping associated with menstruation. However, sometimes headaches, nausea, irritability, and that most elusive of all symptoms, premenstrual tension, are subsumed under the label of dysmenorrhea. Even different types of dysmenorrhea have been proposed. The most popular distinction involves spasmodic and congestive dysmenorrhea (Dalton 1969); the former referring to "spasms of pain similar to labor pain which begin the first day of menstruation," and the latter to "a symptom of the premenstrual syndrome with dull, aching pains accompanied by lethargy and depression prior to the onset of menstruation" (Chesney and Tasto 1975, p. 237). Dalton suggests that the two are distinguished physiologically by different hormone imbalances.

To test this prediction, Chesney and Tasto (1975) have developed a questionnaire to distinguish between the two, finding two distinct factors. The authors found that 61 percent of their sample could be characterized as experiencing spasmodic dysmenorrhea and 39 percent congestive dysmenorrhea, although individual differences with regard to severity existed within classifications. However, Webster et al. (1979), in attempting to replicate the Chesney and Tasto findings, did not find two factors, although the spasmodic-dysmenorrhea factor did appear. Rather than a congestive-dysmenorrhea factor, Webster et al. found that premenstrual and menstrual symptoms were somewhat separate. Several possibilities may explain these differences. First, women in the Chesney and Tasto sample were selected for their menstrual discomfort, which may have introduced an artifact or may suggest that the two components only exist in women with severe symptoms. Second, spasmodic dysmenorrhea may be a relatively separate (and perhaps biologically linked) condition, while congestive dysmenorrhea is not. Third, qualitative distinctions (for example, spasmodic) may not exist at all. Perhaps dysmenorrhea should be conceptualized as quantitative (for example, severity) instead. No comparable data on adolescents have been collected to address this issue.

Dysmenorrhea in Adult Women

Most of the research on severity and prevalence of dysmenorrhea relies on retrospective self-report data, which often are dissimilar from prospective data. Taking the findings of several studies using variations of the same self-report instrument, the Moos (1968) Menstrual Distress Questionnaire (MDQ), we examined dysmenorrhea in retrospective and prospective studies as well as studies measuring general knowledge or stereotypes about cyclic differences (Ruble and Brooks-Gunn 1979). Several findings are of interest. First, the magnitude of the mean cycle-phase differences is small, between .50 and 1.00 on a six-point scale; this measure translates into severity ratings of *experience the symptom mildly or somewhat*. Second, of the five prospective studies looking at pain, two found significance differences, two did not, and one did not report significance levels. Third, reports of dysmenorrhea retrospectively are more severe than prospectively. Fourth, reports of dysmenorrhea for other women indicate that women perceive others to experience more severe dysmenorrhea than they themselves experience (Brooks, Ruble, and Clarke 1977; Parlee 1974). In addition, dysmenorrhea is related to attitudes, as women who believe it is not a particularly debilitating event and believe that women should deny all menstrual effects report less severe pain themselves (Brooks et al. 1977).

In brief, dysmenorrhea is reported fairly consistently but not universally, especially in prospective studies. Cultural beliefs do seem to play a role in the reported experience of dysmenorrhea as seen in general knowledge, retrospective, and attitudinal studies.

Dysmenorrhea in Adolescence

To better understand the meaning of dysmenorrhea and the role of socio-cultural and physiological determinants, we have examined developmental trends in actual or anticipated self-report of menstrual pain in an adolescent sample. By comparing premenarcheal and postmenarcheal girls with age-controlled (in which physiological status varies but presumably sociocultural experiences do not), premenarcheal girls of differing ages (in which physiological status may be similar but sociocultural experiences are not), and postmenarcheal girls of differing ages (in which physiological status of girls who have been menstruating several years may not vary systematically while sociocultural experiences presumably will vary greatly); the contribution of experience, culture and physiology to reports of dysmenorrhea might better be elucidated. We caution to add that these comparisons are inferential in nature. In addition, if we assume interactions among determinants, it is impossible to assess the precise contribution of physical and psychological variables (an example is stress-induced amenor-rhea). However, such an analysis provides some information with regard to the determinants of dysmenorrhea.

Sample Characteristics

We have surveyed several samples of adolescent and college women. In this chapter, data from our large cross-sectional sample of adolescents will be presented. Six hundred and thirty-nine girls ranging in age from ten to nine-teen years were seen. The girls were public-school students, resided in cen-tral New Jersey, and were relatively heterogenous with respect to social class. Approximately 95 percent of the sample were Caucasian; and one-half were first born and one-half later born. Forty percent of the sample were premenarcheal: 85 percent of the fifth-to-sixth graders, 33 percent of the seventh-to-eighth graders, and none of the eleventh-to-twelfth graders.

One hundred and fifty-four college women also were seen. These sub-jects attended one of three public colleges or universities in central New Jersey. These women were divided among the four college classes, with somewhat more being in their freshman or sophomore than their junior or senior year. The social class, race, and birth order of the college sample were the same as those of the adolescent sample.

Menstrual-status comparisons were made in the seventh to eighth grade, premenarcheal comparisons were made between the fifth-to-sixth and the seventh-to-eighth graders. Postmenarcheal comparisons were made among the junior high-school, senior high-school, and college females.

Incidence of Dysmenorrhea

The postmenarcheal adolescents were asked whether or not they experienced cramps, how often they experienced pain, and how often they took medication for dysmenorrhea. Over three-quarters of the adolescents and college students had menstrual cramps, and two-thirds experienced premenstrual cramps. Fewer seventh-to-eighth graders reported cramping than the younger and older students (but only 10 percent less). Of those who reported dysmenorrhea, two-thirds reported experiencing it every month, one-quarter every other month, and one-tenth every six months. The frequency of premenstrual cramps was the same as for menstrual pain. Ten percent more of the senior-high-school girls reported cramps every month than the younger and older students.

The number of girls taking medication for cramping paralleled the incidence and frequency data, suggesting that girls take medication each time they experience pain, even though, as we shall see in the next section, the severity of cramping is rated as quite mild.

Severity of Dysmenorrhea

Severity of pain was determined by asking the girls to rate the incidence of thirty symptoms during their intermenstrual, premenstrual, and menstrual cycle phases on a six-point scale (experience the symptom not at all to experience the symptom a lot). The symptoms were taken from the Moos Menstrual Distress Questionnaire (Moos 1968), but were modified by including more familiar adjectives (that is, *crabby*, as well as *irritable*). Two of the eight factors generated by Moos (1968) are of interest here—pain and water retention. One-half of the sample completed the MDQ according to what they themselves experienced or experience, while the other half rated the MDQ for "girls in general."

Cycle-phase effects were examined for the adolescent sample as well as the college one, with comparisons being made between the premenarcheal fifth-to-sixth and seventh-to-eight graders, the premenarcheal and postmenarcheal seventh-to-eighth graders, and the postmenarcheal junior-high-school, senior-high-school, and college females. Figure 20-1 presents the mean difference MDQ pain-scale scores for the different age and menarcheal groups.

Like the majority of the adult studies, all groups of girls reported experiencing or anticipating cycle phase differences for the two MDQ scales (all one-way analyses of variance (ANOVAs) were significant). The menstrual-intermenstrual and premenstrual-intermenstrual differences were significant across age and menarcheal status. Menstrual pain was reported

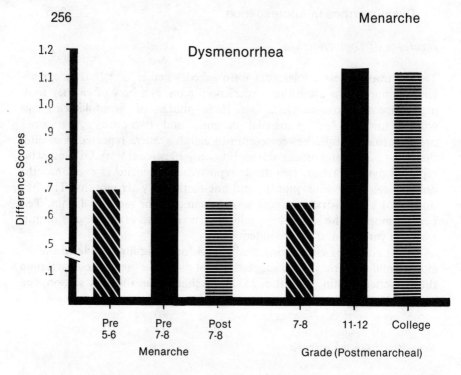

Figure 20-1. Mean-Difference Scores for MDQ Pain Factor (Menstrual-Intermenstrual) by Grade and Menarcheal Status

to be significantly more severe than premenstrual pain by all but the premenarcheal seventh-to-eighth graders.

When looking at the age and menarcheal effects, the premenarcheal fifth-to-sixth graders expected to experience the same pain as the premenarcheal seventh-to-eighth graders. The premenarcheal seventh-to-eighth graders expected to experience more pain than the postmenarcheal junior-high students reported experiencing. Finally, the older postmenarcheal adolescent girls reported more severe pain than the younger postmenarcheal girls (two-way ANOVA and t-test differences were significant). The college and senior-high-school women's symptom-severity scores were similar.

Thus, in the younger girls, dysmenorrhea is related to age and menarcheal status, with the premenarcheal girls expecting more severe symptoms than what their postmenarcheal peers actually experience. With increasing age, however, postmenarcheal adolescents report more severe symptomatology, which may be related to actual physical experience or socialization. By late adolescence, severity seems to have stabilized as the college and high-school females' self-reports are the same. The findings for general knowledge of what others are believed to experience were quite similar to those reported above for self-reports. However, others were believed to experience more severe dysmenorrhea than oneself (Brooks-Gunn and Ruble in press, b).

Onset of Menarche and Dysmenorrhea

Dysmenorrhea is believed not to appear at menarche, presumably because early cycles are anovulatory and because the onset of ovulation is necessary for dysmenorrhea. The research relating to this set of beliefs is somewhat contradictory. In support of them, early cycles do seem to be anovulatory; for example, one retrospective study reports that fourteen months is the average length of time for regular cycles to become established (Zacharias, Wurtman, and Schatzoof 1970). Girls may experience anovulatory cycles interspersed with ovulatory cycles for the first several years postmenarche. Hormonal studies of postmenarcheal girls suggest that early cycles may be anovulatory or have short luteal phases (Penny et al. 1977; Winter and Faiman 1973). Thus, hormonal fluctuations alone probably do not account for dysmenorrhea. In addition, ovulation does not necessarily lead to dysmenorrhea (not all women or girls experience dysmenorrhea). Finally, 80 percent of our fifth-to-sixth graders report experiencing cramps, and the majority of these girls had been menstruating less than a year.

To investigate this issue further, we examined the self-reports of dysmenorrhea in our adolescent sample in relation to onset of menarche. We would expect those who have menstruated longer to report more severe or a higher incidence of dysmenorrhea than girls the same age who have menstruated a shorter time. The senior-high girls were divided into those who have been menstruating more than four years (60 percent) and less than four years (40 percent), the seventh-to-eighth-grade girls into those who had been menstruating more than two years (22 percent) and less than two years (88 percent). Mean-difference scores on the MDQ Pain Scale were compared for an estimate of severity, the number of subjects reporting cramps, and the number of subjects using medication for incidence estimates.

The senior-high-school girls who had been menstruating longer reported more severe pain both menstrually and premenstrually than those whose menarche was later (Pain: P-I, 2.08 versus 1.48, $p < .05$ and M-I, 2.30 versus 1.57, $p < .02$). In the junior-high-school sample, no significant differences appeared (although girls with an earlier menarche reported somewhat more severe premenstrual pain, $p < .07$, than girls with a later menarche). In terms of incidence, somewhat more early menarcheal senior-high-school girls reported menstrual cramps and taking medication for them than did those with later menarche ($p < .10$).

Thus, length of time menstruating affected dysmenorrhea more in the older adolescents, all of whom had been menstruating at least two years, than in the younger adolescents, none of whom had been menstruating more than four years. Since the onset of dysmenorrhea is believed to occur twelve to eighteen months after the onset of menarche (Lennare and Lennare 1973), the junior-high-school girls menstruating for over two years might have been expected to experience more pain than those menstruating for less than two years. These data suggest that the experience of dysmenorrhea is the result of various factors, not just physiology (Ruble and Brooks-Gunn in press).

Dyemenorrhea during the First Menstrual Period

The incidence of symptoms during the first menstrual period also was examined retrospectively. Approximately one-half of the elementary and junior-high-school girls reported experiencing cramps at menarche, while one-third of the senior-high-school girls reported cramps with the first period.

Dysmenorrhea and Psychological Factors

We also have examined the relationship of psychosocial factors and dysmenorrhea, looking at correlations and mean differences between the MDQ Pain Scales and other variables (Ruble and Brooks-Gunn 1979). In terms of the first menstrual experience, the girls who began early, who reported having cramps during the first period, who remembered their explanation of menstruation as poor, who did not feel prepared, who felt surprised, and who felt negative reported more severe pain than those with the opposite characteristics (r's range from .20 to .27, p's < .01).

Daughters' perceptions of their mothers' menstrual experience was examined. Three-quarters of the mothers were believed to experience cramping and to take medication for it. Those who believed their mothers experienced dysmenorrhea reported more severe premenstrual and menstrual pain scores themselves, but not a higher incidence of dysmenorrhea, than those who did not believe their mothers had menstrual cramps (t test comparisons).

Finally, daughters' perceptions of parental attitudes and knowledge about the first menstrual period were examined. Parent's positive, negative, and surprised feelings were not related to daughter's dysmenorrhea although parental knowledge of the first period was. Whether or not the father knew about the daughter's menarche was related to menstrual pain

$(r = .31, p < .01)$; girls who reported that their father did not know about their menarche (from either the mother or the daughter) reported significantly more severe dysmenorrhea.

References

Brooks-Gunn, J. and Ruble, D.N. 1980a. Menarche: The interaction of physiological, cultural and social factors. In A.J. Dan, E.M. Graham, and C. Beecher, eds., *The menstrual cycle: Synthesis of interdisciplinary research*. New York: Springer.

_____ . 1980b. The Menstrual Attitude Questionnaire. *Psychosomatic Medicine* 42:503-512.

_____ . 1982a. The experience of menarche from a developmental perspective. In J. Brooks-Gunn and A. Petersen, (eds.), *Girls at puberty: Biological and psychosocial perspective*. New York: Plenum.

_____ . 1982b. The development of menstrual-related attitudes and beliefs in adolescence. *Child Development*.

Brooks, J., Ruble, D.N., and Clarke, A. 1977. College women's attitudes and expectations concerning menstrual-related changes. *Psychosomatic Medicine* 39:288-298.

Chan, W.Y., Dawood, M.Y., and Fuchs, F. 1979. Relief of dysmenorrhea with prostaglandin synthetase inhibitor ibuprofen: Effect on prostaglandin levels in menstrual fluid. *American Journal of Obstetrics and Gynecology* 135:102.

Chesney, M.A., and Tasto, D.L. 1975. The development of the menstrual symptom questionnaire. *Behavior/Research/and Therapy* 13:237-244.

Dalton, K. 1969. *The menstrual cycle*. New York: Pantheon Books.

Englander-Golden, P., Whitmore, M.R., and Dienstbier, R.A. 1978. Menstrual cycle as a focus of study and self-reports of moods and behaviors. *Motivation and Emotion* 2:75-86.

Golub, S., and Harrington, D.M. 1981. Premenstrual and menstrual mood changes in adolescent women. *Journal Personality and Social Psychology* 41:961-965.

Halbert, D.R., Demers, L.M., and Jones, D.E. 1976. Dysmenorrhea and prostaglandins. *Obstetrics and Gynecology* 31:77.

Klein, J.R., and Litt, I.F. In press, a. The effect of aspirin on dysmenorrhea in adolescents. *Journal of Pediatrics*.

_____ . In press, b. Epidemiology of adolescent dysmenorrhea. *Pediatrics*.

Lennare, M.B., and Lennare, R.J. 1973. Alleged psychogenic disorders in women—a possible manifestation of sexual prejudice. *New England Journal of Medicine* 288:288-292.

Moos, R.H. 1968. The development of the Menstrual Distress Questionnaire. *Psychosomatic Medicine* 30:853-867.

Novak, E.R., Jones, G.S., and Jones, H.W. 1965. *Novak's textbook of
gynecology*, 7th ed. Baltimore: Williams and Wilkins.

Paige, K.E. 1973. Determinants of menstrual distress: Stress, femininity, and religion. Paper presented at the American Sociological
Association, September, New York City.

Parlee, M.B. 1974. Stereotypic beliefs about menstruation: A methodological note on the Moos Menstrual Distress Questionnaire.
Psychosomatic Medicine, 36:229-240.

————. 1978. Psychological aspects of menstruation, childbirth, and
menopause. In J.A. Sherman and F.L. Denmark, eds., *Psychology of
women: Future directions of research*. New York: Psychological
Dimensions.

Penny, R., Parlow, A.F., Olambiwonnie, N.O., and Frasier, S.D. 1977.
Evolution of the menstrual pattern of gonadotropin and sex steroid
concentrations in serum. *Acta Endocrinology* 84:79.

Petersen, A.C., and Taylor, B. 1980. The biological approach to adolescence: Biological change and psychological adaptation. In J. Adelson,
ed., *Handbook of adolescent psychology*. New York: John Wiley and
Sons.

Ruble, D.N., and Brooks-Gunn, J. 1979. Menstrual symptoms: A social
cognition analysis. *Journal of Behavioral Medicine* 2:171-194.

————. In press. A developmental analysis of menstrual distress in adolescence. In R.C. Friedman, ed., *Behavior and the menstrual cycle*. New
York: Marcel-Dekker.

Sherif, C.W. 1980. A social psychological perspective on the menstrual
cycle. In J.E. Parsons, ed., *The psychbiology of sex differences and sex
roles*. Washington: Hemisphere.

Sommer, B. 1973. The effect of menstruation on cognitive and perceptual-
motor behavior: A review. *Psychosomatic Medicine* 35:515-534.

Webster, S.K., Martin, H.J., Uchalik, D. and Gannon, L. 1979. The
menstrual symptom questionnaire and spasmodic/congestive dysmenorrhea: Measurement of an invalid construct. *Journal of
Behavioral Medicine* 2:1-19.

WHO Task Force on the Acceptability of Fertility Regulating Methods.
1975. *Patterns and Perceptions of Menstrual Bleeding in Ten Regions*.
Devon, Eng.: Exeter University.

Widholm, O. 1979. Dysmenorrhea during adolescence. *Acta Obstetrica et
Gynaecologica Scandininavica* 87:61-66.

Winter, J.S.D., and Faiman, C. 1973. The development of cyclic pituitary
and gonadal function in adolescent females. *Journal of Clinical Endocrinology and Metabolism* 37:714.

Zacharias, L., Wurtman, R.V., and Schatzoff, M. 1970. Sexual maturation in contemporary American girls. *American Journal of Obstetrics and Gynecology* 108:833.

21 Steroidal Contraceptive Use and Subsequent Development of Hyperprolactinemia

Shawky Z.A. Badawy,
Frances Rebscher,
Lawrence Kohn,
Honor Wolfe,
Richard P. Oates, and
Arnold Moses

Steroidal oral contraceptives were introduced over twenty years ago as a solution to the world's population problem. This method became the most prevalent means of family planning. Various studies since, have focused on cardiovascular effects, metabolic actions, and the incidence of genital and liver tumors. In addition, the suppressive effect of these steroidal contraceptives on gonadotropins has been well-documented. Hence, the contraceptive effect is due to suppression of ovulation.

During the past decade, the diagnosis of many cases of hyperprolactinemia and prolactin-secreting pituitary tumors suggest that there is an increase in the incidence of these tumors. It has also been suggested that this increase actually is due to the development of more sophisticated means of diagnosing such conditions; for example, sensitive roentgenographic techniques of hypocycloidal polytomography and computerized axial tomography. In addition, the hormone prolactin was identified as a separate hormone from growth hormone in 1970-1971 (Hwang, Guyda and Friesen 1972). Shortly thereafter, a specific radioimmunoassay procedure was developed and became available to study such hormones. It is conceivable that such pituitary tumors were prevalent but undiagnosed in the past, before the era of the contraceptive pill, but the relationship between the use of steroidal contraceptives and the development of hyperprolactinemia and pituitary tumors could not be totally excluded (Sherman et al. 1978; Anngers et al. 1978).

Before I deal with this relationship, I would like to discuss briefly the physiology of the hormone prolactin. Prolactin is a polypeptide made of about 198 amino acids. It is secreted from the anterior pituitary lactotropes

Supported in part by Grant RR-229 from the General Clinical Research Centers Program; Division of Research Resources, National Institutes of Health.

263

under the tonic inhibitory effect of prolactin-inhibiting factor, which is secreted from the hypothalamus. This factor is believed to be dopamine (Takahara, Arimura and Schally, 1974). Dopamine is delivered to the anterior pituitary gland via the portal circulation. Factors that interfere with this dopaminergic mechanism lead to the development of hyperprolactinemia. For example, the administration of phenothiazines, tricyclic antidepressants, α Methyl dopa (Aldomet), or reserpine lead to either blockage of dopamine receptors or depletion of hypothalamic dopamine, all of which lead to hyperprolactinemia. Similarly, conditions of stress and administration of estrogens could lead to the development of hyperprolactinemia.

The dopaminergic mechanism is not the only mechanism controlling prolactin secretion. The serotonins are known to stimulate prolactin secretion. Indeed, it has been suggested that the disturbance in balance between the serotonins and dopamines lead to hyperprolactinemia if the serotonin mechanism in the hypothalamus gains the upper hand (Kamberi, Mical and Porter 1971). In addition, the effect of B-endorphins on this system is significant. Studies in this field are presently in progress in various research centers.

It has been suggested that both estrogens and progestins stimulate prolactin secretion (Dericks-Tan and Taubert, 1976). Indeed, prolactin levels are high in the serum during pregnancy due to the high levels of circulating estrogens. In addition, studies have demonstrated that 30 percent of women using the steroidal contraceptive pill have hyperprolactinemia (Reyniak et al. 1980). The relationship between the use of the steroidal contraceptive pill and the subsequent development of hyperprolactinemia prompted us to conduct a study in the Reproductive Endocrinology Unit at Upstate Medical Center, Syracuse, New York. In this study, 123 patients who came to the unit because of infertility or menstrual dysfunction served as subjects. The following information was recorded for every patient: age at presentation, age at which the steroidal contraceptive pill was used, and duration of use. Patients were excluded if they were hypothyroid, had a history of intake of medications that were known to increase prolactin, or if they had a history of menstrual irregularities before going on the contraceptive pill.

In the patient population examined, 63 patients (age sixteen to forty) had hyperprolactinemia (prolactin levels of 26 to 843 ng/ml); and 60 patients (age fifteen to thirty-six) had normal prolactin levels (prolactin levels 3-22 ng/ml). The results of this study revealed that the patients who used steroidal oral contraceptives for more than one year when under the age of twenty-five years had a 6.25 times greater relative odds of developing hyperprolactinemia than did nonusers of comparable age ($x^2 = 8.04$, $p < 0.005$). This figure did not hold true for women who used the steroidal oral contraceptives after the age of twenty-five.

In this work, we use the term *relative odds* rather than *risk factor* because it is difficult in studies such as the one discussed in this chapter to have control groups of patients matched for type of pill used and for age, height, and weight. This work also differs from studies published in various other publications, in which the relationship between oral contraceptive use and the development of pituitary tumors has been examined. In some of these studies, the control groups consisted of a very limited number of patients, thus making the conclusion difficult to interpret. In addition, in some studies a large number of patients used the pill to regulate periods. This use might stimulate the growth of a pre-existing tumor. For that reason the present study focused only on patients who used the oral contraceptive pill without prior history of menstrual irregularities, thus removing any error due to a pre-existing pituitary lesion.

Since it is sometimes difficult to diagnose clinically pituitary tumors despite modern evaluation technology, we chose to study the relationship of steroidal oral contraceptives to the problem of hyperprolactinemia. The finding of a significantly increased risk of developing hyperprolactinemia among users of the contraceptive pill under the age of twenty-five years is an important one. Perhaps young women have a labile hypothalamic pituitary system that is vulnerable to various environmental factors. A study, in which girls who took the steroidal contraceptive pill close to menarche were found to take longer to resume normal menses following discontinuation of such treatment, would seem to support this view (Evrad, Buxton and Erickson 1976). In addition, this study raises several points of concern to the primary care physician and to counselors in the field of family planning in relation to the use of the steroidal contraceptive pill. Proper counseling of patients as to the dangers in using such compounds—not only to the cardiovascular, genital, and liver-tumor risks but also to the risk of developing hyperprolactinemia with or without pituitary tumors—is essential. It is interesting to note that various studies demonstrated that 30 to 80 percent of patients with prolactin-secreting pituitary tumors have a history of use of steroidal oral contraceptives (Badawy, Nusbaum and Omar 1980; Chang et al. 1977).

If the patient decides to use the contraceptive pill as her method of birth control, she must also be advised about follow-up care. The question of how long a patient can remain on the pill is still an unanswered one. However, a serum prolactin-level study every six months would be advisable, enabling detection of those women who develop hyperprolactinemia while on the pill. This group of patients might need close follow-up. One might argue that this kind of supervision could lead to increased expense. However, we believe that this hormone study is an important aspect of the follow-up care of a patient using these steroids. It is necessary to monitor the patients not only for tumors related to the uterus or liver, but also for pituitary dysfunction and tumor process.

References

Anngers, J.F., Coulam, C.B., Laws, E.R., and Kurland, L.T. 1978. Pituitary adenomas and oral contraceptives. *Lancet 2:1384.*

Badawy, S.Z.A., Nusbaum, M.L., and Omar, M. 1980. Hypothalamic pituitary evaluation in patients with galactorrhea-amenorrhea and hyperprolactinemia. *Obstetrics and Gynecology* 55:1.

Chang, R.J., Keye, W.R., Jr., Young, J.R., Wilson, C.B., and Jaffe, R.B. 1977. Detection, evaluation, and treatment of pituitary microadenomas in patients with galactorrhea-amenorrhea. *American Journal of Obstetrics and Gynecology* 128:356.

Dericks-Tan, J.S.E., and Taubert, H.D. 1976. Elevation of serum prolactin during application of oral contraceptives. *Contraception* 14:1.

Evrard, J.R., Buxton, B.H., Jr., and Erickson, D. 1976. Amenorrhea following oral contraception. *American Journal of Obstetrics and Gynecology* 124:88.

Hwang, P, Guyda, H., and Friesen, H. 1972. Purification of human prolactin. *Journal of Biological Chemistry* 247:1955.

Kamberi, I.A., Mical, R.S., and Porter, J.C. 1971. Effects of melatonin and serotonin on the release of FSH and prolactin. *Endocrinology* 88:1288.

Reyniak, J.V., Wenof, M., Aubert, J.M. and Stangel, J.J. 1980. Incidence of hyperprolactinemia during oral contraceptive therapy. *Obstetrics and Gynecology* 55:8.

Sherman, B.M., Harris, C.E., Schlechte, J., Duello, T.M., Halmi, N.S., Van Gidler, J., Chapler, F.K., and Gvanner, D.K., 1978. Pathogenesis of prolactin secreting pituitary adenomas. *Lancet* 2:1019.

Takahara, J., Arimura, A., and Schally, A.V. 1974. Suppression of prolactin release by a purified porcine PIF preparation and catecholamines infused into a rat hypophysial portal vessel. *Endocrinology* 95:462.

**Part VII
Psychiatric Issues**

Introduction to Part VII

Psychoanalytic theory has been maligned and dismissed by many feminists as irrelevant today. Yet despite its flaws psychoanalysis has contributed greatly to our understanding of human behavior and serves as an important theoretical orientation for much of contemporary psychiatry. Usually the critics focus on traditional Freudian theory, ignoring the fact that Freud modified his theories during the course of his lifetime and failing to recognize that psychoanalytic thought has changed and evolved over time. Psychoanalysis is no longer only Freud, if it ever was. And there is certainly no one psychoanalytic view of women. Over the years women analysts such as Horney, Deutsch, Benedek, and Thompson, among others, have both criticized Freud and added differing perspectives to our understanding of the female personality (Strouse 1974).

Malkah Notman notes that psychoanalytic views regarding female development are still changing and that they have been modified because of new findings in the biological and social sciences as well as by clinicians' observations. In her chapter the normal developmental tasks of adolescence are described and presented in contrast with earlier theories of castration anxiety and female masochism. Notman observes that the more recent view of menarche is a positive one; it is seen as a so-called organizer for the young woman and leads to her acceptance of her feminine identification. It is also a time of diminished dependence on mother, a time of increased interest in father and boys, and a time when other women serve as role models. For some, menarche also serves to clarify the composition of the female genitals, particularly the existence of the vagina. Notman also discusses some of the disturbances associated with menarche, particularly denial of menstruation, which may be related to conflicts regarding acceptance of the female role or to an attempt to delay adulthood.

Jaine Darwin applied psychoanalytic theory in her research. Using projective techniques as well as a structured interview, she explored the range of affective and cognitive responses to menarche by focusing on a sample of normal and psychiatrically ill adolescents. Darwin hypothesized that menarche might be a contributing factor in the psychiatric hospitalization of girls between eleven and thirteen. Her research generally supported the psychoanalytic view of menarche as a time of concern with dependency, separation, aggression, and body integrity. She found differences between the pre- and postmenarcheal girls, as well as between the inpatient and control groups. Perhaps most interesting was Darwin's finding that the issues surrounding menarche were the same for both the sick and the well groups but they handled the developmental stresses differently: the control subjects used fantasy, whereas the inpatients tended to act out in a self-destructive way.

Anorexia nervosa is a psychosomatic condition seen most often in young women. It is characterized by prolonged inability or refusal to eat and is sometimes accompanied by amenorrhea, extreme emaciation, binge eating, induced vomiting, and/or the abuse of purgatives. James Falk and his associates have been studying anorexia nervosa for some time; in their chapter they focus on the amenorrhea often seen in these patients. Falk et al. tested the critical body-weight hypothesis proposed by Frisch and found that body weight alone did not explain menstrual disturbances in this population. The authors suggest that other factors, such as stress, may interact with physiological changes in delaying menses in this group. Patients with more severe symptoms were also found to be more likely to have prolonged menstrual disturbances.

Richard Friedman and his colleagues are studying the relationship between psychopathology and the menstrual cycle. In their chapter they look at premenstrual affective syndrome (PAS) in adolescent and adult psychiatric patients. The authors note that the literature regarding psychiatric illness and PAS is contradictory, with some studies indicating a relationship between psychopathology and the menstrual cycle while others do not. They also note the absence of reports of PAS among adolescent psychiatric patients. Using structured interviews, Friedman et al. found PAS to be as common among the adolescent psychiatric inpatients as it was among the adults. Moreover, in both the adolescent and adult samples a relationship was found between PAS and traumatic sexual experiences such as rape or incest. These data stand in contrast to other studies of mood changes in normal adolescent and adult women (Golub & Harrington 1981; Golub 1976) and point up the need for research among different populations.

References

Golub, S. 1976. The magnitude of premenstrual anxiety and depression. *Psychosomatic Medicine* 38:4-14.

Golub, S., and Harrington, D.M. 1981. Premenstrual and menstrual mood changes in adolescent women. *Journal of Personality and Social Psychology* 41:961-965.

Strouse, J. ed. 1974. *Women and analysis*. New York: Dell.

22 Menarche: A Psychoanalytic Perspective

Malkah T. Notman

Psychoanalytic views of the psychology of women and of adolescent development are changing. They were not actually as uniform and monolithic as is sometimes assumed, and early on Freud had his critics in Horney (1973) and Jones (1935) among others. However, at present, in attempting to formulate a psychoanalytic understanding of these experiences and events, questions arise in relation to a literature on puberty, adolescent development, and reproductive functioning and its significance that still do not fully reflect recent changes. Kestenberg (1976) one of the few writers who has addressed menarche in some detail first in 1961 and in a more recent paper in 1975, still preceded the wide publication of the changed psychoanalytic views.

Freud's original formulations and those of his early colleagues, have been modified with the growth of information from the biological sciences, from social science, from direct observations of children, and from the increase of treatment experience with children and adults. The importance of socialization and the influences of early experiences with parents and of the pre-oedipal period have been more fully recognized. The concept that women have a *primary femininity* not based on modification or deviation from male development, which precedes the oedipal conflict and is based on many elements, including biological influences, physical sensations, and identification with the pre-oedipal mother, has been proposed (Stoller 1976). In this view, the resolution of the oedipal period brings a richer, although conflicted, addition to the earlier femininity. Penis envy is not seen as the pivotal experience for feminine development but is instead related to loss, envy, and the stability and character of object relations (Galenson and Roiphe 1976; Blos 1980). In the adult woman, emotional maturity is not necessarily thought to be attained only if she bears a child. The relationship between femininity and reproduction is being re-evaluated (Notman and Nadelson in press).

In this context it is important to take a contemporary look at psychoanalytic views of menarche. Menarche occurs as one of the major events within the complex changes of puberty. Data from a variety of sources (Tanner 1974) indicates that it is one of the latest events of puberty, although there are wide individual variations. The hormonal, physical, and psychological changes of adolescence have by and large already begun, with

271

changes in relationships and in ego development. Although correlations between endocrine status and psychological changes have not been conclusive or fruitful to date, the endocrine changes have affected growth and body development, so menarche occurs when the development and awareness of adult femininity is already in process.

Where is the preadolescent and young adolescent developmentally at this time? To understand the psychological meaning of menarche for the young girl, one must look at the adolescent in whom menarche occurs, including the developmental tasks and experiences that are taking place. It is also important to include the symbolic meaning as well as the actual implications of menarche.

The developmental tasks of early adolescence involve the detachment from early ties to parents and the capacity to form relationships with peers, eventually to establish an integrated identity as a female and then as a woman, with later consolidation of identity, and the development of the capacity for intimacy and potential commitment to a person and a life course.

In the early process of separation and individuation from parents, there is a withdrawal of investment from them and their values. In the past this process was conceptualized as having an effect of increasing self-preoccupation and narcissism. The loss of old ties was compared with mourning and expected to be difficult. This process does occur, but it is less disintegrating than was thought (Blos 1980). The literature tended to emphasize the pathology and the dangers to the body image because of the changes produced by a growth spurt and development of secondary sex characteristics. The effects are indeed profound. However, if a cohesive self has been established in childhood, fragmentation does not occur, and the adolescent can make a shift to nonincestuous figures with whom to form relationships. Turmoil does not appear inevitable.

Another change in conceptualization about adolescent development is the assessment as to the degree to which the superego is weakened and its capacity to support the ego also weakened in the shift away from the the parents and their values. This process does occur to some extent, with some sense of emptiness and loss of self-esteem, but this development can also proceed more smoothly than had been thought. The ego ideal may also be projected and others can be idealized as the parents are deidealized, resulting in adolescent crushes.

In feminine development, the earlier views (Blos 1979; Deutsch 1944) held that the activity of the preadolescent girl represented a denial of femininity, because of unresolved conflicts about penis envy, and that new sensations accentuated this conflict, because they focused the prepubertal girl's castration complex (Harley 1961). The girl was thought to turn away from her mother in disappointment and her so-called feminine concerns—namely preoccupation with boys, were seen as substitutive. The current view is that these concerns represent a real move toward new interests and fulfillment of a girl's "feminine self" consistent with cultural patterns (Barglow and Schaefer 1979). The girl is drawn to the father, as in the oedipal period, for a variety of reasons, including the father's interest in the girl, her maturation, and her attractiveness. She also seeks closeness and partial identification.

In the young adolescent girl at the time of menarche there is still a shifting back and forth between her infantile attachment to both parents and her moves toward her adult personality. This fluctuation appears normally to be more fluid in girls than in boys, where a resolution of the oedipus complex is thought to be more complex and abrupt before the boy can move on developmentally. This sex difference is partly explained by the force of castration anxiety.

The girl thus remains ambivalently attached to the pre-oedipal mother, who is both a rival and an object of longing. Sometimes if these longings and dependent wishes are too great, the girl throws herself defensively into heterosexual relationships to ward them off. Another interference in the development away from the early attachments can be the mother's pull toward the girl because of her own needs. In the adolescent struggle for autonomy the girl must free herself from this attachment. When she moves further away from the attachments to her parents she seeks support and security in relationships with peers.

Kestenberg (1975) has observed that in early adolescence physical internal sensations as well as bodily changes are anxiety provoking. They are unlocalized and in some ways, particularly for inner sensations, undefined. Because of the shifting body image associated with the growth spurt, the changes in shape, the development of axillary and pubic hair, and the other events of adolescents, anxiety and concern about one's normality result, and the conformist attachment to peers and their validation of one's own worthwhileness and normality becomes particularly important—and their influence can be intense.

It is clear that the timing of puberty and menarche in relation to a girl's psychosocial development and age is important. Menarche in a younger girl comes at a point of less social and cognitive maturity than in an older one, although the relationship is reciprocal and the timing of puberty can have effects on psychosocial development as well. The psychoanalytic literature relating pubertal development to psychosocial development is still scanty.

Having considered the psychological state of the early adolescent, one can return to menarche itself. Earlier writers, (Deutsch 1944) saw the complex experience of menstruation as traumatic. The mother's role in relation to the girl and the lack of preparation that was the rule were cited as important. Male attitudes towards menstruation were considered negative—including concern about the blood, which activated castration anxiety. Cross-cultural attitudes reflected fear and danger associated with this period. Deutsch summarized much of the literature in her formulation that each period was a new disappointment at not being pregnant and revived ideals of genital injury with reactivation of old fears and conflicts about sexuality and masturbation.

Kestenberg (1975) recognized the gamut of adult reaction to menstruation but questioned the traumatic aspect. She saw menarche as a potentially positive experience and as a turning point in the acceptance of femininity. Menstruation provided an "organizer and cornerstone of feminine identification" that was better than the undefined inner sensations prior to it. She cited clinical evidence of diminished anxiety with the onset of menarche.

The relationship with mother she also felt to be important at this time. Most observers found that menarche normally stimulates a diminished dependency on mother and an identification with her as a reproductive prototype, with a renewed interest in father and boys. In prepuberty the girl's interest in her body expressed itself in a variety of fantasies. Menarche brings relief, providing the girl with fixed points of reference upon which she can organize her experience. Her genitals are also more defined and specific.

Kestenberg states that in the past socialization was different. Mothers either did not inform or prepare their daughters or stressed the trauma or the sexual danger. The blood and its connection to injury does however remain a potential stimulus for concern.

At the same time, in 1975, Kestenberg still wrote about normal "feminine masochism," which is no longer currently regarded as universal nor normal—nor is femininity equated with passivity. Early adolescent relationships are not regarded as more masochistic for girls than for boys. Menarche is only one of the organizers of adolescence. Other people are important, not only the girl's mother but other models of womanhood.

Another role of menarche is in confirming the existence of the vagina. In a child there may be confusion about female genitalia (Lerner 1976; Ash 1980). The vagina or uterus is often the name the little girl is given when the vulva is what she sees if she looks at herself. It is difficult to "check out" what there is.

Freud and others believed that for girls the vagina was a "silent area" a part of themselves of which they were not aware. Vaginal awareness came with adult femininity. Child observations have contradicted this view (Galenson and Roiphe 1976; Clower 1976). Sensations from the vagina do occur and some little girls masturbate vaginally, but there may be considerable confusion as to exact relationships.

When menses begin it is clear that the menstrual flow comes from some internal source. It needs to be distinguished from excretions. Some young adolescents who are still unclear about their anatomy have a cloacal concept of the vagina; they have not differentiated the openings. Some authors (Shopper 1979; Whisnant, Brett, and Zegans 1979) regard learning to use a tampon as a helpful experience in defining and learning the anatomy of the vagina. The mother's instructions are important and convey support for femininity and adulthood (Shopper 1979; Whisnant, Brett, and Zegans 1979). The way in which a girl is trained and instructed involves her relationships with her mother and peers. Shopper feels that mothers tend to inhibit girls' perineal exploration in toileting and reinforce this inhibition at menarche.

Disturbance Associated with Menarche

For some girls the onset of menarche is accompanied by ambivalence or distress. It is not uncommon for a girl to deny to herself or others that she has actually begun to menstruate. This denial may be conscious concealment or the unconscious refusal to recognize that she has begun her periods, and since the first period may be light and consist of no more than staining she may attribute this bleeding to some other cause. Some girls associate it with trauma and feel they have injured their genitals. Sometimes guilt from some other source, such as aggressive wishes or forbidden sexual fantasies or masturbation, becomes associated with the bleeding and the girl may feel that she is being punished or has caused some damage to herself, until she recognizes this is the beginning of her periods. Some guilt may remain nevertheless.

For example, one twelve-year-old girl had been a tomboy, accepted by the boys in their games. When they entered junior high school she was excluded, since the games were strictly gender segregated. She turned to other girls, but with some regret that she was not there to continue the more active athletic involvement that was not available at that time to the girls. One day the boys asked her to join them. She was delighted, played, had a good time after the first moments of feeling somewhat ill at ease. On her return home she climbed over a fence rather awkwardly and tore her jeans. Later that day she noticed her underwear was stained. Although she had learned about menstruation she did not at the moment think about it but rather her first thought was that she had been hurt when she climbed the fence; and she connected this thought with some conflicts she had been momentarily aware of when joining the boys for the game. It was as if she had to pay a price for stepping out of the conventional bounds of what was expected of girls. Later she realized with some pride that she had begun to menstruate.

Some girls carry the denial to the extent of hiding the fact of their menstruating from everyone; they hide stained underwear, make excuses for it, refuse to wear pads or tampons. They may not be ready for or rebel against sexuality or motherhood, or they may feel frightened or uncomfortable being like the women they know. This reaction is particularly likely if the girl's relationship with her mother is not so good, the girl's mother is ambivalent or hostile, if the mothering was inadequate, or the girl's mother was chronically depressed (Benedek 1970; Weisman and Paykel 1974). In using the defense of denial the girl regresses to a more primitive adaptation, which involves a compromise with reality. It is as if by refusing to recognize it the process will stop.

Some do actually stop their menstruating by becoming anorexic. Although this disorder is complex, with many determinants, it does give the girl some control of her body functions—albeit in a self-destructive way. The anorexia is not necessarily a conscious goal but is part of a process that also leaves the girl with a less "feminine" shape.

Although for some girls who are disturbed by menarche the central issue is a conflict about femininity or the feminine role as they perceive it; for others it is an attempt to delay adulthood with its problems and decisions. The menses themselves require some adaptation and special skills to manage.

Cultural expectations and family patterns may add to the girl's experience of her menses as a time of distress (Parlee 1973; Parlee 1976). The existence of cleansing or purifying rituals, such as in Orthodox Judaism, implies dirtiness rather than normality, which can reinforce the girl's own conscious or unconscious feelings about her body. Whisnant and Zegans (1975) found that the white middle-class summer campers they studied had little conception of what their bodies were like or what menstruation involved, despite superficial knowledge. They emphasize that the culture ignores the affective importance of menarche. They also found that those girls experienced menarche as an "affectively charged event" related to emerging adult identity. They were "frightened and ashamed in spite of their stated belief that they should not be." It seemed difficult for them to integrate the information they had received. They did strongly associate menses with excretory soiling, and some clearly associated menarche with a wound or cut. At the same time their relationships to their mothers changed, with both manifestation of dependent regressive aspects and indications of identification with womanhood and motherhood.

The importance of menstruation in stimulating the girl to recognize some perception of her inner organs—her vagina and uterus, and to integrate these into her body image, which was discussed earlier as a positive effect—may also arouse fears connected not only with sexuality but with childbirth. Whisnant, Brett, and Zegans (1979) and Shopper (1979) studied the influence of mothers and peers on the reactions to menarche. The girls were influenced by their perceptions of their mother's attitudes in relation to various aspects of menstruation, and also in the use of napkins or tampons.

Initially most did not use tampons, nor was this encouraged by mothers. Many girls began to use tampons in any event one or two years after menarche. The mother's acceptance of the tampon could be seen as acknowledging the vagina and the potential for adult sexuality (Whisnant, Brett, and Zegans 1979). The use of the tampon also provides a socially accepted opportunity for girls to touch their genitals. This experience in turn helps a girl develop a clearer idea about her vagina and its relationship to her external genitals and confirms by her own experience and perception what she has been taught. The activity and explanation in relation to her genitals may have an important effect on her later sexuality.

Reactions of parents to a child's menarche are complex (Anthony 1970) and reflect not only responses to the child's sexuality but also serve as a reminder of their own aging. They may remember their own sexual struggles; there may be some recapitulation of these and the parent may provoke the adolescent to some acting out, or, if anxiety or depression is stirred up, it may precipitate sadistic behavior in the parent. Resolution of the conflicts aroused, acceptance and support, provide an important step toward the girl's maturity.

Research in this area is just beginning to expand. One can look forward to increased understanding of this very important experience in women's development.

References

Anthony, E.J. 1970. The reaction of parents to adolescents and to their behavior. In E.J. Anthony and T. Benedek, eds., *Parenthood*. Boston: Little, Brown.

Ash, M. 1980. The misnamed female sex organ. In M. Kirkpatrick, ed., *Women's sexual development*. New York: Plenum.

Benedek, T. 1952. *Psychosexual functions in women*. New York: Ronald Press.

_____ . 1970. Mothering and nurturing. In E. Anthony and T. Benedeck, eds., *Parenthood*. Boston: Little Brown.

Barglow, P., and Schaefer, M. 1979. The fate of the feminine self in normative adolescent regression. In M. Sugar, ed., *Female adolescent development*. New York: Brunner/Mazel.

Blos, P. 1979. The second individuation process of adolescence. In P. Blos, ed., *The adolescent passage*. New York: International Universities Press.

_____ . 1980. Modifications in the traditional psychoanalytic theory of female adolescent development. In S. Feinstein et al., eds., *Adolescent psychiatry*. Chicago: University of Chicago Press.

Clower, V. 1976. Theoretical implications in current views of masturbation in latency girls. *Journal of the American Psychoanalytic Association* 74:109-125.

Deutsch, H. 1944. *Psychology of women.* New York: Grune and Stratton.

Galenson, E., and Roiphe, H. 1976. Some suggested revisions concerning early female development. *Journal of the American Psychoanalytic Association* 24:269-283.

Harley, M. 1961. Some observations on the relationship between genitality and structural development in adolescence. *Journal of the American Psychoanalytic Association* 9:434-460.

Horney, K. 1973. The flight from womanhood. In J. Miller, ed., *Psychoanalysis and women.* New York: Brunner/Mazel.

Jones, E. 1935. Early female sexuality. *International Journal of Psychoanalysis* 6:263-273.

Kestenberg, J. 1975. Menarche. In Lorand and Schneer, eds., *Children and parents, psychoanalytic studies in development.* New York: J. Aronson.

Lerner, H. 1976. Parental mislabeling of female genitals as a determinant of penis and learning inhibitions in women. *Journal of American Psychoanalytic Association* 24:269-283.

Notman, M., and Nadelson, C. 1981. New views of femininity and its relation to reproduction. *Journal of the Hillside Hospital.*

Parlee, M. 1973. The premenstrual syndrome. *Pscyhological Bulletin* 80: 454-465.

———— . 1976. Social factors in the psychoanalysis of menstruation, birth and menopause. *Primary Care* 3:447-490.

Shopper, M. 1979. The (re)discovery of the vagina and the importance of the menstrual tampon. In M. Sugar, ed., *Female adolescent development.* New York: Brunner/Mazel.

Stoller, R. 1976. Primary femininity. *Journal of the American Psychoanalytic Association* 24:59-78.

Tanner, J.M. 1974. Sequence, tempo, and individual variation in the growth and development of boys and girls age 12-16. *Daedalus* 100:12-16.

Weisman, M., and Paykel, E. 1974. *The depressed woman.* Chicago: University of Chicago Press.

Whisnant, L., Brett, E., and Zegans, L. 1979. Adolescent girls and menstruation. In S. Feinstein and P. Giovacchini, eds., *Adolescent psychiatry,* vol. VII. Chicago: University of Chicago Press.

Whisnant, L., and Zegans, L. 1975. A study of attitudes toward menarche in white, middle-class American adolescent girls. *American Journal of Psychiatry* 132:809-820.

23 The Psychological Concomitants of Menarche in Psychiatric Patients

Jaine L. Darwin

Menarche is a developmental milestone in the lives of women, a discrete event often subsumed in the psychological literature under the rubrics of puberty and adolescence. The psychological literature is sparse despite the strong feelings and memories evoked when one speaks with girls and women about their menarche. These reactions suggest confirmation of Benedek's observation (Benedek 1952) that "it is as if menarche were a puberty rite cast upon woman by nature itself."

The study described in this chapter sought to begin to articulate the affective and cognitive responses to menarche that could be understood as falling within an adaptive range of functioning. The intent was to generate hypotheses and to begin to explore possible causal relationships between menarche and other aspects of preadolescent psychological functioning; to better understand the developmental and environmental skills necessary or sufficient to successfully negotiate the onset of menstruation. Clinical observation led me to speculate that menarche might be a contributing factor in the first psychiatric hospitalizations of a population of girls aged eleven to thirteen; that the symptoms that necessitated the hospitalization—agitation, hypervigilance, suicidal ideation and gesturing, cognitive disorganization—might be a manifestation of an exaggerated reaction to normal development rather than the early onset of a more severe psychiatric illness. However, the dearth of normative data on menarche has created a vacuum that complicates the task of understanding these girls.

The existing literature consists largely of theoretical articles supported by anecdotal reports emanating from the psychoanalytic community and of a growing body of empirical studies about attitudes toward menarche by developmental psychologists. Psychoanalytic theorists (Blos 1962; Deutsch 1944; Fraiberg 1955; Greenacre 1958; Harley 1971; Hart and Sarnoff 1971; Kestenberg 1975; Laufer 1968; Ritvo 1977; Shainess 1961) view menarche as a crisis of normal development occurring amidst the work of adolescence. The girl struggles to manage heightened sexual and aggressive impulses to cope with a reascendence of unresolved psycho-sexual conflicts, many of which are pregenital, and to separate from the primary object. The psychoanalytic writers view menarche as an organizing event, one that aids in the establishment of a female sexual identity, and as an anxiety-provoking event because of associations to castration and genital damage feared to stem from masturbation.

Empirical studies (Clarke and Ruble 1978; Harrison 1975; Koff, Rierden, and Silverstone 1978; Rierden and Koff 1980; Whisnant and Zegans 1975) have explored attitudes toward menarche and toward changes in a girl's sense of body integrity and sexual identity. Girls' attitudes differed with changes in their menarcheal status. The study described here used projective techniques to compare the feelings, fantasies, and adaptation of hospitalized pre- and postmenarcheal girls with a control group.

Method

Subjects

Four samples were selected for comparison: Five postmenarcheal girls ($\overline{X}$ age 12.3) for whom symptoms of behavioral disturbance appeared within one year of onset of menarche and resulted in a first psychiatric hospitalization were compared to a postmenarcheal control group ($N = 6$, $\overline{X}$ age 12.3) matched on the basis of age, number of months postmenarcheal, grade, socioeconomic status, and, when possible, religion and marital status of parents. Four premenarcheal girls ($\overline{X}$ age 11.5) for whom symptoms of behavioral disturbance appeared and a first psychiatric hospitalization ensued coincidental to the development of secondary sexual characteristics— breast budding, pubic/axial hair, or vaginal discharge— were compared to a premenarcheal control group ($N = 5$, $\overline{X}$ age 11.6) matched on the same demographic criteria as the postmenarcheal samples. Postmenarcheal groups were also compared to premenarcheal groups.

Inpatient subjects were selected by reading charts and identifying girls whose menarcheal or prepubescent status was documented, who lacked prior psychiatric hospitalization or confounding conditions like major neurological deficit, and for whom test and psychosocial data were available. The control groups were selected from a pool of girls solicited via newspaper ads and notices sent through organizations such as schools and girl scouts asking for participants in a study of normal development without mention of menarche, menstruation, or physical development. That information was obtained during phone conversations with mothers after the initial response. The controls were chosen on the basis of demographic match with members of the inpatient groups. Controls were paid for their time.

Procedure

For both inpatient groups, test data were collectd retrospectively from the charts. The Rorschach, the Thematic Apperception Test (TAT), cards 1,

3BM, 5, 16, and 18GF, the Draw-a-Person Test (DAP, and the psychosocial summaries were used. The controls were tested individually in their homes, by me. The mothers of the controls were asked to complete the Social Readjustment Rating Scale (Holmes and Rahe 1968) and to respond to a structured interview.

Each insrument was scored by two independent raters who did not know to which group any subject belonged. The Rorschach was scored utilizing Klopfer's system (1954). I then compiled summary sheets to ascertain ratios from these scorings. Four content scales were also used: Barrier and Penetration (Cleveland and Fisher 1958) and Anxiety and Hostility (Elizur 1949). Interrater agreeement spanned from 83 to 99 percent on the Rorschach measures. The TAT was scored using the Fine Manifest Content Scale (Fine 1955), which rates for the presence of a possible thirty-three feelings, ten types of interpersonal interactions, and for favorable, unfavorable, or indeterminant outcome of stories. The DAP was scored replicating the procedures used by Rierden and Koff (1980). Two trained social workers computed Social Readjustment Rating Scale scores for the inpatient groups on the basis of the information provided by the psychological summaries.

Results

The data were analyzed in a series of one-way analyses of variance for each of nineteen independent variables in the study. The material was also studied clinically. On the basis of most Rorschach measures, only the premenarcheal inpatients could be differentiated from the other groups. The postmenarcheal inpatients did not differ significantly in terms of quantitative measures from the control groups. When all the postmenarcheal girls were compared to all the premenarcheal girls on the basis of the Experience Balance, a Rorschach ratio thought to be related to the ability to attend to the demands of inner and outer reality, the postmenarcheal girls were significantly different, t (18) = 2.46, p = .02. Menarche appears to be an event that enhances a girl's ability to negotiate and balance internal and external demands.

The TAT data differentiated inpatients from controls without regard to menarcheal status. Both control groups could articulate a wider range of feelings and a greater frequency of feelings in their stories, $F(3,16)$ = 9.17, $p > .001$. Control groups also depicted more interpersonal interactions in their stories, $F(3,16)$ = 4.69, $p < .02$. The controls were significantly better able to tell stories with favorable endings than the inpatients $F(3,16)$ = 9.34, $p < .001$. The Social Readjustment Scale, a measure of objective stress in the environment, failed to distinguish among groups.

When the Rorschach and TAT data were examined from a clinical perspective, the postmenarcheal controls produced graphic fantasy materials, while the postmenarcheal inpatients were more constricted in their production. Both sets of protocols reflected similar concerns, but the postmenarcheal controls were better elaborated. Both postmenarcheal groups showed a high level of concern about aggression and about genital damage. Premenarcheal controls tended to be better defended and premenarcheal inpatients produced protocols that reflected a significant level of ego deficiency.

Discussion

Quantitative measures of intrapsychic structure failed to distinguish between postmenarcheal inpatients and postmenarcheal controls. The differences may lie in the manner in which the same conflicts are expressed. While the postmenarcheal inpatients often presented as markedly disturbed, their symptoms remitted rapidly in the hospital and the data obtained from psychological testing did not reflect the level of disturbance suggested by the behavior. The postmenarcheal controls gave Rorschach responses replete with blood and violence; all the postmenarcheal controls gave at least one Rorschach response in which they used color shading as a determinant. Color shading is thought to represent a heightened sensitivity to affect and a potential suicidal indicator (Appelbaum and Holzman 1962). None of these girls appeared suicidal or expressed suicidal ideation. These signs were absent in the protocols of the postmenarcheal inpatients, all of whom had expressed suicidal ideation or made gestures. The postmenarcheal controls appear to utilize fantasy as a mode in which to work through intrapsychic issues, allowing multiple opportunities to wrestle with the conflicts—in this case around the separation from the internalized representation of the mother. The postmenarcheal inpatients appear to act out these conflicts, limiting the chances to practice because of the dangerous consequences of some of these actions. Fantasy themes are dominated by aggressive content-reflecting concerns about separation and genital mutilation. The highly descriptive and graphic manner in which some of the postmenarcheal girls fantasize may be indicative of the same loosening ego boundaries thought to occur during pregnancy (Bibring 1959). Postmenarcheal girls also appear to show more flexible cognitive-affective balances, the ability to shift attention between demands from within and demands from without, than the premenarcheal girls.

Premenarcheal controls are able to elaborate their fantasies, but tend to avoid aggressive content and to be less pulled by phallic stimuli than the postmenarcheal groups. On TAT stories, the premenarcheal controls expressed feelings rated under *pain* with very high frequency. This finding may confirm Kestenberg's (1975) observation that premenarcheal girls may seek painful solutions in an effort to find boundaries. Premenarcheal inpatients are barely able to respond to the demands of the tasks. They lack sufficient ability to organize intrapsychic energies, to manage affect and, at times, to reality test. While a first psychiatric hospitalization shortly after menarche is not necessarily indicative of a serious mental illness, a first psychiatric hospitalization during prepubesence is a poor prognostic indicator. Why the premenarcheal inpatients are different from the postmenarcheal inpatients will need further exploration; if the difference between the two hospitalized groups is a function of menarcheal status, it may be the organizing, progressive aspects of menarche that make the postmenarcheal inpatients look healthier and recompensate faster.

Girls hospitalized within one year of menarche shared many similarities with the postmenarcheal controls, but they lacked the capacity to utilize fantasy as a predominant mode in which to practice and work through issues of development and were prone to revert to action. At this time, it is difficult to understand why the ability to utilize fantasy is lacking. At a time in development when many of the concerns relate to aggression, the tendency to express in action may have serious consequences; that is, behavior destructive to oneself or to others. The control group showed a capacity for a wider range of response than the inpatient girls. They could be more labile and more reactive; at the same time they could exercise better control over which behavior they chose to demonstrate at which time.

The postmenarcheal girls from both groups were impressive in their preoccupations with issues of aggression and with issues of body integrity. Both groups also suggest they may have shifted in their cognitive-affective balance to being oriented both inward and to the external world.

The premenarcheal girls appeared more global in their preoccupations and less focused on issues of aggression. While these findings cannot be attributed to menarcheal status conclusively, the menarcheal status must be considered as a possible cause, reflecting Kestenberg's (1975) perception of premenarcheal girls as overstimulated and unable to focus.

Menarche, as Ritvo (1977) suggested, is a crisis of development with the potential for both progression and regression. Girls in preadolescence are confronted with a surge of instinctual energies by which they are, at times, confused and frightened. Postmenarcheal girls in this study appear to be dealing with concerns about body intactness, about aggression, about separation from mother. Postmenarcheal hospitalized girls appear to differ in the manner in which they deal with these issues rather than in the content of the issues with which they are dealing. Whether menarche serves to disrupt functioning significantly may be a function of ego modes available to the girl in which to work through the issues. A hospitalization shortly after menarche may indicate an ultimately regressive result of menarche or may be reactive in nature and eventually facilitate growth and consolidation. Though menarche raises anxiety, it suggests itself as facilitating the developmental work of preadolescence.

The most salient fact emerging from this study in terms of implications for education is the discrepancy between the girl's understanding of what is happening physiologically and her own way of making meaning out of the event. Articulate girls who could explain intellectually what was happening to their bodies produced fantasies that implied they felt castrated or genitally mutilated. These girls gave few overt signs of their fantasies; and these were girls who had available mothers who at least professed to be enlightened and accepting of their daughters' sexuality. What must it be like for girls who are provided with little factual information and for whom mothers are unavailable as resources? Does the discrepancy exist because the information was not presented in a way that was cognitively helpful to the girl at her specific level of development?

In therapeutic work with menarcheal girls, a therapist might view the fantasy productions of these girls as reminiscent of the fantasy productions of pregnant women, where there is a loosening of ego boundaries and a primary process-like quality. In fact it may be helpful to view menarche as having a psychology of its own, much like pregnancy, which is superimposed on the developmental tasks going on when it occurs. One would expect some aspects to remain constant whether a girl began to menstruate at age eleven, fourteen, or seventeen; and some aspects would change because of the different developmental work required at age eleven, fourteen, or seventeen. A therapist may need to pay special attention to depression in girls of this age because of the concerns they have about aggression and the potential for self-destruction as an expression of those concerns. Mainly, a case may be made for focusing a special lens on menarcheal status and its potential for disruption in functioning in some preadolescent girls.

The task for the future is to compile empirical data that support theoretical and clinical data on menarche. As our society becomes focused on issues of female development, it must look at the point at which the physiological transition from girl to woman is made.

References

Applebaum, S.A., and Holzman, P.S. 1962. The color shading response and suicide. *Journal of Projective Techniques* 26:151-161.
Benedek, T. 1952. *Psychosexual functions in women.* New York: Ronald Press.

Bibring, G.L. 1959. Some considerations of the psychological processes in pregnancy. *Psychoanalytic Study of the Child* 14:113-121.

Blos, P. 1962. *On adolescence.* New York: Free Press.

Clarke, A., and Ruble, D. 1978. Young adolescents' beliefs concerning menstruation. *Child Development* 49:231-234.

Cleveland, S., and Fisher, S. 1958. *Body image and personality.* New York: Van Nostrand.

Deutsch, H. 1944. *The psychology of woman,* vol. 1. New York: Grune and Stratton.

Elizur, A. 1949. Content analysis of the Rorschach with regard of anxiety and hostility. *Journal of Projective Techniques* 13:247-284.

Fine, R. 1955. A scoring system for the TAT and other verbal projective techniques. *Journal of Projective Techniques* 19:306-316.

Fraiberg, S. 1955. Some considerations of the introduction to therapy in puberty. *Psychoanalytic Study of the Child* 10:264-286.

Greenacre, P. 1958. The sense of identity. *Journal of the American Psychoanalytic Association* 6:612-627.

Harley, M.J. 1971. Some reflections on identity problems in prepuberty. In J. McDevitt, ed., *Separation-individuation, essays in honor of Margaret S. Mahler.* New York: International Universities Press.

Harrison, S. 1975. The body experience of prepubescent, pubescent, and postpubescent girls and boys. Unpublished doctoral dissertation, Yeshiva University.

Hart, M., and Sarnoff, C. 1971. The impact of the menarche: A study of two stages of organization. *American Journal of Child Psychiatry* 10:257-271.

Holmes, T., and Rahe, R. 1968. The social readjustment rating scale. *Journal of Psychosomatic Research* 11:213-218.

Kestenberg, J.S., and Robbins, E. 1976. *Children and parents: Psychoanalytic studies in child development.* New York: J. Aronson.

Klopfer, B., Ainsworth, M., Klopfer, W., and Holt, R. 1954. *Developments in the Rorschach technique,* vol. 1. New York: Harcourt and Brace.

Koff, E., Rierden, J., and Silverstone, E. 1978. Changes in representation of body images as a function of menarcheal status. *Developmental Psychology* 14:635-664.

Laufer, M. 1968. The body image: Problems of ownership of the body. *Psychoanalytic Study of the Child* 23:114-137.

Rierden, J., and Koff, E. 1980. The psychological impact of menarche: Integrative versus disruptive changes. *Journal of Youth and Adolescence* 9:49-58.

Ritvo, S. 1977. Adolescent to woman. In H.P. Blum, ed., *Female psychology: Contemporary psychoanalytic views.* New York: International Universities Press.

Shainess, N. 1961. A re-evaluation of some aspects of feminity through a study of menstruation: A preliminary report. *Comprehensive Psychiatry* 2:20-26.

Whisnant, L., and Zegans, L. 1975. A study of attitudes toward menarche in white middle-class American adolescent girls. *American Journal of Psychiatry* 132:809-814.

24 Primary and Secondary Amenorrhea in Anorexia Nervosa

James R. Falk,
Katherine A. Halmi,
Elke Eckert,
and *Regina Casper*

A prominent symptom of anorexia nervosa in women is amenorrhea. Several investigtors have proposed that there are critical body weights (depending on height) for onset of menstruation or recovery from secondary amenorrhea (Frisch 1977; Frisch and McArthur 1974; Frisch and Revelle 1970). Perhaps the relation of primary and secondary amenorrhea in anorexia nervosa would be better explained by nutritional or caloric deficits since it has been observed that menstruating obese women on low-calorie diets may become amenorrheic (Russell and Beardwood 1970). Moreover, Fries (1977) in his study of secondary amenorrhea in anorexia nervosa has noted, by averaging data from the literature, that secondary amenorrhea in anorectics precedes other symptoms (for example, weight loss) an average of 16.2 percent of the time and is coincident with other symptoms an average of 55 percent of the time.

Frisch and McArthur (1974) note that other factors, including emotional stress, can affect the onset and continuation of the menstrual cycle. Therefore, menstrual cycles may cease without weight loss, and may not resume in some women even after the minimum-required weight is reached. Frisch and McArthur (1974) continue their statement by emphasizing that "this does not negate the finding that a critical minimum weight appears to be necessary for the onset and maintenance of normal menstrual cycles in the human female" (p. 951). This interesting hypothesis stimulated a number of investigations, with results both supporting and not supporting the hypothesis.

For example, Trussell (1978) reexamined the studies of Frisch and others, which led to the formulation of the critical-body-weight hypothesis. His conclusions were that the work of Frisch and her colleagues did not supply evidence that conclusively supports the hypothesis. In an interesting Monte-Carlo test of weight as a critical factor in menarche, Van't Hof and Roede (1977) found that weight and height were only moderately related to menarche—not the critical factor.

There is a great deal of evidence in support of the critical-body-weight hypothesis. For example, Boyar et al. (1974) have shown that the circadian secretion of luteinizing-hormone (LH) in emaciated anorectics resembled that of prepubertal and pubertal children. Frisch (1977) notes that the nine anorectic patients of Boyar et al. (1974), who were amenorrheic with prepubertal LH secretory patterns, were below the minimal weights required for recovery of menses. However, Katz et al. (1977) found that anorectic women who had regained their weight and continued an abnormal eating pattern, continued to have an "immature" LH secretory pattern.

Pirke et al. (1979) found that the adult circadian LH secretory pattern returned only in those anorectics at greater than 80 percent of ideal body weight (IBW). Pirke et al. (1979) also noted that the older the patients and the longer they are ill, the slower the normalization of the LH pattern. The data of Frisch (1977; table 2, p. 155) suggest that both the onset of menarche and recovery from secondary amenorrhea occur when the patient weighs approximately 87 percent of average weight for height for these events (with approximately 10 percent of the population falling below this value). Since normalization of adult LH secretion (at 80 percent IBW) is necessary for normalization of menstruation (at ≈ 87 percent IBW), the body-weight figures appear to be in accord.

To test the critical-body-weight hypothesis we examined the menstrual history of 105 female anorexia-nervosa patients seen at three collaborating hospitals. The body weights of patients with primary amenorrhea and those of patients having recovered from secondary amenorrhea (that is, from a previous episode of anorexia nervosa) were compared. We examined the relationships of menstrual history with weight history and other variables to test a second hypothesis that patients having symptoms typical of poor prognosis in anorexia (that is, self-induced vomiting, purgative abuse, and bulimia) would also have a history of a more severe menstrual disorder.

Method

In three collaborating hospitals, data regarding age of menarche and menstrual history of 105 female anorexia-nervosa patients were obtained as part of a structured interview conducted prior to treatment by a social worker with the patient's family and the patient. This interview was designed to examine the clinical characteristics of the patients just prior to hospitalization including: (a) behavior typical of anorexia nervosa and sexual attitudes, (b) mental status, (c) menstrual history, and (d) previous medical history and premorbid personality. Included in the interview was the parent's or spouse's rating of the patient's anorectic behavior using the Slade Anorectic Behavior Scale (Slade 1973), which examines items such as vomiting, purgative abuse, hyperactivity, and aberrant food handling.

Subjects

All subjects participating in this study were female and met the diagnostic criteria of anorexia nervosa as outlined in Halmi et al. (1977, table 1, p. 44). Patient participation in this study was strictly voluntary and contingent on their informed consent. The mean age of the 105 patients at time of admission to the study was twenty years (SD ± five years). All subjects were amenorrheic at the time of the interview.

Results and Discussion

The mean (± SD) age of menarche was found to be 13 ± 1.2 years with fifteen patients having never menstruated. Having never menstruated will be referred to as *primary amenorrhea*, although in a stricter sense primary amenorrhea implies that the patient is older than the upper normal age limit for menarche (that is, 18 years) and has never menstruated. The range of ages of those patients with primary amenorrhea (loosely defined) was 12 to 18 years (Mean = 14.9 ± 1.9 years). The range of ages at which anorexia nervosa became apparent in these fifteen patients was 10 to 14 years (Mean = 12.4 ± 1.5 years; that is, covering a range of years normal for menarche).

A comparison of the highest weight and height of those patients with primary amenorrhea with the minimal weight for height for menarche as tabulated in Frisch (1977) was performed. Two patients had episodes of anorexia nervosa at ten years old (roughly at the lower normal age limit for menarche) and their data were not included in the comparison. All but three of the remaining thirteen patients with primary amenorrhea had sufficient weight (according to the critical-body-weight hypothesis) prior to anorexia nervosa for menarche to have occurred. Figure 24-1 illustrates this comparison.

The mean percent of the average weight for menarche of the ten eligible primary-amenorrhea patients prior to anorexia nervosa was 99.15 ± 10.96 percent (using as normative, the fiftieth percentile as tabulated in Frisch 1977). Mean percent of average weight for those three patients not eligible for onset of menarche was 82.13 ± 5.32 percent. A t-test of the mean percent of average weight of the thirteen patients with primary amenorrhea against Frisch's 86.71 ± .09 percent figure for menarche yielded a t = 2.503 (p<.013 one-tailed test). It would appear that body weight was not the major cause of the primary amenorrhea in this group, but further investigation is warranted for a definitive conclusion.

The remaining ninety patients who were menstruating prior to the onset of anorexia nervosa were asked questions that examined the regularity of

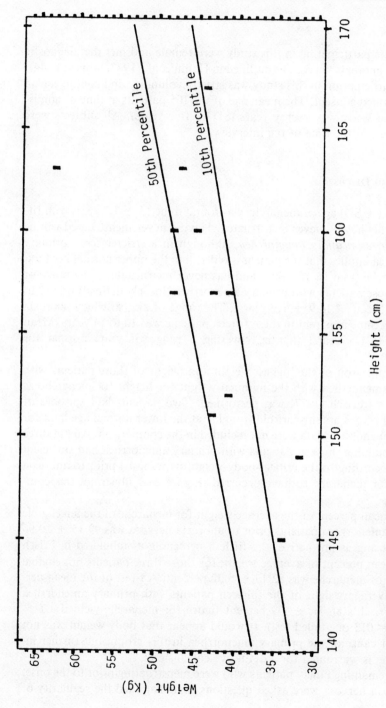

Height (cm)

Weight (kg)

50th Percentile

10th Percentile

Note: The 10th and 50th percentiles for onset of menses were obtained from the data presented in Frisch (1977). *Anorexia nervosa*, New York: Raven Press.

Figure 24-1. Highest Weight and Height of Thirteen Anorexia-Nervosa Patients with Primary Amenorrhea (represented as ■)

their menstrual cycles, frequency of occurrence of amenorrhea lasting three or more months, time of secondary amenorrhea relative to onset of anorexia nervosa, and whether secondary amenorrhea occurred before or after ten pounds of weight loss. Also, information regarding time from onset of anorexia and weight at recovery of menses was obtained from thirteen patients (14.9 percent) who had resumed menstruating at least once since the first episode of secondary amenorrhea *and* anorexia.

Before the onset of anorexia nervosa, 60 percent of the ninety patients reported that their menstrual cycles were fairly regular (that is, the same number of days ± 3). The remaining 40 percent reported that their cycles were only moderately irregular, varying 4 to 10 days. Regarding the frequency of occurrence of amenorrhea lasting three or more months, 28.9 percent of the patients reported that they were never amenorrheic before their present episode, 52.2 percent reported having been amenorrheic once before, and 18.9 percent reported having been amenorrheic twice before.

The majority of the patients (65.5 percent) claimed that their current episode of amenorrhea first occurred after the onset of anorexia nervosa; 18.4 percent of the patients claimed they became amenorrheic before anorexia (ranging one to fourteen months before anorexia) and 16.1 percent said amenorrhea occurred at onset of anorexia. (Three of the ninety postmenarcheal patients were not certain of their menstrual history and were not included in this analysis or the following analyses.) Menstruation stopped after 10 pounds of weight loss in 57.5 percent of the patients, and the remaining 42.5 percent of the patients claimed menstruation stopped before ten pounds of weight loss.

These results, in general, agree with the results of other studies of secondary amenorrhea in anorexia nervosa as reported in Fries (1977). However, our results show a greater occurrence of secondary amenorrhea after manifest eating disorder or significant weight loss rather than before or coincident with these symptoms (compare table 1 in Fries 1977).

Thirteen (14.9 percent) of the postmenarcheal patients had recovered menses at least once since the first episode of amenorrhea and anorexia prior to the current episode of anorexia. We were able to obtain the weight of twelve of these patients at return of menses; however, our height record was available for only eight of the twelve patients. Frisch (1977) tabulates the minimal weight for height at the tenth percentile of recovery from secondary amenorrhea, which is 87.08 ± .07 percent of average weight for recovery (that is, the fiftieth percentile). Three of the eight recovered from secondary amenorrhea with weights above the 87 percent threshold point (Mean = 93.16 ± 7.77 percent). The remaining five patients (62.5 percent or five-eighths) in the comparison had recovered from secondary amenorrhea well below the 87 percent threshold value (Mean = 73.7 ± 10.82 percent). This comparison is illustrated in Figure 24-2.

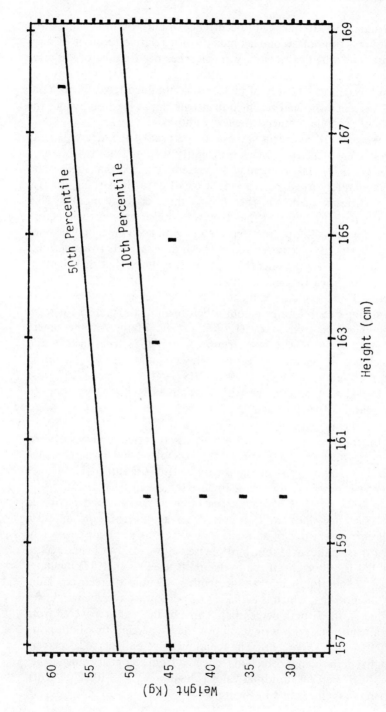

Note: The 10th and 50th percentiles for restoration of menses were obtained from the data presented in Frisch (1977). *Anorexia nervosa*, New York: Raven Press.

Figure 24-2. Weight at Restoration of Menstrual Cycles and Height of Eight Anorexia-Nervosa Patients Who Had Recovered from a Previous Episode of Secondary Amenorrhea (represented as ■)

If Frisch (1977) is correct, we would have expected only 10 percent of our eight patients, or one person, to have recovered below the threshold value. Thus, there would appear to be a mechanism superseding weight as a critical factor in recovery from secondary amenorrhea. Perhaps it is calorie intake, but unfortunately we do not have the patient's calorie records prior to their admission to the study. Of interest, however, is that higher caloric intake at the end of the seven-day pretreatment period was negatively correlated with greater frequency of occurrence of amenorrhea ($r = -.1839$, $p<.05$ one-tailed test) prior to the current episode of anorexia nervosa. Nevertheless, we must emphasize using caution in interpreting these results since the menstrual history was obtained in retrospect.

In our examination of the relationship of the patients' menstrual history with other symptoms of anorexia nervosa we found greater use of purgatives ($t = 2.28$, $p<.014$) and self-induced vomiting ($t = 1.80$, $p<.038$) with greater frequency of occurrence of amenorrhea before the current episode of anorexia nervosa (one-tailed tests).

Bulimia in these patients did not contribute significantly to occurrence of amenorrhea; however, in those patients that recovered from secondary amenorrhea before the current episode (seven patients were bulimic and six were nonbulimic) the bulimic group took an average of sixteen months (from onset of illness) to recover, while the nonbulimics recovered in an average of eight months ($t = 1.8$, $p<.05$ one-tailed test). Self-induced vomiting also played a role in recovery from secondary amenorrhea due to anorexia. Six of the patients who recovered from secondary amenorrhea were vomiters and seven were nonvomiters. The vomiters recovered menses in an average of seventeen months while the nonvomiters recovered in an average of eight months ($t = 1.9$, $p<.042$ one-tailed test). These results might simply indicate that bulimics and vomiters continue to suffer the ill effects of anorexia nervosa longer.

Purgative use apparently did not significantly affect time to recovery in these patients (although eight of the thirteen who recovered menses also abused purgatives). Purgative use did affect the length of time from secondary amenorrhea to onset of anorexia in those sixteen patients where amenorrhea occurred before anorexia. The purgative group ($N = 7$) experienced amenorrhea an average of five-and-one-half months before onset of anorexia while the nonpurgative group ($N = 9$) experienced amenorrhea an averge of twenty-two months prior to onset of anorexia ($t = 2.79$, $p<.019$ two-tailed test). This difference between the two groups may simply indicate that purgative users succumb more rapidly to anorexia nervosa.

The results obtained in this study did not support the critical-body-weight hypothesis. That is, the results are inconclusive regarding critical body weight and menarche. The majority of the patients experiencing primary amenorrhea were above the threshold weight for menarche prior to anorexia nervosa; however, other stress factors, perhaps those leading to anorexia nervosa, are likely to have delayed menarche. The results indicate that body weight is not the critical factor in recovery from secondary amenorrhea resulting from anorexia nervosa; however, the use of retrospective data in this analysis make further study of this issue necessary.

Patients having engaged in purging behavior (that is, self-induced vomiting and/or purgative abuse) suffered more episodes of secondary amenorrhea than nonpurgers. Bulimic patients and/or vomiters also took significantly longer to recover menses after onset of illness than non-bulimics and nonvomiters as a result of longer illness. It would be interesting to examine bulimia and purging behavior in a nonanorectic population to more fully understand their effects on menstruation.

References

Boyar, R.M., Katz, J., Finkelstein, J.W., Kapen, S., Weiner, H., Weitzman, E.D., and Hellman, L. 1974. Anorexia nervosa: Immaturity of the 24-hour luteinizing hormone secretory pattern. *New England Journal of Medicine* 291:861-865.

Fries, H. 1977. Studies on secondary amenorrhea, anorectic behavior, and body-image perception: Importance for the early recognition of anorexia nervosa. In R. Vigersky, ed., *Anorexia nervosa*. New York: Raven Press.

Frisch, R.E. 1977. Food intake, fatness, and reproductive ability. In R. Vigersky, ed., *Anorexia nervosa*. New York: Raven Press.

Frisch, R.E., and McArthur, J.W. 1974. Menstrual cycles: Fatness as a determinant of minimum weight for height necessary for their maintenance or onset. *Science* 185:949-951.

Frisch, R.E., and Revelle, R. 1970. Height and weight at menarche and a hypothesis of critical body weights and adolescent events. *Science* 169:397-399.

Halmi, K.A., Goldberg, S.C., Eckert, E., Casper, R., and Davis, J.M. 1977. Pretreatment evaluation in anorexia nervosa. In R. Vigersky, ed., *Anorexia nervosa*. New York: Raven Press.

Katz, J.L., Boyar, R.M. Roffwarg, H., Hellman, L., and Weiner, H. 1977. LHRH responsiveness in anorexia nervosa: Intactness despite prepubertal circadian LH pattern. *Psychosomatic Medicine* 39:241-251.

Pirke, K.M., Fichter, M.M., Lund, R., and Doerr, R. 1979. Twenty-four hour sleep-wake pattern of plasma LH in patients with anorexia nervosa. *Acta Endocrinologica* 92:193-204.

Russell, G.F.M., and Beardwood, C.J. 1970. Amenorrhea in the feeding disorders: Anorexia nervosa and obesity. *Psychotherapy and Psychosomatics* 18:358-364.

Slade, P.D. 1973. A short anorexic behavior scale. *British Journal of Psychiatry* 122:83-85.

Trussell, J. 1978. Menarche and fatness: Reexamination of the critical body composition hypothesis. *Science* 200:1506-1509 (with a reply from R. Frisch).

Van't Hof, M.R., and Roede, M.J. 1977. A Monte-Carlo test of weight as a critical factor in menarche compared with bone age and measures of height, width and sexual development. *Annals of Human Biology* 4:581-585.

25 Premenstrual Affective Syndrome in Adolescent and Adult Psychiatric Patients

Richard C. Friedman,
John F. Clarkin,
Stephen W. Hurt,
Ruth Corn, and
Michael S. Aronoff

Menarche has often been written about as if it were a single event: the first occasion of menstrual bleeding. From another point of view, menarche is the beginning of a cyclical process. The onset of rhythmical changes in the internal environment that begin with menarche have been underemphasized in the clinical literature on adolescent psychopathology.

Our interest in menarche originally stemmed from retrospective observations of relationships between psychopathology and the menstrual cycle in adults. Initially, we found the literature difficult to interpret. On the one hand, a variety of psychopathological or otherwise deviant acts occur premenstrually and menstrually with greater frequency than would be expected by chance (Friedman et al. 1980; O'Conner, Shelly, and Stern 1974; Glass et al. 1971; Janowsky, Gorney, and Castelnuovo-Tedesco 1969). On the other hand, the few studies done of symptomatic excerbation occurring regularly premenstrually and/or menstrually in psychiatric patients had not yielded uniformly positive results. Thus, Coppen (1965) reported that patients with affective disorders did not experience increased depression premenstrually or menstrually. Diamond et al. (1976) found that patients with primary affective disorders did not differ from controls with regard to the occurrence of premenstrual affective symptomatology. These negative studies of patients with affective disorders appeared particularly puzzling in view of the evidence that suicide (MacKinnon, MacKinnon and Thomson 1959), and suicide attempts (Wetzel and McClure, 1972), as well as calls to suicide prevention centers (Wetzel, Reich, and McClure 1971) occur more frequently premenstrually and menstrually than expected by chance, at least in some studies. These data, as well as abundant literature indicating that mood frequently fluctuates with the cycle, suggested to us that Premenstrual Affective Syndrome (PAS) might actually be more common in adult psychiatric patients than had been previously realized.

The authors would like to acknowledge the most helpful assistance of Ms. Madeline C. Murphy and Ms. Pat Cobb in the preparation of this chapter.

There have been no reports to date in which PAS has been described in adolescent patients suffering from psychiatric illnesses, however. The little data about PAS in psychiatric patients presently available comes from studies of women above the age of thirty (Coppen 1965; Diamond et al. 1976; Kashiwagi, McClure, and Wetzel 1976; Endicott, Halbreich, and Schacht 1981). PAS has been reported to peak in incidence and severity in women between the ages of twenty-five and forty (O'Conner, Shelly, and Stern 1974). Thus, although the clinical literature is extremely scant, it might appear that the subject of PAS is far removed from the psychological aspects of menarche.

If, however, the complex set of symptomatic behaviors subsumed under the rubric PAS actually occurred earlier in the life cycle than previously realized, its relevance for furthering the understanding of menarche would be more apparent. It is possible, for example, that associated with the onset of the cycling process could be the onset of cyclical psychopathology in some adolescent patients. It is noteworthy that the literature on psychological difficulties associated with the menstrual cycle in normal girls is also sparse. However, in a study of 5,485 normal Finnish adolescent girls, Widholm and Kantero (1971) found that 32.7 percent complained of premenstrual tension and 59.4 percent complained of premenstrual fatigue and/or irritability.

In the absence of reports of PAS in adolescent psychiatric patients, it seems important to ascertain its occurrence in this age range. If PAS does exist in adolescents who are already vulnerable to stressors because of psychiatric illness, it may exacerbate the pre-existing illness and behavioral difficulties. Conversely, if PAS does not exist in such adolescents to any significant degree, the intermediate psychophysiological mechanisms responsible for the age disparity and occurrence would become an important focus for future research. As a pilot step in investigating the relationship between age, psychopathology, and PAS, we compared the prevalence of PAS between a small number of adolescent and adult psychiatric inpatients.

Method

The study described in this chapter was carried out on the inpatient service of the Westchester Division of New York Hospital. Patients were interviewed by a research nurse if they were between fourteen and forty-five years of age, were not pregnant or on oral contraceptive medication, and were given a diagnosis on admission to the hospital of major affective disorder, borderline personality disorder, or schizophrenia. All patients were interviewed on a single occasion by a research nurse who completed a menstrual history to determine the physical characteristics of the menstrual cycle. A structured interview was administered to determine the presence of PAS according to the (slightly modified) criteria of Kashiwagi, McClure, and Wetzel (1976). (See table 25-1.) Patients were asked about the premenstrual and menstrual phases of their last three cycles. For probable PAS, dysphoric mood of at least moderate severity, plus at least one somatic symptom during the premenstrual week were required. We note that in no case was a patient assigned to the PAS positive category on the basis of increased mood or energy (5 on table 25-1) as the only behavioral criterion. In addition, patients either had to rate the overall severity of symptomatic impairment as being moderate or severe, or judge that someone else would be able to recognize when they were about to have a period. For definite PAS, both of these latter two criteria were required. Patients with probable or definite PAS are referred to as *positive PAS patients* in the remainder of this chapter. In addition the Menstrual Attitude Questionnaire (MAQ) (Brooks, Ruble, and Clark 1977) was administered. Scores on each dimension were calculated by dividing the sum of all items in a dimension by the number of items.

Table 25-1
Criteria for Premenstrual Affective Syndrome (PAS)

Criteria of Kashiwagi, McClure, and Wetzel (1976)[a]	*Current Criteria*[b]
A. At least one of the following psychological symptoms:	A. At least one of the following psychological symptoms:
1. Sad, blue, depressed	1. Sad, blue, depressed
2. Tense or nervous	2. Tense, on edge, irritable
3. Crying easily	3. Nervous, agitated, pacing
4. Decreased energy	4. Tired, listless, decreased energy
5. Increased mood or energy	5. Increased mood, felt more positive or better
	6. Worried, fearful, panicky
	7. Hostile, quarrelsome, assaultive
B. At least one of the following somatic symptoms:	B. At least one of the following somatic symptoms:
1. Swelling of legs	1. Swelling of legs or ankles
2. Swelling of abdomen	2. Swelling of abdomen
3. Tenderness of breasts	3. Swelling or tenderness of breasts
4. Weight gain	4. Weight gain
C. Subjective rating of symptoms (moderate or severe)	C. Subjective rating of symptoms (moderate or severe)
D. Objective recognition	D. Objective recognition

[a]Time interval: at any point during the last three premenstrual days.
[b]Time interval: at any point during the week preceding the onset of the last three menses.

Subsequently, a chart review for definitive DSM-III diagnosis was conducted by judges blind to the menstrual data. In equivocal cases, a second, independent chart review was done. In rare cases of disagreement, a third reviewer independently reviewed the chart and the diagnosis chosen by two of three reviewers was used. If all three disagreed, the patient was dropped from the study ($N = 3$). Fifteen patients met criteria for Axis I major depression and concommitant Axis II borderline personality disorder, eleven patients met criteria for major depression alone, thirteen patients met criteria for schizophrenia and nine patients manifested borderline personality disorder only.

Results and Discussion

In analyzing the results of this study, we found the menstrual histories of these patients in the year preceding their hospitalizations were remarkable for the absence of abnormalities. In general, no significant differences due to either age or PAS status were found. Average cycle length was approximately twenty-eight days and was not influenced by age or presence of PAS. Seventy-six percent of the adolescents and 58 percent of the adults reported regular cycles of twenty-five to thirty-five days in length for the same period. As with average cycle length, the regularity of the cycle was not significantly affected by either age or presence of PAS. Dysmenorrhea was reported as sometimes present by 70 percent of the adolescent sample in contrast to only 58 percent of the adult sample. While slightly higher for the adolescents, the difference is not significant and for either group is not affected by the presence or absence of PAS. In both age groups, no one reported dysmenorrhea of at least moderate severity among the PAS negative group. In the PAS positive group, dysmenorrhea of at least moderate severity was reported by 20 percent and 26 percent of the adolescents and adults, respectively.

In a previous report (Hurt et al. in press) we described a relationship between prevalence of PAS and DSM-III diagnosis. To exclude the possible confounding influence of diagnosis on the relationship between prevalence of PAS and age group, we analyzed our current data for differences in the diagnostic make-up of the two age groups. We found no significant relationship between diagnosis and age group in these data. This fact was true for the total sample, for the positive PAS, and the negative PAS groups considered separately. No differences in prevalence of symptoms of PAS were found between the adolescent and adult age groups for either positive PAS or negative PAS groups.

Table 25-2 shows the comparison of the total behavioral-symptom severity for the premenstrual and menstrual phases of these patients' last

Table 25-2
Total Behavioral-Symptom Scores by Age Group and PAS Status Determined by Modified Kashiwagi Criteria

Age Group	Positive PAS				Negative PAS			
	Premenstrual Phase	Menstrual Phase	t	$p <$	Premenstrual Phase	Menstrual Phase	t	$p <$
Adolescents	(n = 10)				(n = 7)			
Mean	17.70	14.30	2.02	.05	9.00	12.71	-2.28	n.s
Standard deviation	5.40	4.24			2.89	5.28		
Adults	(n = 19)				(n = 12)			
Mean	18.53	13.79	4.37	.0005	11.67	9.58	1.18	n.s.
Standard deviation	3.63	3.68						
t	-0.49	0.34			-1.47	1.42		
p	n.s.	n.s.			n.s.	n.s.		

n.s. = not significant.

three cycles. For both the adolescent and adult PAS groups, irrespective of diagnosis, total behavioral-symptom severity was significantly lower (one-tailed t tests) during the menstrual phase of the cycle in comparison to the premenstrual phase of the cycle. For the PAS negative groups, no significant changes were found in total behavioral-symptom severity when the premenstrual and menstrual phases of the cycle were compared. Thus, both the adolescent and adult positive PAS groups show a significant diminution of total behavioral symptomatology following the onset of menstruation. Comparisons of the mean levels of total behavioral symptomatology within cycle phase but across age groups revealed no significant age effects on these levels for either the positive PAS or negative PAS groups.

Table 25-3 gives the mean item values and percent of patients who agree (mean item value > 4.00) for the five attitude dimensions of the MAQ. We found no significant age effects for either the comparisons of the adolescent and adult positive PAS or negative PAS groups. In general, however, the positive PAS adolescents tended to view menstruation as a more debilitating and bothersome event than the adults.

These results, albeit from a small number of patients, suggest that PAS, as manifested by specific criteria, is as common among adolescent psychiatric inpatients as it is among adults, and therefore might not be age dependent. Moreover, symptoms that regularly fluctuate with the cycle are

Table 25-3
Menstrual Attitude Questionnaire

	Adolescents		Adults	
	Positive PAS (n = 10)	No PAS (n = 7)	Positive PAS (n = 19)	No PAS (n = 12)
Debilitating				
Percent agree	80%	43%	47%	42%
Mean-item value	4.19	4.00	3.99	3.78
Bothersome				
Percent agree	90%	57%	79%	58%
Mean-item value	4.77	4.59	4.30	4.20
Positive				
Percent agree	90%	71%	79%	83%
Mean-item value	4.87	4.20	4.86	4.75
Predictable				
Percent agree	90%	71%	84%	67%
Mean-item value	4.84	4.37	4.86	4.33
Denial				
Percent agree	10%	29%	0%	17%
Mean-item value	2.67	2.84	2.68	3.11

associated with significant distress in both adolescent and adult inpatient samples and are, therefore, of clinical significance. These data are at variance with the findings of other investigators that Premenstrual Affective Syndrome is more likely to occur in older women (Kramp 1968).

The cycle may be associated with psychopathological behavior in adolescents. Endo et al. (1978) described seven cases of periodic psychosis associated with the menstrual cycle. Six of these patients were nineteen years of age or younger. Williams and Weekes (1952) reported on sixteen such patients, four of whom were nineteen or younger. Douvan (1970) has emphasized that adaptive strain is normatively imposed on the adolescent girl as a function of the menstrual cycle. The fact that PAS is common among adolescent psychiatric inpatients is also compatible with the frequency of premenstrual-symptom reports among adolescent girls generally (Widholm and Kantero 1971).

Our data from the MAQ are in keeping with the historical information we obtained. Interestingly, adolescent and adult PAS patients found menstruation to be positive, despite being debilitating and bothersome. The positive responses of our patients might be understandable in light of the improvement of premenstrual symptoms that occurred with menstruation.

One set of potential influences contributing to the occurrence of PAS that interested our group was that deriving from deviant psychosexual development. Some data reported by previous investigators had suggested that menstrual symptomatology might be related in some fashion to sexual pathology (Coppen 1965; Glass et al. 1971).

We found that in our sample of adolescent and adult patients described above, there did in fact seem to be a relationship between grossly abnormal psychosexual development and the occurrence of PAS. Of twenty-eight patients who satisfied criteria for PAS, sixteen, or 57 percent, had grossly abnormal sexual histories as determined by our reviewerrs blind to PAS status. In contrast, of seventeen patients who did not meet criteria for PAS, only one, or 5 percent, had a comparably abnormal sexual history. These data are statistically significant ($X^2 = 9.74$; $p < .005$) and seem clinically quite relevant.

Six patients, all from the positive PAS group, reported that they had been raped. One patient from the PAS group had been traumatically sexually molested by an adult when she was five. In two additional cases, incest with older brothers, and sexual contact with their friends as well, began during the early juvenile period. In another case, sex with a stepfather and prostitution both allegedly began at age twelve. As adults, these patients were undeniably pained and conflict-ridden about their earlier sexual activities. Three patients, all from the positive PAS group, met DSM-III criteria for ego dystonic homosexuality. Two other patients met DSM-III criteria for gender identity disorder. The remaining patient suffered from inhibited sexual desire following gynecological surgery in early adulthood. These findings suggested to us that the subjective context within which menarche (and subsequently, menstruation) occurred might influence the capacity of some females to respond positively or negatively to the events of the cycle.

Furthermore, it appeared to us that psychodynamic models derived from the study of the free association of psychoanalytic patients (Benedek & Rubenstein 1939) might have wider applicability among younger patients suffering from more severe psychopathology than had been realized generally. We were aware of recent evidence that the sexual behavior of females may be influenced by the menstrual cycle (Adams, Gold, and Burt 1978). We have elsewhere pointed out how diverse types of behavioral symptoms could theoretically be associated with sexual behavior. For example, if intensity of sexual desire fluctuated with the cycle, so presumably would symptoms resulting from unconscious conflicts exacerbated by the desire (Friedman et al. 1980; Hurt et al. in press). Space does not allow detailed psychodynamic discussion here. However, we speculated that if the subjective meaning of sexual events is extremely negative, for a variety of reasons, and if the adaptive capacities of females are already impaired because of psychiatric illness, then many patients will regularly experience premenstrual symptoms to the degree that criteria for PAS are fulfilled. Our data, therefore, seemed of interest not only with regard to the etiology of premenstrual symptoms but also suggested that these symptoms might constitute evidence that conflicts about earlier sexual traumata had not been resolved. The type of model we used was not meant to account for the occurrence of PAS in general but seemed relevant to understanding menstrual cycle and behavioral relationships in subgroups of patients who already were severely impaired psychiatrically. We were unable to study biological variables such as hormones. Our data (from a different level of organization of the organism) neither support nor contradict biological studies.

The data we have presented in this chapter highlight the need for more detailed study of the *beginning* of the complex biopsychosocial processes associated with the menstrual cycle than has previously been the case. The absence of such data, a dramatic fact in itself, suggests that a focus on menarche in psychiatric patients will be an important area for research in the future. Our feeling is that the most productive overall approach to furthering knowledge in this area would be a multifaceted one in which psychodynamic and psychobiological levels of behavioral organization are integrated.

References

Adams, D.B., Gold, A.R., and Burt, A.D. 1978. Rise in female-initiated sexual activity at ovulation and its suppression by oral contraceptives, *New England Journal of Medicine* 229:1145-1150.

Benedek, T., and Rubenstein, B.B. 1939. Correlations between ovarian activity and psychodynamic process; II. The menstrual phase. *Psychosomatic Medicine*, 1:461-485.

Brooks, J., Ruble, D., and Clark, A. 1977. College women's attitudes and expectations concerning menstrual-related changes. *Psychosomatic Medicine* 39:288-293.

Coppen, A. 1965. The prevalence of menstrual disorders in psychiatric patients. *British Journal of Psychiatry* 3:155-167.

Diamond, S.B., Rubenstein, A.A., Dunner, D.R., et al. 1976. Menstrual problems in women with primary affective illness. *Comprehensive Psychiatry* 17:541-548.

Douvan, E. 1970. New sources of conflict in females at adolescence and early adulthood. In J.M. Bardwick, ed., *Feminine personality and conflict*. Monterey, Cal.: Brooks-Cole.

Endicott, J., Halbreich, U., and Schacht, S. 1981. Premenstrual changes and affective disorders. *Psychosomatic Medicine* 43:88.

Endo, M., Daiguji, M., Asano, Y., Yamashita, I. and Takahaski, S. 1978. Periodic psychosis recurring in association with menstrual cycle. *Journal of Clinical Psychiatry* 39:456-466.

Friedman, R.C., Hurt, S.W., Aronoff, M.S., and Clarkin, J. 1980. Behavior and the menstrual cycle. *Signs-Journal of Women in Culture and Society* 5:719-738.

Glass, G.S., Heninger, G.R., Lansky, M., and Talan, K. 1971. Psychiatric emergency related to the menstrual cycle. *American Journal of Psychiatry* 128:61-67.

Hurt, S.W., Friedman, R.C., Clarkin, J., Corn, R., and Aronoff, M.S. In press. Psychopathology and the menstrual cycle. In R. Friedman, ed., *Behavior and the menstrual cycle*. New York: Marcel Dekker, Inc.

Janowsky, D.S., Gorney, R., and Castelnuovo-Tedesco, P. 1969. Premenstrual-menstrual increases in psychiatric hospital admission rates. *American Journal of Obstetrics and Gynecology* 103:189-191.

Kashiwagi, T., McClure, J.N., and Wetzel, R.D. 1976. Premenstrual affective syndrome and psychiatric disorder. *Diseases of the Nervous System* 37:116-119.

Kramp, J.L. 1968. Studies on the premenstrual syndrome in relation to psychiatry. *Acta Psychiatrica Scandinavica. Supplement* 203:261-267.

MacKinnon, I.L., MacKinnon, P.C.B., and Thomson, A.D. 1959. Lethal hazards of the luteal phase of the menstrual cycle. *British Medical Journal* 1:1015-1017.

O'Conner, J.F., Shelly, E.M., and Stern, L.O. 1974. Behavioral rhythms related to the menstrual cycle. In M. Ferin et. al., eds., *Biorhythms and human reproduction*. New York: John Wiley and Sons.

Wetzel, R.D., and McClure, J.N., 1972. Suicide and the menstrual cycle: A review. *Comprehensive Psychiatry* 12:369-374.

Wetzel, R.D., Reich, T., and McClure, J.N. 1971. Phase of the menstrual cycle and self-referrals to a suicide prevention service. *British Journal of Psychiatry* 119:523-524.

Widholm, O., and Kantero, R. 1971. A statistical analysis of the menstrual patterns of 8,000 Finnish girls and their mothers. *Acta Obstetricia et Gynecologica Scandinavica. Supplement* 14:1-36.

Williams, E.Y., and Weekes, L.R. 1952. Premenstrual tension associated with psychotic episodes. *Journal of Nervous and Mental Disease* 116:321-329.

**Part VIII
Epilogue**

26 Future Directions for Research

Mary Brown Parlee

The term *future directions for research* has two meanings. One, the familiar concluding theme of conferences and textbooks, refers to the directions research questions and problems may take as they develop in the future. The other, less usual, meaning refers to the directions research findings may take as they move beyond the domain of the research community.

Researchers undoubtedly have fairly decided views on the first of these two meanings: because of individual training, skills, experience, and even personality, each investigator pursues a line of research that he or she believes is most promising for the future development of knowledge about menarche. While we peruse each other's data with pleasure and profit, the interdisciplinary interchange rarely prompts a fundamental change in a researcher's perspective.[1]

What I would like to address, instead, in this chapter is the second reading of *future directions for research:* the directions our research can take as we move it beyond the research community. Here, I believe, in spite of our very great diversity of perspectives, we are on common ground. My underlying assumption is that research is only one stage in a much larger process. In addition to their research, scientists have a responsibility to play an active role, however limited, in this larger process.

First a prefatory note. The various chapters of this book make it especially clear that research problems and ideas do not arise in a vacuum. Perhaps more than general research on the menstrual cycle, the variety of research on menarche reported here conveys an image of the individuals who are the subjects of the investigations. While there are many important gaps, and perhaps some distortions, in the descriptive picture of young adolescent girls that arises from the research, the fact that the research problems and questions are rooted in real lives comes through very clearly. The athlete's concern over her "failure" to begin menstruating when her friends do, the premenarcheal girl's increasing awareness of bodily configurations as she moves to postmenarcheal status, the young unmarried schoolgirl who is pregnant almost as soon as she becomes sexually active—such investigations illuminate and clarify experience and behavior in a way that research based largely on academic theories applied to "social issues" generally does not. The relatively close connection in investigations of menarche between research questions and the settings in which they arise seems to me to be one reason for optimism that the research-based knowledge will have meaning as it is taken in various directions beyond the research community. Without this base, consideration of the impact of research findings in broader public arenas would be pointless.

There are three general directions in which movement of research into broader domains occurs. These directions are what have typically been referred to as *application* of research, its *popularization,* and its implications for *policy.* I want to discuss each of these very briefly and to point to ways in which researchers can, depending on their skills and interests, play an active role in determining the future, public impact of their work.

One way in which research findings traditionally have had an impact beyond the scientific community is in their direct application. That is, theory-based research is used to modify the clinical treatment or social environments of those who are the subjects of the research. Most obvious and traditional are clinical applications of research. (Research on the role of prostaglandins, for example, is used in the treatment of dysmenorrhea). A somewhat less obvious but equally important area of application of research findings lies in their impact on the content of various curricula and training programs. Thus, research on the ratio of body fat/lean and age of menarche could be incorporated in the curriculum for training future physical-education teachers. Research-based information of preadolescents' beliefs about the effects of menstruation could be used to design appropriate science or health-education curricula or could be incorporated into training programs for counselors or teachers.

We must not allow the traditional and narrow academic disinterest in this sort of applied work to blind us to the importance of doing it well; of doing problem-centered, theoretically based (or theory-building) research that we then feed into channels where it can be applied to some useful social end. Of course research as an end in itself can be a passionately absorbing enterprise, and of course doing research does not entail a committment or the ability to carry out its applications. But researchers do need to assume at least some responsibility for thinking about future applications of their research, and, if approprite, for taking the first steps necessary to bring their work to the attention of those who are interested in applying it. Such steps might include participation in conferences and publication in journals primarily directed toward biomedical and mental-health practitioners, or to those involved in vocational education or in teacher training.

A second direction research can take as we move it outside the traditional academic and clinical audiences and functions is into the arena of public information. Research findings can be communicated in nontechnical language (popularized) to various segments of the general public through mass media such as newspapers, magazines, radio, and television. A major aim of such communication is to increase public awareness of research on significant topics in a way that will promote the welfare of individuals.[2] A not inconsiderable side effect of such general public awareness, however, is that it often leads indirectly to effective pressure for changes in social institutions. An informative newspaper article about research on menarche, for example, might prompt a local parent group to pressure their school board for expanded athletic programs for preadolescent and adolescent girls. Politicians at the national level, too, are often more responsive to a constituent's awareness of research findings (and subsequent political pressure) than to the scientists' report of the data themselves, even as framed in policy-relevant position papers. In times of sharply reduced federal funding for social-science research, an aware and supportive public may also be one of the research community's best allies.

It is not always easy to disseminate research findings through the popular media, however, and I want to mention just two traditional academic beliefs or values that may make it more difficult. One is the notion that if a piece of work is comprehensible by the general public, or popularized, it cannot, by definition, be good science. (I think I exaggerate this view only slightly.) While it is certainly true that all good research cannot be made accessible to the general public, it does not follow that understandable work is necessarily thereby inferior. The other belief that interferes with serious popularization of research is the traditional academic assumption that what is entailed in disseminating research findings to the general public through the mass media is the researcher's "translating" the findings "down to the level" of a lay audience. An effective meshing of academic and journalistic perspectives and skills is a good deal more complicated than that, and once again researchers need to assume responsibility for taking some active steps, correctly, to enable these interactions to occur. An important step in this direction would be for researchers to educate themselves in the skills necessary to deal effectively with media representatives.[3]

A third direction for research, at least for social science research as it moves out beyond academic and clinical settings, is into the arena of public policy. For those who do not engage in research that is explicitly policy-related, the transition involved in moving from an audience of fellow researchers to an audience of policymakers at various levels of government can be a difficult one. The researcher's notion of the kinds of policy decisions to which a particular study is relevant is often much broader than the scope of the work warrants. Furthermore, policymakers do not read research reports, special issues of journals, or any of the familiar vehicles for exchange of information within the research community. Yet they do want to know about the availability and substance of research on different topics as the need arises in the legislative and decision-making process. (Usually, what they want to know is who is doing what and what's their phone number.) They want a summary of the research on a three-by-five-inch card yesterday. If we researchers are not able to draw attention to our work in a form they can use, and at their time schedule, our opportunity to have an impact will be missed.

While it may not be possible for the individual researcher to identify precisely the arenas in which his or her work is related to issues of public policy, it is possible for the researcher to take some first steps to make the data available to policymakers in a form they can use. One simple step might be to develop the habit of sending summaries of work to those organizations whose function it is to provide policymakers with access to research they need.[4] As in the case of *applied* and *public-information* uses of research data, the investigator may not want to or be able to implement the findings in the broader domain of policymaking, but he or she can take responsibility for ensuring that the results at least reach the channels through which they can have a wider impact.

Effective use of the channels through which data-based knowledge moves beyond the research community requires that researchers be aware of the activities, values, and skills of those professionals whose job it is to use research in broader public arenas. A clinician or someone who develops high-school curricula, a science writer, a congressional aide—all are highly skilled professionals whose interests lie in finding and using the best research currently available. They are not, professionally speaking, interested in the future directions of research in the internal, theory-development sense. They are vitally interested, however, in the future directions of research as it reaches audiences and serves purposes outside the research community. Sometimes we the researchers and they the users are the same people. Sometimes we are not. But when we are not, researchers concerned with the future of our work should take responsibility for those first steps of communication with at least some of the other groups and professions that are concerned with the uses of research. This first step will increase the likelihood that we do not simply talk to ourselves about the research, interesting though it might be, but that what we do will be heard by others as well—and may make a difference in people's lives.

Notes

1. I think the reasons for this tenacity of focus go beyond disciplinary parochialism or sheer cussedness and are in fact important for the development of scientific knowledge. There is unfortunately not enough time to consider these issues here.

2. The assumption in all such public-information activities is that awareness is preferable to ignorance. Serious questions do arise, however, when public awareness of only part of the research findings, out of context,

would contribute to, rather than modify, widely shared social beliefs or pre-judices.

3. The American Psychological Association has developed a *Media Guide* to enable researchers to begin educating themselves in this way. It is available from the APA Public Information Office, 1200 Seventeenth Street, N.W., Washington, D.C. 20036.

4. One such group is the Women's Research Education Institute of the Congresswomen's Caucus, 400 South Capitol Street, Washington, D.C. 20003. Another is the APA Public Information Office, mentioned above.

27

Implications for Women's Health and Well-Being

Sharon Golub

The purpose of this book was to assess the impact of menarche on the physical, psychological, and social development of adolescents. For the first time, researchers from a variety of fields focused attention on menarche. We identified gaps in our knowledge and clarified research directions. Now it seems appropriate to ask what we have learned that can be used to foster women's health and well-being.

Menarche is a focal point in a continuum of pubertal development that includes hormonal changes, breast development, and the growth of body hair; it generally follows a growth spurt and a rapid gain in fat. Gradually, the adolescent establishes a regular menstrual cycle. During this period, adolescents are very concerned about "being normal," which they equate with being the same as their peers. Therefore, it is important for those working with this age group to be aware of some of the factors that influence when menarche occurs and of those conditions that may cause menstrual disturbances.

The physiological data presented indicate that many things can influence the onset of menstruation or interfere with menstrual regularity; some of these factors are benign, others serious. These factors include: race; heredity; weight—either obesity or excessive thinness (a weight loss of 10 to 15 percent can cause amenorrhea); stress—ranging from going off to camp to a death in the family; blindness; and diseases such as ulcerative colitis, cystic fibrosis, uremia, congenital heart disease, anorexia nervosa, and sometimes diabetes mellitus and leukemia.

Nutrition and exercise appear to be critical factors. Frisch (chap. 1) proposed that a certain ratio of fat to lean is an important determinant of fertility in the human female. She has found that girls who are involved in athletic training before the onset of menstruation are more likely to have delayed menarche and irregular or absent menstrual cycles. Female athletes in general have an increased incidence of oligomenorrhea and amenorrhea as compared with the general population and ballet dancers are similarly affected by their training.

In recent years girls and women have been encouraged to increase their participation in athletic activities both to foster physical fitness and to gain the psychological benefits found to be associated with participation in sports. If unaware of the relationship between body fat and menstruation, athletic girls and young women may be unduly disturbed by their menstrual irregularities. After physical examination has ruled out the presence of serious illness or pregnancy, it is reassuring for these women to know that an increase in caloric intake, cessation of training, or a reduction in the intensity of training generally results in menarche or a return of cycles that have been interrupted. At this time we do not know if this kind of interruption of menstrual function has any long-term deleterious or advantageous effect. (There is some recent evidence that fewer cycles over the course of one's life is correlated with a lower incidence of breast cancer: we should not think of missed periods as being only harmful.) Longitudinal studies comparing the menstrual lives and health of athletic and nonathletic women are needed to address this question.

The weight issue is an important one. In our culture thinness is equated with beauty and we focus inordinate prejudices on fat people. This concern apparently comes through quite clearly to the young female who is defining herself as a woman. Both Petersen (chap. 4) and Warren (chap. 18) point out that adolescent girls, particularly postmenarcheal girls, are more concerned about their weight than are their younger peers. Preoccupation with diet is common and diet-related amenorrhea, particularly among girls who are involved in ballet, gymnastics, and modeling is also common. When preoccupation with thinness and diet is carried to extremes, anorexia nervosa may result. Anorexia nervosa is a psychophysiologic disorder characterized by severe and prolonged inability or refusal to eat. It is sometimes accompanied by binge eating and vomiting. The etiology is unclear. However, Warren (chap. 18) suggests that it is increasing in incidence and the peak age of onset is right around puberty—in girls between ten and fifteen. Thus we need not only to focus some attention on the basic principles of good nutrition but also to foster a healthy acceptance of individual differences in body shape. And, since some theorists have suggested that anorexia represents an attempt to avoid menstruation, delay adulthood, and deny the female role, some attention to the psychological aspects of menarche is also important.

The psychological research reported by Petersen, Koff, and Danza shows that menarche affects a girl's perception of herself as well as her behavior and family relationships. She begins to see herself as more feminine, as a more sexual person. She is more grown-up. She generally demands and is given increasing responsibilities and privileges. However, the transition is not necessarily a smooth one.

Some girls have difficulty with menarche itself. They are frightened at the onset of menstruation or they experience feelings of disgust or shame. Unconsciously some may associate menstruation with loss of control and excretory functions. Some deny that they are menstruating. In part, lack of preparation is to blame. Milow (chap. 10) points out that even today one-third of women report that they were not prepared for menstruation. And Rierdan (chap. 9) suggests that even the preparation that is given is not adequate. Menarche needs to be explained not just as something normal that happens to everyone but also as something that is happening now—to an individual, with whatever meaning it has for that individual and the people around her. Perhaps we do need a contemporary ritual celebration of menarche. I am currently studying recollections of menarche and some of the most positive memories reported are those of girls whose parents sent them flowers, took them out to dinner, or gave them a gift, thereby recognizing their new status. More primitive cultures than ours have puberty rites. Perhaps all of the secrecy that enshrouds menstruation—our increase in so-called civilization—has caused us to lose something.

In recent years other taboo topics have been taken on and desensitized. First it was sex; then, death. The time has come to talk more openly about menstruation. The contradictory messages conveyed by our culture in literature and the media could be changed and reinterpreted. Menstruation could be explained realistically, not unduly glorified while ignoring the nuisance aspects, nor hidden away as something shameful that must be concealed at all cost. Some progress has already been made. For example, there are commercials on television that describe products and discuss the need for absorbancy in sanitary napkins or tampons. And The TAMPAX Report (1981) showed that Americans are overwhelmingly in favor of continuing menstrual education in the schools. But two-thirds of Americans still believe that menstruation should not be discussed in the office or socially.

It seems very likely that our hush-hush attitude toward menarche is due in part to the relationship between menarche and the capacity to reproduce. Paige (chap. 13) points this relationship out in cultures where chastity control and economics are strongly intertwined. The relationship is no less true in our own culture.

But just what is the relationship between menarche and sexual behavior? And what role do hormones play? Apparently sexual behavior among adolescents is very variable. And the role of hormones in triggering sexual feelings is not clear. No direct relationship has been found between hormone levels and sexual interest or behavior. However, Gagnon (chap. 16) did find that socio-sexual behavior was indirectly influenced by hormones. Increasing hormone levels led to sexual maturation; concomitant body changes led to dating and sexual activities. The emphasis here seems to be on the changes in self-perception and others' perception and on the differing expectations of others that occur at the time of puberty. This finding has profound implications for the girl who deviates noticeably from the norm.

The early-maturing girl presents us with a specific set of potential problems. She is less likely to be prepared for puberty and menarche. Hence, she is more likely to be frightened. Her early sexual maturation—the development of breasts and curves—will influence the way in which others react to her and she may be subjected to overtures for which she is not psychologically or socially ready. She is also likely to experience some ambivalent or negative feelings about herself. On the one hand she enjoys having a mature body and being admired; on the other, she would like to be like everyone else. Generally the early maturing girl has lower self-esteem and more behavioral problems than her peers.

Conversely, the late-maturing girl is troubled by her lack of breast development and sex appeal. She worries about not having started to menstruate and thinks that perhaps she is not normal. What can be done for these troubled adolescents? The study of adolescent psychology with emphasis on pubertal changes in body, cognitive function, and social relations would go a long way toward helping adolescents to weather this transition period more comfortably. Courses in adolescent psychology really should be given to adolescents. Barring this structured approach, which has the added advantage of reaching even the shy, unquestioning adolescent, second best would be having people around (teachers, school nurses, psychologists, physicians) who are familiar with the problems of puberty and have the ability to communicate comfortably with this age group. Sex-education courses also hold the potential for filling this need. Which brings us to a major health and social problem of adolescents: teenage pregnancy.

More than a million U.S. teenagers become pregnant every year (New York Times 20 December 1981). Those who decide to have their babies experience a higher incidence of prematurity, anemia, and high blood pressure than do older mothers, not to mention their psychological and social problems. Leppert's finding (chap. 15) that girls can and do conceive within three to nine months following menarche is surprising. It stands in contrast to previous beliefs that girls were mostly anovulatory for about two years after menarche and it has profound implications for sex education.

Mary Calderone, executive director of The Sex Information and Education Council of the U.S. (SIECUS) has said, "It is impossible to keep children innocent but it is possible to keep them ignorant. That is where the danger lies" (Calderone 1982). And that is precisely what is happening. Only 15 percent of U.S. schools offer any planned sex education. Yet teens and their parents need this information. The peer-outreach program Leppert describes and the provision of contraceptive information represent one way of meeting this need. But it is not being met early enough. The need for sex education seems to begin before menarche. If given then it would provide teenagers with the information they need to make responsible decisions about their sexuality. However, early sex-education programs are unlikely to be developed as long as parents deny that their pubertal children are sexual beings.

Although some young women do not experience menstrual cramps until they have been menstruating for some time, some do have dysmenorrhea when their periods begin. Brooks-Gunn and Ruble (chap. 20) report that about half of the elementary and junior-high-school girls they studied experienced cramps at menarche. They also cite a Finnish study that suggested that 23 percent of adolescents were absent from school because of dysmenorrhea. Other data, surveying older women, indicate that about 50 percent of women have dysmenorrhea.

Thus the new treatment of dysmenorrhea warrants the special attention of health professionals. No longer do women have to endure being told, "It's all in your head," by doctors and others with nothing to offer in the way of pain relief. No longer do girls have to sit along the wall during gym because they are menstruating and unable to participate in the days' activities. Though sociopsychological factors play a role in the expectation of symptoms and the perception of pain, today those who endorse a purely psychogenic explanation for dysmenorrhea lack an understanding of its etiology.

Chan (chap. 19) and others have clearly demonstrated that high levels of prostaglandins in the uterus are the cause of primary dysmenorrhea. There are now medications that can be used to alleviate this pain, specifically: Motrin, Ponstel, Naprosyn, and Anaprox. Unlike birth-control pills, which eliminate dysmenorrhea by stopping ovulation, these prostaglandin-inhibiting drugs need not be taken all of the time. They are taken only when there is pain. The medication works quickly and is excreted rapidly. And most women need the medication for only a day or two. There are relatively few side effects, but gastrointestinal symptoms such as nausea, indigestion, vomiting, and diarrhea sometimes do result. Most of these side effects can be prevented by taking the medication with food. The discovery of the relationship between dysmenorrhea and prostaglandin activity also enables us to understand why aspirin, so often used in the past, is effective in treating mild dysmenorrhea: aspirin is a mild antiprostaglandin. However, it is not nearly as effective as the newer drugs in treating severe dysmenorrhea.

There seem to be two important points to be made with regard to the psychiatric studies presented. First, psychiatric patients are not the same as normal adolescents. For example, Friedman and his colleagues (chap. 25) found no differences in the prevalence of symptoms of premenstrual affective syndrome between the adolescents and adults in his sample of psychiatric patients. Differences have been reported among normal women of different ages (Golub and Harrington 1981; Lloyd 1963; Moos 1969). Friedman also suggests, on the basis of psychiatric histories, that there may be a relationship between abnormal psychosexual development and the occurrence of these symptoms. And, in addition, he found a very high incidence of dysmenorrhea among these adolescents, 70 percent as opposed to about 50 percent among normal girls. Darwin (chap. 23) points out that the disturbed adolescents in her sample dealt with the developmental stresses of menarche in a way different from that of the normal girls. Specifically, the inpatients tended to exhibit self-destructive behavior, whereas the normal girls exerted more control over their behavior and used fantasy to resolve their concerns about body integrity, aggression, and separation from mother.

Second, those working with psychiatric patients need to be aware of the possibly disorganizing or disturbing effects of menarche and the menstrual cycle on this population. Perhaps information about menarcheal experiences and menstrual-cycle timing should be a routine part of the psychiatric histories of female patients taken by physicians and nurses.

In sum, the chapters of this book offer new information that can influence educational programs, clinical practice, and the counseling of adolescent girls and their parents. Some suggestions for social action are implicit as well. The next step is implementation. Now these research findings must be disseminated and used to improve women's lives.

References

Calderone, M. 1982. A moral responsibility to the majority. *Sexual Medicine Today* 6:33.

Golub, S., and Harrington, D.M. 1981. Premenstrual and menstrual mood changes in adolescent women. *Journal of Personality and Social Psychology* 41:961-965.

Lloyd, T.S. 1963. The mid-thirties syndrome. *Virginia Medical Monthly* 90:51.

Moos, R.H. 1969. *Preliminary manual for the menstrual distress questionnaire.* California: Stanford University School of Medicine.

Research and Forecasts. 1981. *The Tampax Report.*

Index

About the Contributors

Michael S. Aronoff, M.D., clinical assistant professor of psychiatry, The New York Hospital-Cornell Medical Center, Westchester Division, White Plains, New York.

Shawky Z.A. Badawy, M.D., professor, Department of Obstetrics and Gynecology, and director, Reproductive Endocrinology Unit, State University of New York, Upstate Medical Center, Syracuse.

Jeanne Brooks-Gunn, Ph.D., research scientist, Educational Testing Service, Princeton, New Jersey, and assistant professor of Clinical Pediatric Psychiatry, College of Physicians and Surgeons, Columbia University, New York.

Virginia H. Brown, B.A., Department of Psychology, Montclair State College, Upper Montclair, New Jersey.

Vern L. Bullough, Ph.D., dean, Faculty of Natural and Social Sciences, State University of New York College at Buffalo.

Regina Casper, M.D., associate professor, Department of Psychiatry, Illinois State Psychiatric Institute, Chicago.

W.Y. Chan, Ph.D., professor, Department of Pharmacology, Cornell University Medical College, New York.

John F. Clarkin, Ph.D., associate professor of clinical psychology in psychiatry, The New York Hospital-Cornell Medical Center-Westchester Division, White Plains.

Ruth Corn, M.S.W., lecturer of social work in psychiatry, The New York Hospital-Cornell Medical Center, White Plains.

Roberta Danza, M.S.N., private practice, New Haven, Connecticut, and adjunct professor of psychiatric nursing, School of Nursing, Southern Connecticut State College, New Haven.

Jaine L. Darwin, Psy.D., staff psychologist, Brighton-Allston Mental Health Clinic, Brighton, Massachusetts.

Gretchen Kramer Dery, R.N., M.S.N., associate professor, School of Nursing, Duke University, Durham.

Inge Dyrenfurth, Ph.D., senior research associate. Department of Obstetrics and Gynecology, College of Physicians and Surgeons, Columbia University, New York.

Elke Eckert, M.D., assistant professor, Department of Psychiatry, University of Minnesota, Minneapolis.

James R. Falk, Ph.D., research associate, Department of Psychiatry, Cornell University Medical College, White Plains.

Richard C. Friedman, M.D., associate professor of clinical psychiatry, The New York Hospital-Cornell Medical Center-Westchester Division, White Plains.

Rose E. Frisch, Ph.D., lecturer in population sciences, Center for Population Studies, Harvard University, Cambridge.

John H. Gagnon, Ph.D., professor, Department of Sociology, State University of New York at Stony Brook.

Fred I. Gilbert, Jr., M.D., medical director, Pacific Health Research Institute, and professor, School of Public Health, University of Hawaii, Honolulu.

Sharon Golub, Ph.D., associate professor, Department of Psychology, School of Arts and Sciences and the Graduate School, College of New Rochelle.

Madeleine J. Goodman, Ph.D., associate professor of general science and women's studies, and director, Women's Studies Program, University of Hawaii, Honolulu.

John S. Grove, Ph.D., research associate, Pacific Health Research Institute, Honolulu.

Katherine A. Halmi, M.D., associate professor, Department of Psychiatry, Cornell University Medical College, White Plains.

Stephen W. Hurt, Ph.D., instructor of psychology in psychiatry, The New York Hospital-Cornell Medical Center-Westchester Division, White Plains.

Elizabeth Kincaid-Ehlers, Ph.D., adjunct writer-in-residence, English Department, Trinity College, Hartford.

Elissa Koff, Ph.D., associate professor, Department of Psychology, Wellesley College, Wellesley, Massachusetts.

Lawrence Kohn, M.D., Department of Medicine, State University of New York, Upstate Medical Center, Syracuse.

M. Victoria Larson, M.A., Department of Psychology, Montclair State College, Upper Montclair.

Phyllis C. Leppert, M.D., assistant professor, Departments of Obstetrics and Gynecology and Pediatrics, College of Physicians and Surgeons, Columbia University, New York.

Edna M. Menke, R.N., Ph.D., associate professor, Department of Nursing, Ohio State University, Columbus.

Vera J. Milow, vice president-educational affairs, TAMPAX Incorporated, Lake Success, New York.

Arnold Moses, M.D., professor, Department of Medicine, State University of New York, Upstate Medical Center, Syracuse.

Ada Most, R.N., Ed.D., associate professor, School of Nursing, Duke University, Durham.

Malkah T. Notman, M.D., clinical professor of psychiatry, Tufts University School of Medicine, New England Medical Center Hospital, Boston.

Richard P. Oates, Ph.D., associate professor, Department of Preventive Medicine, State University of New York, Upstate Medical Center, Syracuse.

Karen Ericksen Paige, Ph.D., associate professor, Department of Psychology, University of California at Davis.

Mary Brown Parlee, Ph.D., associate professor, The Graduate School and University Center, City University of New York, New York.

Anne C. Petersen, Ph.D., director, Laboratory for the Study of Adolescence, Michael Reese Hospital and Medical Center, and associate professor, Department of Psychiatry, University of Chicago.

Frances Rebscher, R.N., Clinical Research Center, State University of New York, Upstate Medical Center, Syracuse.

Jill Rierdan, Ph.D., research associate, Center for Research on Women, and lecturer, Department of Psychology, Wellesley College, Wellesley.

Diane N. Ruble, Ph.D., associate professor, Department of Psychology, New York University, New York.

Rhoda K. Unger, Ph.D., professor, Department of Psychology, Montclair State College, Upper Montclair.

Michelle P. Warren, M.D., assistant professor, Department of Obstetrics and Gynecology and Medicine, St. Lukes-Roosevelt Hospital Center, Columbia College of Physicians and Surgeons, New York.

Lenore R. Williams, R.N., M.S.N., outreach nurse educator, Cleveland Regional Perinatal Network, Cleveland.

Honor Wolfe, M.D., Department of Obstetrics and Gynecology, Case Western Reserve University, Cleveland.

Nancy Fugate Woods, Ph.D., associate professor, School of Nursing, University of Washington, Seattle.

About the Editor

Sharon Golub is an associate professor of psychology at the College of New Rochelle and adjunct associate professor of psychiatry at New York Medical College. She received the Ph.D. from Fordham University. Dr. Golub has written extensively about the psychology of women, human sexuality, and women's health. She is currently president of the Society for Menstrual Cycle Research and is editor of the journal *Women and Health*.